Celine Bicquart Ord · Eric K. Hansen
Charles R. Thomas, Jr.

Editors

Radiation Oncology Study Guide

D1420318

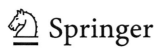 Springer

Editors
Celine Bicquart Ord, MD
Department of Radiation Oncology
Scott & White Memorial Hospital
Temple, TX, USA

Charles R. Thomas, Jr., MD
Department of Radiation Medicine
Knight Cancer Institute
Oregon Health & Science University
Portland, OR, USA

Eric K. Hansen, MD
Department of Radiation Oncology
The Oregon Clinic
Providence St. Vincent Medical Center
Portland, OR, USA

ISBN 978-1-4614-6399-3   ISBN 978-1-4614-6400-6 (eBook)
DOI 10.1007/978-1-4614-6400-6
Springer New York Heidelberg Dordrecht London

Library of Congress Control Number: 2013934977

Printed on acid-free paper

Springer is part of Springer Science+Business Media (www.springer.com)

Charles Schulz once said, "In the book of life, the answers aren't in the back."
I dedicate this book to my patients who inspire me every day. They've taught me so much!

EH

To my wonderful mother and best friend, Farida, a breast cancer survivor, who has taught me compassion, selflessness, and dedication. To my father, Paul, who always put my education above all. Thank you for all the effort and direction. To my amazing husband, Justin, for the daily joy, humor, and enduring support.

CBO

To my supportive wife, Muriel Elleen, our wonderful two children, Julian Franklin and Aurielle Marie, and my parents and siblings for their love and support of my career path.

In memory of my mother, Ruth Marie Wilson Thomas, who fought gallantly in the war against cancer and whose prayers have blessed me over the past five decades.

CRT

Preface

Radiation oncology is a constantly evolving field, with our clinical practice becoming increasingly evidence-based. We hope that this book will be a valuable resource to residents as they learn the fundamentals of radiation oncology. While there are excellent textbooks and "handbooks" in our specialty that serve as day-to-day resources for clinical practice, there is not a comprehensive Q&A book for preparing for the written board exam of radiation oncology conducted by the American Board of Radiology.

It is our intent that this book aids in the study for the board exam and also guides learning of some salient features of clinical oncology. We hope that our questions lead to raising more questions by our readers that would help in further learning. While covering the breadth of radiation oncology is difficult, our hope is that this review covers most of the important concepts of radiation treatment for each disease site. Sources that were used to compile the questions and rationales for each chapter include the following: the primary literature – *Textbook of Radiation Oncology*; *Principles and Practice of Radiation Oncology*; *Biliary Tract and Gallbladder Cancer*; *Cancer: Principles & Practice of Oncology*; *Clinical Pediatric Oncology*; *Principles and Practice of Pediatric Oncology*; *Nelson Textbook of Pediatrics*; *Clinical Target Volumes in Conformal Radiotherapy and Intensity Modulated Radiotherapy*; *Gynecology and Obstetrics*; *Gynecologic Oncology*; the National Comprehensive Cancer Network Guidelines (www.nccn.org); and the American Society for Therapeutic Radiology and Oncology Annual Meeting Educational Sessions. Despite an attempt to concisely summarize studies in each of the rationales, readers are encouraged to refer to the references listed at the end of each answer's rationale (primary literature and aforementioned sources) for further details.

Each chapter covers the clinical features, staging, principles of treatment, and treatment-driving studies of specific disease sites, with an emphasis on radiotherapy studies.

As trials are updated and new studies are published, our long-term goal is to regularly update a high-quality, essential study resource for physicians-in-training in radiation oncology.

We sincerely thank the contributors for their dedication, hours of hard work, and excellent chapters.

Temple, TX, USA   Celine Bicquart Ord, MD
Portland, OR, USA   Eric K. Hansen, MD
Portland, OR, USA   Charles R. Thomas, Jr., MD

Contents

Contributors

Sravana K. Chennupati, MD Department of Radiation Medicine, Oregon Health & Science University, Portland, OR, USA

Patrick J. Gagnon, MD, MS Department of Radiation Oncology, Southeast Centers for Cancer Care, Fairhaven, MA, USA

Eric K. Hansen, MD Department of Radiation Oncology, The Oregon Clinic, Providence St. Vincent Medical Center, Portland, OR, USA

John M. Holland Department of Radiation Oncology, Oregon Health & Science University, Portland, OR, USA

Arthur Y. Hung, MD Department of Radiation Medicine, Oregon Health & Science University, Portland, OR, USA

Charlotte Dai Kubicky, MD, PhD Department of Radiation Medicine, Oregon Health & Science University, Portland, OR, USA

Carol Marquez, MD Department of Radiation Medicine, Oregon Health & Science University, Portland, OR, USA

Subhakar Mutyala, MD Department of Radiation Oncology, Scott & White Healthcare System and Texas A&M College of Medicine, Temple, TX, USA

Celine Bicquart Ord, MD Department of Radiation Oncology, Scott & White Memorial Hospital, Temple, TX, USA

Faisal Siddiqui, MD, PhD Department of Radiation Medicine, Oregon Health & Science University, Portland, OR, USA

Charles R. Thomas, Jr., MD Department of Radiation Medicine, Oregon Health & Science University, Knight Cancer Institute, Portland, OR, USA

Joseph G. Waller, MD, MPH   Department of Radiation Medicine, Oregon Health & Science University, Portland, OR, USA

Kristina H. Young, MD, PhD   Department of Radiation Medicine, Oregon Health & Science University, Portland, OR, USA

Chapter 1
Central Nervous System Tumors: Adult and Pediatric

Celine Bicquart Ord and Charlotte Dai Kubicky

Questions

1. Neurofibromatosis type 1, von Recklinghausen's disease, is most commonly associated with what type of intracranial tumor?
   A. Meningioma
   B. Astrocytoma
   C. Glioblastoma
   D. Oligodendroglioma

2. What type of intracranial tumor is most commonly seen with neurofibromatosis type 2?
   A. Schwannoma
   B. Meningioma
   C. Astrocytoma
   D. Oligodendroglioma

3. All of the following are correct regarding Turcot's syndrome except:
   A. There is an association with familial polyposis of the colon.
   B. There is an association with medulloblastoma.
   C. There is an association with high-grade glioma.
   D. There is an association with low-grade glioma.

C.B. Ord, MD (✉)
Department of Radiation Oncology, Scott & White Memorial Hospital,
Temple, TX 76508, USA
e-mail: cord@sw.org

C.D. Kubicky, MD, PhD
Department of Radiation Medicine, Oregon Health Science University,
3181 SW Sam Jackson Park Road, KPV4 Portland, OR 97239, USA
e-mail: charlottedai@gmail.com

C.B. Ord et al. (eds.), *Radiation Oncology Study Guide*,
DOI 10.1007/978-1-4614-6400-6_1, © Springer Science+Business Media New York 2013

4. All of the following are tumors associated with tuberous sclerosis except:
   A. Hemangioblastoma
   B. Angiofibromas
   C. Hamartomas
   D. Subependymal giant cell tumors

5. Cerebellar, brainstem, and spinal cord hemangioblastomas are frequently seen in which disorder?
   A. Cowden's syndrome
   B. Turcot's syndrome
   C. Von Hippel-Lindau disease
   D. Gorlin's syndrome

6. In which of the following tumors does survival increase with increasing age?
   A. Glioblastoma multiforme
   B. Oligodendroglioma
   C. Anaplastic astrocytoma
   D. Brainstem glioma

7. *MDM2* amplification/overexpression is a genetic event frequently seen in what tumor?
   A. Secondary glioblastoma multiforme
   B. Primary glioblastoma multiforme
   C. Anaplastic astrocytoma
   D. Oligodendroglioma

8. Deletion of *1p* and *19q* in oligodendroglioma is associated with:
   A. Better response to therapy but similar progression-free and overall survival
   B. Better response to therapy with improved progression-free but similar overall survival
   C. Similar response to therapy with improved progression-free and overall survival
   D. Better response to therapy with improved progression-free and overall survival

9. Methylation of the O^6-methylguanine-DNA methyltransferase, *MGMT*, promoter is associated with:
   A. Decreased *MGMT* expression and improved overall survival
   B. Decreased *MGMT* expression and decreased overall survival
   C. Increased *MGMT* expression and improved overall survival
   D. Increased *MGMT* expression with no effects on overall survival

10. The most common presenting symptom of low-grade astrocytoma is:
    A. Headache
    B. Weakness
    C. Personality change
    D. Seizure

11. Which one of the following is *not* a negative risk factor in the prognostic scoring system of low-grade gliomas developed by Pignatti and colleagues?
    A. Astrocytoma histology subtype
    B. Tumor crossing the midline
    C. Age 40 years or less
    D. Presence of neurological deficit before surgery

12. All of the following are true regarding the EORTC 22844 "Believer's Trial" in low-grade glioma except:
    A. Only 25 % of patients underwent gross total resection.
    B. 45 Gy was the radiation dose of one arm in the study.
    C. 50.4 Gy was the radiation dose of one arm in the study.
    D. Overall survival did not improve with dose escalation.

13. According to the long-term results of EORTC 22845 in which early versus delayed radiotherapy for resected low-grade gliomas was compared, which of the following is not true?
    A. Progression-free survival improved in the early radiotherapy group.
    B. Overall survival was not different between the early versus delayed groups.
    C. Seizures were better controlled at 1 year in the delayed radiotherapy group.
    D. Total dose of radiotherapy given was 54 Gy.

14. In the EORTC 26951 trial, patients with low-grade glioma were randomized after surgery and radiation to +/− chemotherapy. Which statement regarding this trial is false?
    A. Chemotherapy consisted of PCV (procarbazine, lomustine, and vincristine).
    B. The initial published results showed only a progression-free survival benefit.
    C. The most recent results still show no overall survival benefit.
    D. Median survival has not yet been reached in those with *1p19q* deletion that received adjuvant PCV chemotherapy.

15. Regarding magnetic resonance spectroscopy (MRS), which of the following is NOT true?
    A. Brain tumors are characterized by an elevated choline to creatine ratio.
    B. Radiation change on MRS is characterized by decreased choline levels.
    C. The MR spectrum of brain tumors is characterized by an increasing Hunter's angle from left to right.
    D. Radiation change on MRS is characterized by decreased N-acetylaspartate.

16. In a four-arm ECOG/RTOG trial for high-grade gliomas comparing a standard 60 Gy to 3 experimental arms, which is NOT true?
    A. A 10 Gy boost in addition to the standard 60 Gy WBRT improved survival.
    B. 40–60 year olds in the 60 Gy + BCNU arm had significantly increased survival.
    C. The 60 Gy + methyl-CCNU and DTIC arm was more toxic than the 60 Gy + BCNU arm.
    D. Age was found to be the most important prognostic factor.

17. In a dose escalation study of malignant gliomas performed by Lee et al. at the University of Michigan, which of the following is NOT true?
    A. Dose-limiting toxicity was not seen.
    B. There was no trend in improved overall survival despite dose escalation.
    C. Despite dose escalation, the majority of tumors progressed "in-field."
    D. In addition to local progression, there was extensive distant progression.

18. Regarding RTOG 90-05, a radiosurgery dose-finding study, which of the following is true?
    A. Dose-limiting toxicity was defined as irreversible grade 2 neurotoxicity.
    B. The maximum tolerated dose for tumors 2–3 cm was 15 Gy.
    C. Patients with gliomas are more likely to fail locally compared to those with metastases.
    D. Approximately two-thirds of patients failed locally.

19. Regarding brachytherapy in the brain for malignant glioma, all of the following are true except:
    A. In a Brain Tumor Cooperative Group study, there was no survival benefit seen with the addition of a brachytherapy boost.
    B. The GliaSite RT system uses an intracavitary device filled with an ^{192}Ir solution.
    C. In using an intracavitary balloon for brachytherapy, there is not a true point source.
    D. Smaller balloon fill volumes may result in higher doses at the balloon surface, possibly leading to increased radiation necrosis.

20. All of the following regarding temozolomide are true except:
    A. It is an alkylating agent with a half-life of minutes.
    B. Hypermethylation of the *MGMT* promoter leads to increased sensitivity to temozolomide.
    C. It was first approved as a single agent in recurrent glioma.
    D. Concurrent with radiation for newly diagnosed glioblastoma, it is given daily at 150mg/m^2.

21. What were the 5-year overall survivals with and without temozolomide, respectively, reported in the latest (2009) update of the Stupp trial?
    A. 10 %, 2 %
    B. 2 %, 10 %
    C. 27 %, 10 %
    D. 10 %, 27 %

22. According to the 2009 update of the Stupp trial, radiation +/− temozolomide for glioblastoma, what was the strongest predictor of outcome?
    A. Extent of resection
    B. Age
    C. Performance status
    D. *MGMT* status

23. Which of the following targets/therapies for glioblastoma multiforme is incorrect?
    A. EGFR/erlotinib
    B. Farnesyl transferase/tipifarnib
    C. EGFR/trastuzumab
    D. VEGF/bevacizumab

24. What was the median survival in those elderly patients treated with radiotherapy as opposed to best supportive care, as reported by Bauman et al.?
    A. 4 months
    B. 6 months
    C. 8 months
    D. 10 months

25. Comparing standard fractionation to hypofractionated radiotherapy for poor prognosis GBM patients aged 60 years or older, Roa et al. found:
    A. Improved survival in the standard fractionation arm.
    B. Improved survival in the hypofractionated arm.
    C. Those receiving standard fractionation were more likely to require an increase in steroids post-treatment.
    D. More patients in the hypofractionated arm did not complete their planned treatment course.

26. What was the prescribed dose of radiotherapy in the randomized glioblastoma multiforme in the elderly study, as reported by Keime-Guibert et al.?
    A. 30 Gy
    B. 45 Gy
    C. 50.4 Gy
    D. 60 Gy

27. All of the following tumors have a propensity for distant dissemination except:
    A. CNS germ cell tumors
    B. Ependymoma
    C. Choroid plexus tumors
    D. Meningioma

28. Maximal resection is an important initial component in therapy in all of the following except:
    A. Glioblastoma multiforme
    B. Meningioma
    C. CNS germinoma
    D. Chondrosarcoma

29. All of the following are risk factors for the development of meningioma except:
    A. Female sex
    B. Neurofibromatosis type 2
    C. Prior exposure to ionizing radiation
    D. Asian race

30. What pathological feature is frequently present in meningioma?
    A. Psammoma bodies
    B. Rosenthal fibers
    C. Pseudorosettes
    D. Gemistocytes

31. Which of the following pathways of spread of meningioma is least common?
    A. Growth along the base of skull
    B. Growth along meningeal surfaces
    C. Growth with invasion into the brain
    D. Growth with invasion of adjacent dural or superior sagittal sinuses

32. Which statement is incorrect regarding 5-year progression-free survival (5-year PFS) of meningioma, as reported by Goldsmith et al.?
    A. Gross totally resected benign meningioma has a 5-year PFS of >80 %.
    B. Subtotally resected benign meningioma has a 5-year PFS of approximately 50 %.
    C. The addition of radiation after subtotally resected benign meningioma raises progression-free survival to >85 %.
    D. The addition of radiation after resection of malignant meningioma raises progression-free survival to >70 %.

33. Which is the most typical appearance of meningioma on magnetic resonance imaging?
    A. Isointense on pre-contrast T1, no enhancement with gadolinium contrast
    B. Isointense on pre-contrast T1, uniform enhancement with gadolinium contrast
    C. Hyperintense on pre-contrast T1, no enhancement with gadolinium contrast
    D. Hyperintense on pre-contrast T1, uniform enhancement with gadolinium contrast

34. In a low-grade oligodendroglioma, which of the following radiographic patterns would most typically be noted on magnetic resonance imaging?
    A. Enhances on T1 after gadolinium administration, hypointense on T1 pre-contrast
    B. Non-enhancing on T1 after gadolinium administration, hypointense on T1 pre-contrast
    C. Non-enhancing on T1 after gadolinium administration, hyperintense on T1 pre-contrast
    D. Enhances on T1 after gadolinium administration, hyperintense on T1 pre-contrast

35. All of the following are rationales for the use of stereotactic radiosurgery to treat meningioma except:
    A. Lesions are typically well circumscribed.
    B. Alpha/beta ratio is similar to that of late-reacting tissue.
    C. Improvement in local control of subtotally resected lesions.
    D. Treatment side effects are independent of tumor location.

36. In treating parasellar meningiomas with SRS, what dose limit to the optic apparatus is suggested to reduce the risk of optic neuropathy?
    A. 12 Gy
    B. 8 Gy
    C. 6 Gy
    D. 5 Gy

37. Rosenthal fibers are a pathognomic feature of which tumor type?
    A. Pleomorphic xanthoastrocytomas
    B. Oligodendrogliomas
    C. Germinomas
    D. Pilocytic astrocytomas

38. Which one of the following tumor/pathologic feature pairings is incorrect?
    A. Glioblastoma/necrosis
    B. Medulloblastoma/pseudorosettes
    C. Craniopharygioma/cystic areas
    D. Oligodendroglioma/fried egg appearance

39. Comparing the incidence in adults and children, ependymomas tend to be:
    A. Intracranial in adults and supratentorial in children
    B. Spinal in adults and infratentorial in children
    C. Spinal in adults and supratentorial in children
    D. Intracranial in adults and infratentorial in children

40. Which of the following subtypes of ependymoma has the worst prognosis?
    A. Myxopapillary
    B. Anaplastic
    C. Solid squamous papillary
    D. Cellular

41. Which of the following statements about ependymoma is false?
    A. Gross total resection is achieved more commonly in infratentorial compared to supratentorial tumors.
    B. The predominant pattern of failure is local.
    C. Extent of resection is the most important prognostic factor.
    D. Radiotherapy dose is typically 59.4 Gy.

42. Which of the following is not a common site of presentation of chordoma?
    A. Base of skull
    B. Lower cervical spine
    C. Lumbar spine
    D. Sacrum

43. Protons are used in place of photons for some chordomas due to all but which of the following:
    A. Steep dose gradients of protons
    B. Excellent 5-year local control rates
    C. Higher RBE of protons
    D. Proximity of tumor to critical structures

44. All of the following are prognostic factors of the RTOG RPA classification for high-grade glioma developed by Curran et al. except:
    A. Age >60
    B. Histology
    C. Performance status
    D. Extent of resection

45. All are true regarding the new RTOG RPA analysis for glioblastoma multiforme developed by Li et al. except:
    A. It includes only 4 variables, compared to the prior RPA analysis, which included 6.
    B. Classes V and VI are combined due to indistinguishable survival.
    C. Extent of resection is no longer one of the four variables in the new RPA analysis.
    D. This new RPA analysis will be used for future RTOG glioblastoma multiforme trials.

46. All of the following are true regarding the RTOG study 94-02 (Cairncross et al.) looking at outcomes in pure and mixed oligodendroglioma receiving postoperative radiotherapy +/− PCV chemotherapy, except:
    A. Progression-free survival was improved with the addition of PCV chemotherapy.
    B. Overall survival was not improved with the addition of PCV chemotherapy.
    C. Those tumors with $1p$ and $19q$ allelic loss had median survival times > 7 years.
    D. There was no increased toxicity with the addition of PCV chemotherapy to radiotherapy.

47. How many mitoses per 10 high-powered fields constitute anaplastic meningioma?
    A. 5
    B. 10
    C. 15
    D. 20

48. What is the grading system used to describe completeness of resection of meningiomas?
    A. Simpson
    B. Brooker
    C. Bloom-Richardson
    D. Kadish

49. What is the most common site for a CNS germ cell tumor?
    A. Anterior pituitary
    B. Posterior pituitary
    C. Pineal gland
    D. Suprasellar region

50. What syndrome is commonly seen with pineoblastoma?
    A. Eaton-Lambert
    B. Parinaud's
    C. Limbic encephalitis
    D. Cushing's

51. Which of the following pineal tumors has the LEAST propensity for craniospinal dissemination?
    A. Pineoblastoma
    B. Germinoma
    C. Non-germinomatous germ cell tumor
    D. Pineocytoma

52. All of the following statements regarding hemangioblastomas and hemangiopericytomas are true except:
    A. While hemangioblastomas are indolent and slow growing, hemangiopericytomas are locally aggressive.
    B. Hemangioblastomas and hemangiopericytomas are both associated with Von Hippel-Lindau.
    C. Hemangiopericytoma, in contrast to hemangioblastoma, shows a propensity for local recurrence after resection.
    D. Surgical resection is the primary therapy for both tumors.

53. Regarding craniopharyngiomas, all of the following are true except:
    A. They are derived from remnants of Rathke's pouch.
    B. There is a bimodal incidence.
    C. Calcification is infrequently seen.
    D. Diabetes insipidus is a frequent complication of surgery.

54. What percent of pituitary adenomas are nonsecretory?
    A. 30 %
    B. 40 %
    C. 50 %
    D. 60 %

55. Which of the following hormones is secreted by the neurohypophysis?
    A. ADH
    B. ACTH
    C. GH
    D. TSH

56. Which one of the following hormones secreted by a pituitary adenoma has no effective medical therapy?
    A. Prolactin
    B. Thyroid-stimulating hormone
    C. Adrenocorticotropic hormone
    D. Growth hormone

57. After radiation to the pituitary axis, which is most likely to be the first hormone to be affected?
    A. Gonadotropin-releasing hormone
    B. Thyroid-stimulating hormone
    C. Adrenocorticotropic hormone
    D. Growth hormone

58. What is the most caudal structure transmitted through the cavernous sinus?
    A. CN III
    B. CN V1 (V one)
    C. CN V2
    D. CN VI (six)

59. What is the most frequent primary ocular tumor?
    A. Melanoma
    B. Lymphoma
    C. Retinoblastoma
    D. Optic nerve sheath meningioma

60. Which of the following primary ocular tumors occurs more frequently in women than men?
    A. Melanoma
    B. Lymphoma
    C. Retinoblastoma
    D. Optic nerve sheath meningioma

61. Which is the most common tumor type to metastasize to the orbit?
    A. Non-small-cell lung cancer
    B. Hepatocellular carcinoma
    C. Breast cancer
    D. Small-cell lung cancer

62. Which of the following Collaborative Ocular Melanoma Study (COMS) classifications is incorrect?
    A. Small melanoma: 1–3 mm thick
    B. Small melanoma: < 10 mm in largest tumor dimension
    C. Medium melanoma: 3–8 mm thick
    D. Large melanoma: > 16 mm in largest tumor dimension

63. Which of the following is true regarding the COMS study for large choroidal melanomas?
    A. Patients were randomized to enucleation versus plaque brachytherapy.
    B. Patients were randomized to enucleation versus external beam radiotherapy.
    C. Patients were randomized to enucleation +/− plaque brachytherapy.
    D. Patients were randomized to enucleation +/− preoperative external beam radiotherapy.

64. Acoustic neuromas most commonly affect which cranial nerve?
    A. Cranial nerve V
    B. Cranial nerve VII
    C. Cranial nerve VIII
    D. Cranial nerve IX

65. Which of the following is not an embryonal CNS tumor?
    A. Medulloblastoma
    B. Atypical teratoid/rhabdoid tumor
    C. Germinoma
    D. Pineoblastoma

66. What is the typical radiotherapy regimen for embryonal CNS tumors?
    A. None
    B. Craniospinal irradiation
    C. Focal radiation
    D. Whole ventricular radiation

67. Which of the following molecular subtypes of medulloblastoma has the best prognosis?
    A. *Wnt*-pathway-associated subtype
    B. *Hh*-pathway-associated subtype
    C. *c-MYC*-pathway-associated subtype
    D. Other subtypes

68. What is the superior border of the posterior fossa?
    A. Clivus
    B. Tentorium cerebelli
    C. Calvarium
    D. Occipital bone

69. What would be the recommended radiotherapy regimen for standard-risk medulloblastoma?
    A. Craniospinal radiation to 36 Gy, followed by a boost to the posterior fossa to a total of 54 Gy in combination with multiagent chemotherapy
    B. Craniospinal radiation to 54 Gy in combination with multiagent chemotherapy
    C. Craniospinal radiation to 23.4 Gy, followed by a boost to the posterior fossa to a total of 54 Gy in combination with multiagent chemotherapy
    D. Craniospinal radiation to 23.4 Gy in combination with multiagent chemotherapy

70. In a St. Jude Children's Research trial prospectively evaluating focal treatment of the tumor bed, as opposed to treatment of the entire posterior fossa, all of the following are true except:
    A. Dose to the entire posterior fossa was 36 Gy, followed by a conformal tumor bed boost to 54 Gy.
    B. 3-year posterior fossa failure was 6.3 %.
    C. Chemotherapy was given after radiation.
    D. Dose reduction to the posterior fossa was over 10 %.

71. Which is not a component of therapy for children<3 years with medulloblastoma?
    A. Surgery
    B. Chemotherapy
    C. Craniospinal irradiation
    D. Posterior fossa irradiation

72. Which is the least common site of ependymoma in children?
    A. Posterior fossa arising from roof of fourth ventricle
    B. Parenchyma of cerebral hemispheres
    C. Cerebellopontine angle
    D. Spinal cord

73. All of the following are true regarding ependymomas except:
    A. Most recurrences are local.
    B. The most common histology in the cauda equina is myxopapillary.
    C. More ependymomas occur supratentorially, rather than infratentorially.
    D. Extent of surgery is the most important predictor of outcome.

74. What is the most appropriate radiotherapy dose after gross total resection of a localized ependymoma?
    A. 50.4 Gy
    B. 54 Gy
    C. 55.8 Gy
    D. 59.4 Gy

75. What is the most appropriate next step in management of a completely resected low-grade astrocytoma of the cerebellum in children and young adults?
    A. Focal radiotherapy
    B. Chemotherapy
    C. Observation
    D. Posterior fossa radiotherapy

76. All of the following are true regarding germinomas except:
    A. Diagnosis does not require a biopsy.
    B. Germinomas are radiosensitive.
    C. Germinomas are chemosensitive.
    D. Whole ventricular radiation is appropriate for localized germinoma.

77. All of the following are true regarding craniopharyngiomas except:
    A. Endocrine abnormalities are infrequent.
    B. Derived from embryonic remnant of the anterior pituitary.
    C. Commonly present with mixed solid/cystic components.
    D. Possesses a bimodal age of incidence.

78. All of the following are true regarding management of craniopharyngiomas except:
    A. Subtotal resection + radiation and gross total resection alone have equivalent outcomes.
    B. Radical surgery has been shown to be associated with loss of more IQ points compared to subtotal surgery.
    C. There is no radiation dose–response in terms of local control of craniopharyngioma.
    D. Hypopituitarism at presentation predicts for treatment-related morbidity.

79. What is the next best step in management of an asymptomatic optic glioma in a 7-year-old child?
    A. Close observation
    B. Surgery
    C. Fractionated radiation
    D. Chemotherapy

80. What gene mutation is seen in over 80 % of atypical teratoid/rhabdoid tumors?
    A. *INI-1*
    B. *Wnt*
    C. *Hh*
    D. *c-MYC*

81. Impingement of what structure results in Parinaud's syndrome, commonly seen
    in pineoblastoma?
    A. Optic nerve
    B. Optic chiasm
    C. Superior colliculi
    D. Inferior colliculi

82. What other tumor can be seen in children that have bilateral retinoblastomas?
    A. Pineocytoma
    B. Pituitary adenoma
    C. Pineoblastoma
    D. Anaplastic ependymoma

Answers and Rationales

1. The correct answer is B. Intracranial astrocytomas of any grade can be seen. Pilocytic astrocytomas (WHO I) are particularly common. Brown PD, Shaw EG, van den Bendt MJ. Low-grade gliomas. In: Gunderson LL, Tepper JE, editors, Clinical radiation oncology. 3rd ed. Philadelphia: Elsevier Saunders; 2012. p. 443–59.

2. The correct answer is A. Although meningiomas and astrocytomas can be seen with NF2, schwannomas, particularly bilateral acoustic neuromas are most commonly seen. Chan MD, Rogers CL, Anderson BM, Khuntia D. Benign brain tumors: meningiomas and vestibular schwannomas. In: Gunderson LL, Tepper JE, editors, Clinical radiation oncology. 3rd ed. Philadelphia: Elsevier Saunders; 2012. p. 473–91.

3. The correct answer is D. Turcot's is an inherited syndrome associated with the biallelic DNA mismatch repair mutations, with an association between familial polyposis of the colon and brain tumors (medulloblastoma, malignant glioma). Turcot J et al. Malignant tumors of the central nervous system associated with familial polyposis of the colon and bright green urine which may be related to vegetables in the diet: report of two cases. Dis Colon Rectum. 1959;2:465–8.

4. The correct answer is A. Tuberous sclerosis is associated with angiofibromas, hamartomas, and subependymal giant cell tumors, but not hemangioblastomas. The latter are associated with Von Hippel-Lindau.

5. The correct answer is C. Von Hippel-Lindau is an autosomal dominant disorder, caused by a tumor suppressor gene on chromosome 3. Cerebellar, brainstem, and spinal cord hemangioblastomas are associated with VHL. Cowden's syndrome (multiple hamartoma syndrome) is an autosomal dominant inherited syndrome resulting from mutation in the *PTEN* gene on arm *10q* that causes hamartomatous neoplasms of the skin, mucosa, GI tract, bones, CNS, eyes, and genitourinary tract. The skin is involved in 90–100 % of cases; the thyroid is involved in 66 % of cases. Turcot's is an inherited syndrome associated with the biallelic DNA mismatch repair mutations, with an association between familial polyposis of the colon and brain tumors (medulloblastoma, malignant glioma). Gorlin's is an autosomal dominantly inherited disorder also known as nevoid basal cell carcinoma syndrome, caused by mutations in the *PTCH* gene on chromosome *9q*. In addition to the development of basal cell carcinomas, benign odontogenic keratocysts of the jaw are seen in 75 % of patients, usually occurring at a young age. Less commonly seen are ovarian or cardiac fibromas, and/or medulloblastomas (seen in children ≤ 2 years). Liaw D et al. Germline mutations of the PTEN gene in Cowden disease, an inherited breast and thyroid cancer syndrome. Nat Genet. 1997;16(1):64–7. Lloyd KM II, Dennis M. Cowden's disease. A possible new symptoms complex with multiple system involvement. Ann Intern Med. 1963;58:136–42. Turcot J et al. Malignant

tumors of the central nervous system associated with familial polyposis of the colon and bright green urine which may be related to vegetables in the diet: report of two cases. Dis Colon Rectum. 1959;2:465–8. Gorlin R, Goltz R. Multiple nevoid basal-cell epithelioma, jaw cysts and bifid rib. A syndrome. N Engl J Med. 1960;262(18):908–12.

6. The correct answer is D. Whereas survival decreases with increasing age in glioblastoma multiforme, oligodendroglioma, and anaplastic astrocytoma, it improves in brainstem glioma with increasing age. Freeman CR, Farmer JP. Pediatric brain stem gliomas: a review. IJROBP. 1998;40:265–71. Guillamo JS, Monjour A, Taillandier L, et al. Brainstem gliomas in adults: prognostic factors and classification. Brain 2001;124:2528–39.

7. The correct answer is B. *MDM2* overexpression is frequently seen in primary glioblastoma, while loss of *19q* and *IDH1* positivity is associated with secondary glioblastoma. Genetics of glioma progression and the definition of primary and secondary glioblastoma. Brain Pathol. 1997;7:1131–36. The next generation of glioma biomarkers: *MGMT* methylation, *BRAF* mutations, and *IDH1* mutations. Von Diemling A, Korshunov A, Hartmann C. Brain Pathol. 2011;1:74–87.

8. The correct answer is D. *1p* and *19q* deletion is an established prognostic factor for anaplastic oligodendrogliomas. Hoang-Xuan et al. described their prospective trial results, which showed loss of *1p* correlated with objective tumor response. In analyzing *1p19* status of 100 low-grade glioma patients enrolled on two North Central Cancer Treatment Group Protocols, Buckner et al. found that *1p* and *19q* deletions were associated with superior 5-year progression-free and overall survival. Hoang-Xuan K, Capelle L, et al. Temozolomide as initial treatment for adults with low-grade oligodendrogliomas or oligoastrocytomas and correlation with chromosome *1p* deletions. J Clin Oncol. 2004;22:3133–8. Bucker JC, Ballman KV, et al. Diagnostic and prognostic significance of *1p* and *19q* deletions in patients (pts) with low-grade oligodendroglioma and astrocytoma. J Clin Oncol. 2005;23:1145.

9. The correct answer is A. *MGMT* is a DNA repair enzyme that repairs damage induced by alkylating agents, such as temozolomide. Methylation of the *MGMT* promoters results in epigenetic silencing and thus decreased *MGMT* expression. After determining the methylation status of glioblastoma patients randomized to radiation +/– temozolomide, Hegi et al. found *MGMT* promoter methylation to be associated with improved survival. Hegi ME et al. MGMT gene silencing and benefit from temozolomide in glioblastoma. N Engl J Med. 2005;352:997–1003.

10. The correct answer is D. Seizure is the most common presenting symptom, occurring in approximately two-thirds of patients. Brown PD, Shaw EG, van den Bendt MJ. Low-grade gliomas. In: Gunderson LL, Tepper JE, editors, Clinical radiation oncology. 3rd ed. Philadelphia: Elsevier Saunders; 2012. p. 443–59.

11. The correct answer is C. Pignatti et al. used the databases of low-grade glioma patients from EORTC trials 22844 and 22845 to develop a prognostic scoring system using imaging, patient, and tumor characteristics. The following were found by Cox regression to be negative risk factors: age 40 years or more, astrocytoma histology subtype, largest diameter of the tumor ≥6 cm, tumor crossing the midline, and presence of neurological deficit before surgery. Two or more risk factors comprised the low-risk group, with a median survival of 7.7 years. Three or more risk factors defined a high-risk group with a median survival of 3.2 years. Pignatti F, van den Bent M, et al. Prognostic factors for survival in adult patients with cerebral low-grade glioma. J Clin Oncol. 2002;20:2076–84.

12. The correct answer is B. In EORTC 22844, the "Believer's Trial," patients with low-grade glioma were randomized to immediate postoperative RT with either 45 Gy or 59.4 Gy. Only 25 % underwent gross total resection prior to radiation. Dose escalation did not result in improved survival, nor progression-free survival. Karim AB et al., A randomized trial on dose–response in radiation therapy of low-grade cerebral glioma: European Organization for Research and Treatment of Cancer (EORTC) Study 22844. Int J Radiat Oncol Biol Phys. 1996;36(3):549–56.

13. The correct answer is C. Long-term results of the EORTC 22845 randomized trial that compared early versus delayed radiotherapy for low-grade gliomas were published in the Lancet in 2005. While progression-free survival improved in the early radiotherapy arm (5.3 years vs. 3.4 years), there was no difference in overall survival (7.4 vs. 7.2 years). There was better seizure control in the early radiotherapy group at 1 year (25 % with seizures in early group vs. 41 %, $p=0.03$). Median dose delivered was 54 Gy in 30 fractions. Van de Bent MJ. et al. Long-term efficacy of early versus delayed radiotherapy for low-grade astrocytoma and oligodendroglioma in adults: the EORTC 22845 randomised trial. Lancet. 2005;355:985–90.

14. The correct answer is C. The EORTC 26951 trial randomized 368 patients with anaplastic oligodendroglioma after surgery and radiation to either observation or adjuvant PCV chemotherapy (procarbazine, lomustine, vincristine). The initial published 5-year results in 2006 showed only a progression-free survival benefit (1.9 years vs. 1.1 years). *1p19q* deletion was subsequently evaluated, and those with 1p19q deletion had a 5-year overall survival of 74 % versus 30 % without the deletion. With 12 years of follow-up, the addition of PCV chemotherapy not only improves progression-free survival, but also improves overall survival. Median survival is significantly prolonged (42.3 months vs. 30.6 months) in those that received adjuvant PCV. In those with *1p19q* deletion that received adjuvant PCV, median survival has not been reached. Van den Bent MJ et al. First analysis of EORTC 26951, a randomised phase III study of adjuvant PCV chemotherapy in patients with highly anaplastic oligodendroglioma. J Clin Oncol. 2006;24(18):2715–22. Van den Bent MJ et al. Long-term follow-up results of EORTC 26951 a randomised phase III study of adjuvant

PCV chemotherapy in anaplastic oligodendroglial tumors (AOD). J Clin Oncol. 2012;(Suppl;abstr 2).

15. The correct answer is C. Magnetic resonance spectroscopy is a method to monitor biochemical changes in the brain. The most commonly used brain metabolites in MRS are choline, a measure of increased cell turnover, which is elevated in tumors and inflammatory processes; creatine, a measure of energy stores, decreased in tumors; and N-acetylaspartate (NAA), a neuronal marker which decreases in processes that adversely affect neuron integrity. The MR spectrum shows various peaks of these metabolites, displayed from left to right—choline, creatine, and NAA. Hunter's angle is a line drawn along the peaks of the white matter metabolites and is generally downward in brain tumors (denoting an increased choline to creatine ratio). Radiation necrosis on MRS is usually denoted by low levels of NAA, creatine, and choline. Nelson SJ et al. Characterization of untreated gliomas by magnetic resonance imaging. Neuroimag Clin. 2002;12:599–613. Graves EE et al. Serial proton MR spectroscopic imaging of recurrent malignant gliomas after gamma knife radiosurgery. AJNR. 2001;22:613–24.

16. The correct answer is A. To attempt to determine an optimal radiation dose for malignant gliomas, ECOG/RTOG performed a four-arm study, comparing 3 experimental arms:(1) 60 Gy WBRT + 10 Gy partial brain boost, (2) 60 Gy WBRT + BCNU, and (3) 60 Gy WBRT + CCNU + dacarbazine (DTIC) against a standard 60 Gy WBRT arm. There was no survival benefit seen with the 10 Gy boost. Age was found to be the most important prognostic factor, with 18-month survival 64 % in those <40 years, versus 20 % in those 40–60 years, and 8 % in those >60 years. Among the 40–60 year-old group, the addition of BCNU did improve survival compared to 60 Gy WBRT alone. Not unexpectedly, the combination of CCNU + DTIC was more toxic than BCNU, producing a higher incidence of thrombocytopenia. Chang CH et al. Comparison of postoperative radiotherapy and combined postoperative radiotherapy and chemotherapy in the multidisciplinary management of malignant gliomas. A Joint Radiation Therapy Oncology Group and Eastern Cooperative Oncology Group Study. Cancer. 1983;(6):997–1007.

17. The correct answer is D. Lee et al. reported on the patterns of failure following high-dose 3-D conformal radiotherapy of high-grade astrocytomas. All patients were treated to either 70 or 80 Gy. An "in-field" recurrence was defined as 80 % or more of the volume of the recurrence lying within the 95 % isodose region. It was termed as "outside" when 20 % or less of the volume of the recurrence was inside the 95 % isodose region. Of the 36 evaluable patients, 89 % failed "in-field," with only 1 failing outside the high-dose region. Despite the dose escalation, there was no improvement in overall survival. No dose-limiting toxicity was seen. Lee SW et al. Patterns of failure following high-dose 3-D conformal radiotherapy for high-grade astrocytomas: a quantitative dosimetric study. Int J Radiat Oncol Biol Phys. 1999;43:79–88.

18. The correct answer is C. RTOG 90-05 sought to define optimal doses for radio-surgery in patients with recurrence malignant brain tumors, including both gliomas and metastases. Patients were stratified by tumor volume: <2 cm, 2–3 cm, and 3.1–4 cm; dose-limiting toxicity was defined as irreversible grade 3 neurotoxicity or any grade 4/5 neurotoxicity seen within 3 months of SRS. While the maximum tolerated dose was not reached in tumors <2 cm, dose was not escalated beyond 24 Gy. Maximum tolerated dose for the 2–3 cm and 3.1–4 cm tumors was 18 Gy and 15 Gy, respectively. Approximately half (48 %) of patients failed locally, with local failure more likely in those with gliomas compared to those with metastases. Shaw EG et al. Single dose radiosurgical treatment of recurrent previously irradiated primary brain tumors and brain metastases: final report of RTOG protocol 90-05. Int J Radiat Oncol Biol Phys. 1996;34:647–54.

19. The correct answer is B. The Brain Tumor Cooperative Group study 8701 randomized patients with malignant glioma post resection to temporary ^{125}I brachytherapy followed by EBRT + BCNU or EBRT and BCNU alone. No survival benefit was seen in the brachytherapy boost group. The GliaSite RT system uses an ^{125}I solution injected into a closed catheter balloon. With a balloon, there is not a true point source, and with smaller fill volumes, the surface dose can be much higher. This can theoretically lead to higher rates of radiation necrosis. Selker RG et al. The brain tumor cooperative group NIH trial 87-01: a randomized comparison of surgery, external radiotherapy, and carmustine versus surgery, interstitial radiotherapy boost, external radiation therapy, and carmustine. Neurosurgery. 2002;51:343–55.

20. The correct answer is D. Temozolomide is an alkylating agent with a half-life of minutes that leads to methylation of the O-6 position of guanine. Unrepaired, this will lead to double-strand breaks. Although now the standard of care in newly diagnosed glioblastoma multiforme due to the overall survival benefit seen in Stupp's landmark trial, it was first studied and FDA approved in recurrent glioma. Yung and colleagues randomized patients with recurrent glioma to either procarbazine or temozolomide and found that those on the temozolomide arm were more likely to objectively respond and remain progression-free at 6 months. In Stupp's study, temozolomide was given concurrently with radiation (60 Gy), at a daily dose of 75 mg/m^2, and adjuvantly for 6 cycles at 150–200 mg/m^2. The latest update published in 2009 in The Lancet showed that the overall survival benefit persisted: 5-year survival 9.8 % versus 1.9 %. *MGMT* is a DNA repair enzyme that repairs this damage induced by temozolomide. Methylation of the *MGMT* promoters results in epigenetic silencing and thus decreased *MGMT* expression. After determining the methylation status of glioblastoma patients randomized to radiation +/− temozolomide, Hegi et al. found *MGMT* promoter methylation to be associated with improved survival. Hegi ME et al. MGMT gene silencing and benefit from temozolomide in glioblastoma. N Engl J Med. 2005;352:997–1003. Yung WK, Albright RE, et al. A phase II study of temozolomide vs. procarbazine in patients with glioblastoma

multiforme at first relapse. Br J Cancer. 2000;83:588–93. Stupp R et al. Effects of radiotherapy with concomitant and adjuvant temozolomide versus radiotherapy alone on survival in glioblastoma in a randomised phase III study: 5-year analysis of the EORTC-NCIC trial. The Lancet Oncol. 2009;10(5):459–66.

21. The correct answer is A. In Stupp's study, temozolomide was given concurrently with radiation (60 Gy), at a daily dose of 75 mg/m^2, and adjuvantly for 6 cycles at 150–200 mg/m^2. The initial report in 2005 showed an improvement in median survival with the addition of temozolomide: 14.6 versus 12.1 m. Two-year survival was also improved (26.5 % vs. 10.4 %). The latest update published in 2009 in The Lancet showed that the overall survival benefit persisted:5-year survival 9.8 % versus 1.9 %. Stupp R et al. Effects of radiotherapy with concomitant and adjuvant temozolomide versus radiotherapy alone on survival in glioblastoma in a randomised phase III study: 5-year analysis of the EORTC-NCIC trial. The Lancet Oncol. 2009;10(5):459–66.

22. The correct answer is D. The latest update published in 2009 in The Lancet showed that the overall survival benefit persisted: 5-year survival 9.8 % versus 1.9 %. MGMT status was retrospectively determined and found to be the strongest predictor of outcome. The benefit of combined modality therapy extended to all clinical subgroups, even those aged 60–70 years. Stupp R et al. Effects of radiotherapy with concomitant and adjuvant temozolomide versus radiotherapy alone on survival in glioblastoma in a randomised phase III study: 5-year analysis of the EORTC-NCIC trial. The Lancet Oncol. 2009;10(5):459–66.

23. The correct answer is C. EGFR is overexpressed in 50 % of GBMs. Erlotinib and gefitinib, small molecule inhibitors of EGFR tyrosine kinase activity, are currently being tested in combination with radiation for glioblastoma. The farnesyl transferase inhibitor, tipifarnib, has been studied in phase I and II trials of recurrent malignant glioma. Trastuzumab is a monoclonal antibody that interferes with the HER-2 receptor, most commonly used in breast cancer. Bevacizumab has been studied in phase I/II trials in the setting of recurrent glioblastoma. Wong AJ et al. Increased expression of the epidermal growth factor receptor gene in malignant gliomas is invariably associated with gene amplification. Proc Natl Acad Sci USA. 1987;84:6899–903. Volgelbaum M et al. Initial Experience with the EGFR tyrosine Tarceva (OSI-774) for single agent therapy of recurrent/progressive glioblastoma multiforme. Neuro-oncology 2003;5:356. Chakravarti A et al. An update of phase I data from RTOG 0211: a phase I/II clinical study of ZD 1839 (Gefitinib) + radiation for newly diagnosed glioblastoma patients [abstract]. Neuro-oncology. 2004;6:372. Cloughsey TF et al. Two phase II trials of R115777 (Zarnestra) in patients with recurrent glioblastoma multiforme (GBM): a comparison of patients on enzyme-inducing anti-epileptic drugs (EIAED) and not on EIAED at maximum tolerated dose respectively: a North American Brain Tumor Consortium (NABTC) report [abstract]. Neuro-oncology. 2004;5:349.

24. The correct answer is D. In this single-arm prospective trial, elderly patients ≥60 years and KPS ≤50 were treated with short-course radiotherapy (30 Gy/10 fractions). When comparing these patients with historical controls of those receiving only best supportive care, median survival was improved from 1 to 10 m. Bauman GS et al. A prospective study of short-course radiotherapy in poor prognosis glioblastoma multiforme. Int J Radiat Oncol Biol Phys. 1994 29(4):835–9.

25. The correct answer is C. To evaluate different fractionations in poor prognosis glioma patients, Roa and colleagues randomized patients to standard fractionation (60 Gy/30 fx) versus hypofractionation (40 Gy/15 fx). No survival difference was found, with median survival approximately 5 months in both arms. Those in the standard fractionation arm were less likely to complete the entire planned course (74 % vs. 90 % in the hypofractionated arm) and were also more likely to require an increase in steroids post-treatment (49 % vs. 23 % in the hypofractionated arm). Roa W et al. Abbreviated course of radiation therapy in older patients with glioblastoma multiforme: a prospective randomized clinical trial. J Clin Oncol. 2004;22:1583–88.

26. The correct answer is C. In this randomized study, 85 elderly patients (≥ 70 years) with a KPS of ≥ 70 were randomized to either best supportive care or 50.4 Gy in 1.8 Gy fractions. At the first planned analysis, the efficacy of radiotherapy exceeded the preset boundary, closing the study. At a median follow-up of 21 weeks, median survival with RT was 29.1 weeks compared to 16.9 weeks without radiotherapy. Quality of life did not differ between the two groups. Keime-Guibert F et al. Radiotherapy for glioblastoma in the elderly. N Engl J Med. 2007;356(15):1527–35.

27. The correct answer is D. While CNS germ cell tumors, ependymomas, and choroid plexus tumors have a propensity for distant dissemination, meningiomas tend to be more locally aggressive in nature. Chan MD, Rogers CL, Anderson BM, Khuntia D. Benign brain tumors: meningiomas and vestibular schwannomas. In: Gunderson LL, Tepper JE, editors, Clinical radiation oncology. 3rd ed. Philadelphia: Elsevier Saunders; 2012. p. 473–91.

28. The correct answer is C. Due to its histology and chemosensitivity, maximal resection is generally NOT an important component of therapy for CNS germinoma. Merchant TE. Central nervous system tumors in children. In: Gunderson LL, Tepper JE, editors, Clinical radiation oncology. 3rd ed. Philadelphia: Elsevier Saunders; 2012. p. 1409–23.

29. The correct answer is D. The incidence of meningiomas in females is double that of males. Prior exposure to ionizing radiation is a risk factor for the development of meningiomas, as is neurofibromatosis type 2. Individuals with NF2 are also at risk for development of schwannomas and ependymomas. There is no known difference in incidence of meningiomas according to race. Mack EE et al.

Meningiomas induced by high-dose cranial irradiation. J Neurosurg. 1993;79:28. Louis DN et al. Meningiomas. In: Kleihues P, Cavenee WK, editors. Pathology and genetics: tumors of the nervous system. Lyon: IARC Press; 2000. p. 176.

30. The correct answer is A. Psammoma bodies are frequently found in meningioma. Rosenthal fibers and gemistocytes are seen in astrocytomas. Pseudorosettes are a hallmark pathological feature of ependymomas. Chan MD, Rogers CL, Anderson BM, Khuntia D. Benign brain tumors: meningiomas and vestibular schwannomas. In: Gunderson LL, Tepper JE, editors, Clinical radiation oncology. 3rd ed. Philadelphia: Elsevier Saunders; 2012. p. 473–91.

31. The correct answer is C. Meningiomas most commonly grow along meningeal surfaces. They can grow along the base of skull and even invade into adjacent structures, such as the dural or superior sagittal sinuses. Invasion into brain parenchyma is less common and more likely to occur with higher-grade meningioma. Chan MD, Rogers CL, Anderson BM, Khuntia D. Benign brain tumors: meningiomas and vestibular schwannomas. In: Gunderson LL, Tepper JE, editors, Clinical radiation oncology. 3rd ed. Philadelphia: Elsevier Saunders; 2012. p. 473–91.

32. The correct answer is D. In this retrospective review, 140 patients with resected meningioma were treated with a median of 54 Gy radiotherapy. This study included a very mixed population of benign and malignant tumors: Twenty-three patients had malignant meningioma. Five-year progression-free survival was 89 % in those that underwent gross total resection and 48 % in those that underwent subtotal resection. With adjuvant radiotherapy, subtotally resected meningioma 5-year progression-free survival approached that of gross totally resected tumors. Five-year progression-free survival of malignant meningioma after adjuvant radiation was 40–50 %. One of the most important points of the study is that outcomes are worse with total dose <52 Gy. Goldsmith BJ et al. Postoperative irradiation for subtotally resected meningiomas. A retrospective analysis of 140 patients treated from 1967 to 1990. J Neurosurg. 1994;80(2):195–201.

33. The correct answer is B. Meningiomas tend to be hypointense or isointense on pre-contrast T1-weighted images and uniformly enhance with gadolinium contrast. Chan MD, Rogers CL, Anderson BM, Khuntia D. Benign brain tumors: meningiomas and vestibular schwannomas. In Gunderson LL, Tepper JE, editors, Clinical radiation oncology. 3rd ed. Philadelphia: Elsevier Saunders; 2012. p. 473–91.

34. The correct answer is B. The majority (2/3) of low-grade oligogliomas tend to be hypointense on T1 pre-contrast sequences, non-enhancing after gadolinium administration on T1 sequences, but hyperintense on T2-weighted sequences. Brown PD, Shaw EG, van den Bendt MJ. Low-grade gliomas. In: Gunderson LL, Tepper JE, editors. Clinical radiation oncology. 3rd ed. Philadelphia: Elsevier Saunders; 2012. p. 443–59.

35. The correct answer is D. The fact that meningiomas are typically well circumscribed and well demarcated on MRI lends them to treatment with stereotactic radiosurgery (SRS). SRS can be used to improve local control after subtotal resection of meningiomas. One rationale for the use of SRS in treatment of meningiomas is that the alpha/beta ratio of meningiomas is thought to be akin to that of late-reacting tissue and thus may be more sensitive to the larger dose per fraction given with SRS. Despite the steep dose gradients possible with SRS, treatment of a lesion with in a location with significant mass effect may be associated with a higher risk of posttreatment edema. Vernimmen FJ et al. Stereotactic proton beam therapy of skull base meningiomas. Int J Radiat Oncol Biol Phys. 2001;49:99. Vermeulen S et al. A comparison of single fraction radiosurgery tumor control and toxicity in the treatment of basal and nonbasal meningiomas. Stereotact Funct Neurosurg. 1999;72(Suppl 1):60.

36. The correct answer is B. To reduce the risk of optic neuropathy, a dose limit of 8–10 Gy to the visual apparatus is suggested. Shrieve DC et al. Dose fractionation in stereotactic radiotherapy for parasellar meningiomas: radiobiological considerations of efficacy and optic nerve tolerance. J Neurosurg. 2004;S3:390.

37. The correct answer is D. Rosenthal fibers are pathognomic for pilocytic astrocytomas. Oligodendrogliomas have a "fried egg" appearance on microscopy. Germinomas are a round, blue cell tumor. Brown PD, Shaw EG, van den Bendt MJ. Low-grade gliomas. In: Gunderson LL, Tepper JE, editors, Clinical radiation oncology. 3rd ed. Philadelphia: Elsevier Saunders; 2012. p. 443–59. Chan MD, Rogers CL, Anderson BM, Khuntia D. Benign brain tumors: meningiomas and vestibular schwannomas. In: Gunderson LL, Tepper JE, editors, Clinical radiation oncology. 3rd ed. Philadelphia: Elsevier Saunders; 2012. p. 473–91.

38. The correct answer is B. Medulloblastoma is associated with Homer-Wright rosettes, not pseudorosettes. These are associated with ependymoma. Merchant TE. Central nervous system tumors in children. In: Gunderson LL, Tepper JE, editors. Clinical radiation oncology. 3rd ed. Philadelphia: Elsevier Saunders; 2012. p. 1409–23.

39. The correct answer is B. Ependymomas are relatively rare glial tumors. While children tend to present at a median age of 5, adults present in the third and fourth decades. The vast majority (90 %) of ependymomas are infratentorial and intracranial in children. In adults, ependymomas present more commonly in the spine or supratentorially. Stieber VW, Siker ML. Spinal cord tumors. In: Gunderson LL, Tepper JE, editors. Clinical radiation oncology. 3rd ed. Philadelphia: Elsevier Saunders; 2012. p. 511–28.

40. The correct answer is B. Anaplastic ependymomas have a much worse prognosis compared to well-differentiated myxopapillary, solid squamous, and cellular ependymomas. The myxopapillary subtype tends to be found in the cauda equina region. Solid squamous papillary ependymomas have a more favorable

prognosis and are found in adults. Stieber VW, Siker ML. Spinal cord tumors. In Gunderson LL, Tepper JE, editors. Clinical radiation oncology. 3rd ed. Philadelphia: Elsevier Saunders; 2012. p. 511–28.

41. The correct answer is A. Gross total resection is more commonly achieved in supratentorial (50 %) rather than infratentorial tumors (30 %). Extent of resection is the most important predictor of outcome. As recurrences tend to be local, postoperative radiotherapy is typically tumor bed + margin to 59.4 Gy. Stieber VW, Siker ML. Spinal cord tumors. In: Gunderson LL, Tepper JE, editors. Clinical radiation oncology. 3rd ed. Philadelphia: Elsevier Saunders; 2012. p. 511–28.

42. The correct answer is B. One-third of chordomas present in the clivus/craniocervical junction (base of skull). One-third present in the thoracic/lumbar spine, and the remaining third present in the sacrum. Stieber VW, Siker ML. Spinal cord tumors. In: Gunderson LL, Tepper JE, editors. Clinical radiation oncology. 3rd ed. Philadelphia: Elsevier Saunders; 2012. p. 511–28.

43. The correct answer is C. The inherent characteristic of protons that is most useful for the treatment of some chordomas is the Bragg Peak and subsequent steep dose gradient. Protons have been used to treat chordomas with excellent 5-year local control rates. Protons have an RBE of 1.1, while photons have an RBE of 1. Stieber VW, Siker ML. Spinal cord tumors. In: Gunderson LL, Tepper JE, editors. Clinical radiation oncology. 3rd ed. Philadelphia: Elsevier Saunders; 2012. p. 511–28.

44. The correct answer is A. The recursive partitioning analysis for high-grade gliomas developed by Curran et al. describes 6 prognostic groups in which patients are grouped by 8 factors: age >50 years, histology (GBM vs. AA), mental status, KPS, length of symptoms prior to surgery (< or>3 m), extent of resection, neurologic function, and RT dose (< or>54.4 Gy). Curran et al. Recursive Partitioning analysis of prognostic factors in three radiation therapy oncology group malignant glioma trials. J Natl Cancer Inst. 1993;85(9):704–10.

45. The correct answer is C. The new recursive partitioning analysis for high-grade gliomas developed by Li et al. describes 3 prognostic groups (Class III, IV, V + VI) in which patients are grouped by 4 factors: age >50 years, KPS, extent of resection, and neurologic function. Classes V and VI were combined due to indistinguishable survival. This new RPA classification will be used in future RTOG GBM trials. Li et al. Validation and simplification of the radiation therapy oncology group recursive partitioning analysis classification for glioblastoma. Int J Radiation Oncol Biol Phys. 2011;81(3):623–30.

46. The correct answer is D. RTOG 94-02 was a phase III study looking at outcomes in pure and mixed oligodendroglioma receiving postoperative radiotherapy (59.4 Gy) +/− PCV chemotherapy (CRT). Two hundred eighty-nine patients were randomized to receive either postoperative RT alone or PCV x up

to 4 cycles, then RT. With 3-year follow-up, median survival was similar (4.9m CRT vs. 4.7m RT). Progression-free survival however was statistically significantly improved with the addition of PCV: 2.6y versus 1.7y, HR = 0.69, (p = 0.004). The PCV group experienced significantly more toxicity; 65 % experienced grade 3 or 4 toxicity. *1p* and *19q* allelic losses were tested by fluorescence in situ hybridization, and deletion was found to confer improved overall (MS: >7y) and progression-free survival. An update was reported at the 2012 ASCO meeting. With 11.3 years of follow-up, the *1p/19q* deleted patients showed a median survival of 14.7 years with PCV versus 7.3 years without (p = 0.03). Cairncross, JG et al. Phase III trial of chemotherapy plus radiotherapy alone for pure and mixed anaplastic oligodendroglioma: intergroup radiation therapy oncology group trial 9402. J Clin Oncol. 2006;24(18):2707–14. Carincross JG et al. Chemotherapy plus radiotherapy (CT-RT) versus RT alone for patients with anaplastic oligodendroglioma: long-term results of the RTOG 94-02 phase III study. J Clin Oncol. 2012 (Suppl; abstr 2008b).

47. The correct answer is D. The (World Health Organization) WHO published revised grading for meningiomas in 2000, based on clinicopathological series from the Mayo Clinic. The revision of the histological grading of meningiomas resulted in upgrading of previously benign meningiomas to the atypical category. In contrast, the criteria for grading anaplastic or malignant meningiomas became stricter. In the new classification, 20 mitoses per 10 hpf are required for classification of an anaplastic meningioma. Atypical meningioma was classified by at least 4 mitoses in 10 hpf or 3 of the following criteria: increased cellularity, high nuclear-to-cytoplasm ratios, prominent nucleoli, sheet-like growth, and necrosis. The most notable change from the 2007 WHO scheme was that brain invasive meningiomas are classified as WHO grade II based on similar recurrence and mortality rates to those of atypical meningiomas. Louis DN, Scheithauer BW, Budka H, Von Deimling A, Kepes JJ. Meningiomas. In: Kleihues P, Cavenee WK, editors. Pathology and genetics of tumors of the nervous system. Lyon: IARC press; 2000. p. 176–84. Perry A, Louis DN, Scheithauer BW, Budka H, Von Deimling, A. Meningiomas. In: Louis DN, Ohgaki H, Wiestler OD, Cavenee WK, editors. WHO classification of tumours of the central nervous system. Lyon: IARC press; 2007. p. 164–72.

48. The correct answer is A. Simpson classification describes extent of resection of meningiomas. Grade I: complete removal including resection of underlying bone and associated dura. Grade II: complete removal and coagulation of dural attachment. Grade III: complete removal without resection of dura or coagulation. Grade IV: subtotal resection. With increasing Simpson grade, there is increased local recurrence. Brooker classification describes the degree of heterotopic bone formation. Bloom-Richardson is the grading system used for breast carcinomas. Kadish staging is used for esthesioneuroblastoma. Simpson D. The recurrence of intracranial meningiomas after surgical treatment. J Neurol Neurosurg Psychiatr. 1957;20(1):22–39.

49. The correct answer is C. The pineal gland is the most common site for CNS germ cell tumors, followed by the suprasellar region. The most common histology is germinoma. 15–30 % of pineal tumors originate in pineocytes and fall into one of the four following types: pineocytomas, mixed pineal parenchymal tumors, pineal parenchymal tumors with intermediate differentiation, and pineoblastomas. In patients with bilateral retinoblastomas, a pineoblastoma is called trilateral retinoblastoma. Merchant TE. Central nervous system tumors in children. In: Gunderson LL, Tepper JE, editors. Clinical radiation oncology. 3rd ed. Philadelphia: Elsevier Saunders; 2012. p. 1409–23.

50. The correct answer is B. Parinaud's syndrome, associated with pineoblastoma, results from pressure on the superior colliculus in the midbrain. The syndrome consists of vertical gaze palsy, light-near dissociation of the pupils, and convergence retraction nystagmus. Eaton-Lambert and limbic encephalitis are paraneoplastic syndromes seen with small-cell lung cancer. Merchant TE. Central nervous system tumors in children. In: Gunderson LL, Tepper JE, editors. Clinical radiation oncology. 3rd ed. Philadelphia: Elsevier Saunders; 2012. p. 1409–23.

51. The correct answer is D. Of the listed tumors found in the pineal gland, pineocytomas have the least propensity for craniospinal dissemination. Treatment usually consists of at least 50 Gy to the primary tumor alone. Merchant TE. Central nervous system tumors in children. In: Gunderson LL, Tepper JE, editors. Clinical radiation oncology. 3rd ed. Philadelphia: Elsevier Saunders; 2012. p. 1409–23.

52. The correct answer is B. While hemangioblastomas are characterized by mutations in the *VHL* tumor suppressor gene on chromosome *3p*, hemangiopericytomas are not characterized by any specific patterns of genetic change. Hemangioblastomas tend to be slow growing with indolent behavior, whereas hemangiopericytomas tend to be more locally aggressive, recurring even after complete surgical resection. Surgical resection is the mainstay of therapy for both tumors. Radiotherapy can be given after subtotal resection of hemangioblastomas, while radiation is recommended even after complete resection of hemangiopericytomas, given their propensity for LR. Stieber VW, Siker ML. Spinal cord tumors. In: Gunderson LL, Tepper JE, editors. Clinical radiation oncology. 3rd ed. Philadelphia: Elsevier Saunders; 2012. p. 511–28.

53. The correct answer is C. Craniopharyngiomas are benign suprasellar neoplasms derived from remnants of Rathke's pouch. There is a bimodal incidence: children from 5 to10 years then adults from 55 to 65 years. Radiographically, calcification is frequently seen. There are solid nodule and cystic components, which may be filled with cholesterol-laden fluid ("crankcase oil"). Development of diabetes insipidus is a frequent complication from surgery. Merchant TE. Central nervous system tumors in children. In: Gunderson LL, Tepper JE, editors. Clinical radiation oncology. 3rd ed. Philadelphia: Elsevier Saunders; 2012. p. 1409–23.

54. The correct answer is A. Approximately 30 % of pituitary adenomas are nonsecreting. Of the secreting tumors, prolactinomas are most common, followed by GH-secreting tumors. Thapar K et al. Pituitary tumors. Cancer of the nervous system. Cambridge: Blackwell Scientific; 1997. p. 363. Suh JH, Chao ST, Weil RJ. Pituitary tumors. In: Gunderson LL, Tepper JE, editors. Clinical radiation oncology. 3rd ed. Philadelphia: Elsevier Saunders; 2012. p. 493–509.

55. The correct answer is A. The posterior lobe of the pituitary, the neurohypophysis, secretes ADH and oxytocin. The anterior lobe of the pituitary, the adenohypophysis, secretes prolactin, ACTH, FSH, LH, GH, and TSH. Suh JH, Chao ST, Weil RJ. Pituitary tumors. In: Gunderson LL, Tepper JE, editors. Clinical radiation oncology. 3rd ed. Philadelphia: Elsevier Saunders; 2012. p. 493–509.

56. The correct answer is B. There is no effective medical therapy for a TSH-secreting pituitary adenoma. Prolactinomas can be treated with bromocriptine. ACTH-secreting adenomas can be treated with cyproheptadine. GH-secreting adenomas can be treated with either octreotide (long-acting somatostatin analogue) or pegvisomant (GH receptor antagonist). Suh JH, Chao ST, Wei RJ. Pituitary tumors. In: Gunderson LL, Tepper JE, editors. Clinical radiation oncology. 3rd ed. Philadelphia: Elsevier Saunders; 2012. p. 493–509.

57. The correct answer is D. After irradiation of the hypothalamic-pituitary axis, growth hormone deficiency is most commonly seen, followed by deficiency of adrenocorticotropin, gonadotropin, and thyroid-stimulating hormone. Robinson IC et al. Differential radiosensitivity of hypothalamo-pituitary function in the young adult rat. J Endocrinol. 2001;169:519–26. Merchant TE et al. Early neuro-otologic effects of three-dimensional irradiation in children with primary brain tumors. Int J Radiat Oncol Biol Phys. 2004;58:1194–207.

58. The correct answer is C. The cavernous sinus is located lateral to the pituitary and transmits the internal carotid artery, CN III, CN IV, CN VI (six), and the V1 (one) and V2 branches of the trigeminal nerve. The nerves transmitted from the cranial to caudal direction are CN III, CN IV, CN VI (six), CN V1 (V one), and CN V2. CN V2, the maxillary branch of the trigeminal nerve, is the most caudal structure in the cavernous sinus.

59. The correct answer is A. Of the primary ocular tumors, melanoma is the most common. Retinoblastoma is the second most common. Primary orbital lymphomas are rare and account for less than 1 % of diagnosed lymphomas. Greven KM, Greven CM. Orbital, ocular, and optic nerve tumors. In: Gunderson LL, Tepper JE, editors. Clinical radiation oncology. 3rd ed. Philadelphia: Elsevier Saunders; 2012. p. 529–42.

60. The correct answer is D. Of the primary ocular tumors, optic nerve sheath meningiomas occur more frequently in women than men, with a typical age of onset of

40 years. Retinoblastoma and melanoma have no gender predilection. Orbital lymphomas occur more frequently in men. Greven KM, Greven CM. Orbital, ocular, and optic nerve tumors. In: Gunderson LL, Tepper JE, editors. Clinical radiation oncology. 3rd ed. Philadelphia: Elsevier Saunders; 2012. p. 529–42.

61. The correct answer is C. The most common tumor to metastasize to the orbit, as well as to the choroid, is breast cancer. Shields JA et al. Survey of 1264 patients with orbital tumors and simulating lesions: the 2002 Montgomery Lecture, part 1. Ophthalmology. 2004;111:997–1008. Shields CL et al. Survey of 520 eyes with uveal metastases. Ophthalmology. 1997;104:1265.

62. The correct answer is B. The COMS study established a standard size classification for ocular melanomas. Small:1–3 mm thick and <16 mm in largest tumor dimension. Medium:3–8 mm thick and < 16 mm in largest tumor dimension. Large: >8 mm thick and >16 mm in greatest dimension. The Collaborative Ophthalmology Study Group. The collaborative ocular melanoma study randomized trial of iodine-125 brachytherapy for choroidal melanoma, III: initial mortality findings. COMS report No. 18. Arch Ophthalmol. 2001;119:969.

63. The correct answer is D. COMS study for large choroidal melanomas randomized patients to receive or not preoperative external beam radiotherapy to 20 Gy, prior to planned enucleation. The addition of EBRT did not improve overall survival, nor local control. Collaborative Ocular Melanoma Group. The collaborative ocular melanoma study randomized trial or pre-enucleation radiation of large choroidal melanoma, II: initial mortality findings. COMS report No. 10. Am J Ophthalmol. 1998;125:779.

64. The correct answer is C. Acoustic neuromas, commonly seen in neurofibromatosis 2, most commonly affect the vestibular division of CN VIII. Chan MD, Rogers CL, Anderson BM, Khuntia D. benign brain tumors: meningiomas and vestibular schwannomas. In: Gunderson LL, Tepper JE, editors. Clinical radiation oncology. 3rd ed. Philadelphia: Elsevier Saunders; 2012. p. 473–91.

65. The correct answer is C. Of the listed subtypes, germinoma is not a type of embryonal CNS tumor. Embryonal CNS tumors are of two major groups: primitive neuroectodermal tumor (PNET)—medulloblastoma and pineoblastoma—and atypical teratoid/rhabdoid tumors (AT/RT). Germinomas are germ cell tumors. Merchant TE. Nervous system tumors in children. In: Gunderson LL, Tepper JE, editors. Clinical radiation oncology. 3rd ed. Philadelphia: Elsevier Saunders; 2012. p. 1409–23.

66. The correct answer is B. Embryonal CNS tumors have a propensity for neuraxis dissemination. As such, craniospinal irradiation is the mainstay of treatment of these tumors. Merchant TE. Central nervous system tumors in children. In: Gunderson LL, Tepper JE, editors. Clinical radiation oncology. 3rd ed. Philadelphia: Elsevier Saunders; 2012. p. 1409–23.

67. The correct answer is A. At least four molecular subtypes of medulloblastoma and their differential outcomes are known. The *Wnt* pathway, associated with monosomy 6 and occurring in all age groups, has the best prognosis. The *Hh* pathway is associated with desmoplastic histology, occurring in infants and adults, and has a good prognosis. The *c-MYC* subtype occurs in children 3–10 years and has the worst prognosis. Other subtypes occur in all age groups and have a fair prognosis. Monje M et al. Hedgehogs, flies, wnts, and MYCs: the time has come for many things in medulloblastoma. J Clin Oncol. 2011; 29(11):1395–98. Cho Y-J et al. Integrative genomic analysis of medulloblastoma identifies a molecular subgroup that drives poor clinical outcome. J Clin Oncol. 2011;29:1424–30. Northcott PA et al. Medulloblastoma comprises four distinct molecular variants. J Clin Oncol. 2011;29:1408–14.

68. The correct answer is B. The borders of the posterior fossa are superior-tentorium cerebelli, inferior-occipital bone, anterior-clivus, posterior-calvarium, lateral-temporal, parietal, and occipital bones. Merchant TE. Central nervous system tumors in children. In: Gunderson LL, Tepper JE, editors. Clinical radiation oncology. 3rd ed. Philadelphia: Elsevier Saunders; 2012. p. 1409–23.

69. The correct answer is C. The previous approach to standard-risk medulloblastoma was 36 Gy to the craniospinal axis, followed by a boost to the posterior fossa to a total of 54 Gy. POG 8631/CCG 923 compared 36 Gy to the craniospinal axis to 23.4 Gy and showed a higher risk of relapse with the lower craniospinal dose. However, CCG-9892 subsequently showed that the two doses were equivalent if the 23.4 Gy craniospinal dose was given in combination with multiagent chemotherapy. Thomas PR et al. Low-stage medulloblastoma: final analysis of standard-dose with reduced-dose neuraxis irradiation. J Clin Oncol. 2000;18: 3004–11. Packer RJ et al. Treatment of children with medulloblastoma with reduced-dose craniospinal radiation therapy and adjuvant chemotherapy. J Clin Oncol. 1999;17(7):2127–36.

70. The correct answer is A. A St. Jude Children's Hospital prospective trial sought to reduce the volume treated with radiotherapy in order to reduce neurocognitive sequelae. In this prospective trial, 86 patients aged 3–21, with standard-risk medulloblastoma were treated with craniospinal irradiation (23.4 Gy), followed by irradiation to a total of 36 Gy to the posterior fossa and followed by a tumor bed + 2 cm boost to a total of 55.8 Gy. Chemotherapy (4 cycles of cyclophosphamide, cisplatin, vincristine) began 6 weeks after radiation. Three-year posterior fossa failure was 6.3 %, and the reduction in radiotherapy targeting volume resulted in a 13 % decrease in volume of posterior fossa receiving doses >55 Gy. The dose reductions to the temporal lobes, cochleae, and hypothalamus were statistically significant. Merchant TE et al., Multi-institution prospective trial of reduced-dose craniospinal irradiation (23.4 Gy) followed by conformal posterior fossa (36 Gy) and primary site irradiation (55.8 Gy) and dose-intensive chemotherapy for average-risk medulloblastoma. Int J Radiat Oncol Biol Phys. 2008;70(3):782–7.

71. The correct answer is C. Due to neurocognitive sequelae, there has been a push to delay radiotherapy use in children < 3 years. POG 8633 (Baby POG) reported by Duffner et al. showed that progression-free survival with primary chemotherapy with cyclophosphamide/vincristine and cisplatin/VP-16 was 32 %. The Children's Cancer Group "8 in 1" regimen showed a 3-year progression-free survival of 22 %. Subsequently, POG 9233/34 attempted to improve survival of very young children with malignant brain tumors using dose-intensified chemotherapy. Unfortunately, this dose-intensified chemotherapy has not shown an improvement in either event-free survival or overall survival. All these trials highlighted the need for a different chemotherapy approach and the need for improved local control; this formed the basis for COG P9934. Children ≥8 months and < 3 years with non-metastatic medulloblastoma were eligible for the COG protocol, P9934 which includes 16 weeks of chemotherapy (cyclophosphamide, vincristine, cisplatin, oral etoposide) after surgery, a second surgery if needed, then sequential radiation of the posterior fossa and primary site to a total of 45–54 Gy. Neurodevelopment outcomes and event-free survival were compared to POG 9233 results (multiagent chemotherapy without irradiation). The addition of CRT to postoperative chemotherapy was found to improve event-free survival compared to postoperative chemotherapy alone. Four-year event-free survival was improved at 50 %, 4-year overall survival was improved at 69 %. Desmoplastic/nodular subtype was found to be a favorable factor in predicting survival, with a 4-year event-free survival of 58 %. Subsequent studies will stratify patients by histopathologic type (desmoplastic/nodular) for therapy, by risk of relapse. Merchant TE et al. Radiation therapy for the treatment of childhood medulloblastoma: the rationale for current techniques, strategies, and dose-volume considerations. Electromedica. 2001;69:69–71. Duffner PK et al. The treatment of malignant brain tumors in infants and very young children: an update of the Pediatric Oncology Group experience. Neuro-oncology. 1999;1(2);152–61. Geyer JR et al. Survival of infants with primitive neuroectodermal tumors or malignant ependymomas of the CNS treated with 8 drugs in 1 day: a report from the Children's Cancer Group. J Clin Oncol. 1994;12(8):1607–15. Ashley DM et al. Induction chemotherapy and conformal radiation therapy for very young children with nonmetastatic medulloblastoma: children's oncology group study P9934. J Clin Oncol. 2012;30(26):3181–6.

72. The correct answer is D. Of the listed sites, ependymoma in children least commonly occurs in the spinal cord. Merchant TE. Central nervous system tumors in children. In: Gunderson LL, Tepper JE, editors. Clinical radiation oncology. 3rd ed. Philadelphia: Elsevier Saunders; 2012. p. 1409–23.

73. The correct answer is C. Ependymomas in the brain tend to occur more frequently infratentorially (2/3), rather than supratentorially. The most common histology in the cauda equina and filum terminale is WHO grade I myxopapillary. Surgical resection is the mainstay of therapy, with extent of resection being the most important predictor of outcome. Five-year OS after gross total resection

ranges from 70 % to 80 %. Recurrences after resection tend to be local, occurring at a median time of 1–2 years. Merchant TE. Central nervous system tumors in children. In: Gunderson LL, Tepper JE, editors. Clinical radiation oncology. 3rd ed. Philadelphia: Elsevier Saunders; 2012. p. 1409–23.

74. The correct answer is D. After gross total resection of a localized ependymoma, given the propensity for local recurrence, the most appropriate radiation dose is 59.4 Gy given to the tumor bed plus margin. Merchant TE. Central nervous system tumors in children. In: Gunderson LL, Tepper JE, editors. Clinical radiation oncology. 3rd ed. Philadelphia: Elsevier Saunders; 2012. p. 1409–23.

75. The correct answer is C. After gross total resection of a low-grade astrocytoma, the best next step in management is observation. Five-year local control after surgery is over 90 %. The CCG9891/POG 9130 study of 726 patients observed after resection of low-grade astrocytomas showed that those that underwent gross total resection had a 5-year progression-free survival of 92 %. Wisoff JH et al. Impact of surgical resection on low-grade gliomas of childhood: a report from the CCG9891/POG 9130 low-grade astrocytoma study. Proceedings of the 39th American Society of Clinical Oncology meeting, 100 (abstr 401), Chicago; 2003.

76. The correct answer is A. Due to its sensitivity to chemotherapy and radiotherapy, as opposed to non-germinomatous germ cell tumors, diagnosis of a germinomatous germ cell tumor requires biopsy. While radiotherapy is the major curative modality, there has been a controversy in determining the appropriate radiation volume. The most recent COG protocol, ACNS0232, attempted to answer this question and randomized patients with newly diagnosed, histologically confirmed CNS germinoma to either conventional radiotherapy alone (Regimen A) or pre-radiotherapy chemotherapy followed by response-based radiotherapy. On Regimen A, patients with M0 disease are treated with whole ventricular radiotherapy to 24 Gy, with a 21 Gy boost to the primary measurable or presumed (occult multifocal) tumors in patients presenting with diabetes insipidus. Patients with metastatic disease will receive 24 Gy CSI with a 21 Gy boost to all measurable disease. On Regimen B, those with a complete response or minimal residual disease to chemotherapy will receive 30 Gy involved field radiotherapy alone, without a boost. Those with metastatic disease will receive 21 Gy CSI with a 9 Gy boost to pretreatment measurable disease. Unfortunately, the trial closed due to poor accrual. Whole ventricular radiation remains an appropriate approach for localized germinoma. Children's Oncology Group. ACNS0232. Radiotherapy Alone vs. Chemotherapy Followed by Response-based Radiotherapy for Newly Diagnosed Primary CNS Germinoma.

77. The correct answer is A. Craniopharyngioma is a histologically benign tumor that is derived from the embryonic remnant of the anterior pituitary (Rathke's pouch). It possesses a bimodal incidence, occurring in both the pediatric population and adults aged 55–65. It commonly (90 %) presents with endocrine abnormalities,

as well as with both cystic and solid components. Three-quarters of craniopharyngiomas possess at least 1 cyst. Merchant TE. Central nervous system tumors in children. In: Gunderson LL, Tepper JE, editors. Clinical radiation oncology. 3rd ed. Philadelphia: Elsevier Saunders; 2012. p. 1409–23.

78. The correct answer is C. There is evidence of increased morbidity after radical surgery compared to limited resection, with no improvement in outcomes. Merchant et al. reported outcomes of 30 patients with craniopharyngioma treated with either radical surgery ($n = 15$) or limited resection + upfront radiation ($n = 15$). Those that underwent radical surgery lost an average of 9.8 IQ points versus 1.25 points lost in the limited resection group. A report of 24 patients with craniopharyngioma treated with external beam radiation as a part of therapy noted that on multivariate analysis, dose (> 55 Gy) was a significant prognostic factor for local control and that pretreatment hypopituitarism predicted for treatment complication probability. Ten-year actuarial local control in this study was 89 %. Merchant TE et al. Craniopharyngiomas: the St. Jude Children's Research Hospital Experience 1984–2001. Int J Radiat Oncol Biol Phys. 2002;53(3):533–42. Varlotto JM et al. External beam irradiation of craniopharyngioma: long-term analysis of tumor control and morbidity. Int J Radiat Oncol Biol Phys. 2002;54(2):492–9.

79. The correct answer is A. Management of optic gliomas is controversial, as there is no optimal time of surgery. A general consensus is that asymptomatic children should be closely observed. If there is progression, an operable tumor could be resected. Inoperable tumors can be treated at the time of progression with chemotherapy (Packer regimen of carboplatin/vincristine) to delay time to radiation. In 78 children (median age:3 years) with inoperable low-grade gliomas, objective response rate to the Packer regimen was 56 %, with a resulting 68 % progression-free survival rate at 3 years. While there was no difference in progression-free survival between those with or without neurofibromatosis type 1, children < 5 years were found to have improved 3-year progression-free survival (74 % vs. 39 %, $p < 0.01$). Subsequent progression after chemotherapy can be treated with radiotherapy (either proton radiation or stereotactic/conformal radiation). A retrospective review of 50 children treated with fractionated radiation (median dose:52.2 Gy) for progression after surgery/chemotherapy showed a 5-year PFS of 83 % and 5-year OS of 98 %. Packer RJ et al. Carboplatin and vincristine chemotherapy for children with newly diagnosed progressive low-grade gliomas. J Neurosurg. 1997;86(5):747–54. Marcus K et al. Stereotactic radiotherapy for localized low-grade gliomas in children: final results of a prospective trial. Int J Radiat Oncol Biol Phys. 2005;61(2):374–9.

80. The correct answer is A. The *INI-1* mutation is seen in 85 % of atypical teratoid/rhabdoid tumors. Judkins AR et al. INI1 protein expression distinguishes atypical teratoid/rhabdoid tumor from choroid plexus carcinoma. J Neuropathol Exp Neurol. 2005;64(5):391–7.

81. The correct answer is C. Parinaud's syndrome, frequently seen with pineal tumors, is comprised of a vertical gaze palsy, papillary and oculomotor nerve paresis, and is due to impingement of the superior colliculi, which surround the pineal gland. Merchant TE. Central nervous system tumors in children. In: Gunderson LL, Tepper JE, editors. Clinical radiation oncology. 3rd ed. Philadelphia: Elsevier Saunders; 2012. p. 1409–23.

82. The correct answer is C. Pineoblastomas can be seen in conjunction with bilateral retinoblastomas, a syndrome known as trilateral retinoblastoma. Merchant TE. Central nervous system tumors in children. In: Gunderson LL, Tepper JE, editors. Clinical radiation oncology. 3rd ed. Philadelphia: Elsevier Saunders; 2012. p. 1409–23.

Chapter 2
Skin Cancer

Celine Bicquart Ord and John M. Holland

Questions

1. All of the following are true regarding basal cell carcinomas, except:
   A. Basal cell carcinomas typically exhibit an indolent growth pattern.
   B. Regional metastases are infrequent in basal cell carcinoma.
   C. Basal cell carcinomas are twice as common as squamous cell carcinomas of the skin.
   D. Nasal locations are better treated with radiation than surgery.

2. All of the following syndromes are associated with a higher incidence of skin carcinoma, except:
   A. Ataxia-telangiectasia
   B. Xeroderma pigmentosum
   C. Basal cell nevus syndrome
   D. Epidermodysplasia verruciformis

3. Which of the following is false regarding basal cell nevus syndrome?
   A. Autosomal dominant inheritance
   B. Associated with jaw cysts
   C. Associated with hypotelorism
   D. Associated with palmar pits

_____

C.B. Ord, MD (✉)
Department of Radiation Oncology, Scott & White Memorial Hospital, Temple,
TX 76508, USA
e-mail: cord@sw.org

J.M. Holland
Department of Radiation Oncology, Oregon Health and Science University,
3181 SW Sam Jackson Park Rd, KPV4, Portland, OR 97239-3098, USA
e-mail: hollanjo@ohsu.edu

C.B. Ord et al. (eds.), *Radiation Oncology Study Guide*,
DOI 10.1007/978-1-4614-6400-6_2, © Springer Science+Business Media New York 2013

4. What is the most common variant of basal cell carcinoma?
    A. Nodular
    B. Superficial
    C. Morpheaform
    D. Infiltrative

5. Which of the following cranial nerves is most likely to be affected by a locally aggressive basal cell carcinoma?
    A. III
    B. V
    C. VIII
    D. IX

6. What is the approximate overall incidence of nodal involvement seen with Merkel cell carcinoma at presentation?
    A. 15 %
    B. 20 %
    C. 30 %
    D. 40 %

7. What percent of relapses occurred within 1 year in a pattern-of-failure series of Merkel cell carcinoma treated at M.D. Anderson Cancer Center reported by Morrison et al.?
    A. 50 %
    B. 70 %
    C. 80 %
    D. 90 %

8. All of the following are true regarding sebaceous carcinoma, except:
    A. Most common neoplasm in the eyelid.
    B. Second most lethal neoplasm in the eyelid.
    C. The most common location is in the upper eyelid.
    D. Behave more aggressively than squamous cell carcinoma.

9. A squamous cell carcinoma that arises out of a chronic burn is:
    A. Erythroplasia of Queyrat
    B. Bowen's disease
    C. Gorlin's tumor
    D. Marjolin's ulcer

10. All of the following are true regarding a Nevus of Ota, except:
    A. It results from entrapment of melanocytes in the upper third of the dermis.
    B. It usually involves the first two branches of the trigeminal nerve.
    C. Men are more commonly affected than women.
    D. The sclera is involved in two thirds of cases.

11. What is the correct 7th edition AJCC T stage for a 4.5 cm squamous cell carcinoma of the cheek?
    A. T1
    B. T2
    C. T3
    D. T4

12. A woman presents with four separate foci of squamous cell carcinoma on the face, the largest focus measuring 2.5 cm. What is the correct 7th edition AJCC T stage?
    A. T2
    B. T2 (4)
    C. T3
    D. T4

13. All of the following are true regarding early-stage skin carcinomas treated with definitive radiotherapy alone, except:
    A. Five-year local control is in excess of 90 %.
    B. Size of the primary lesion is the primary determinant of local control.
    C. For tumors of the same size, squamous cell carcinomas have higher control rates due to their increased radiosensitivity.
    D. Fibrosis and atrophy are long-term complications of radiotherapy.

14. Adjuvant radiation is indicated for treatment of each of the following scenarios, except:
    A. Recurrent skin carcinoma after previous surgery
    B. Extracapsular extension on lymph node dissection
    C. Lymph node of 3.5 cm on lymph node dissection
    D. Electively after complete resection of a primary squamous cell carcinoma of the cheek

15. What is the approximate 5-year local control rate of previously untreated T4 skin carcinomas, treated with radiation to 60–75 Gy, as reported by Lee et al.?
    A. 35 %
    B. 45 %
    C. 55 %
    D. 65 %

16. Which of the following is the most appropriate dose regimen to treat the lymph node regions in a resected skin cancer with positive nodal involvement (2.5 cm with + ECE)?
    A. 40 Gy in 10 fractions
    B. 45 Gy in 15 fractions
    C. 63 Gy in 35 fractions
    D. 66 Gy in 33 fractions

17. Which of the following is not a subtype of Merkel cell carcinoma?
    A. Superficial type
    B. Small-cell type
    C. Intermediate type
    D. Trabecular type

18. Which of the following immunohistochemistry profiles best characterizes Merkel cell carcinoma?
    A. S-100 positive, leukocyte antigen positive, neuron-specific enolase positive
    B. S-100 positive, leukocyte antigen negative, neuron-specific enolase positive
    C. S-100 negative, leukocyte antigen positive, neuron-specific enolase positive
    D. S-100 negative, leukocyte antigen negative, neuron-specific enolase positive

19. Which of the following immunohistochemistry profiles best characterizes melanoma?
    A. S-100 positive, HMB-45 positive
    B. S-100 positive, HMB-45 negative
    C. S-100 negative, HMB-45 positive
    D. S-100 negative, HMB-45 negative

20. Which of the following is not a primary determinant of survival from melanoma?
    A. Maximum thickness of primary lesion
    B. Maximum diameter of primary lesion
    C. Tumor ulceration
    D. Status of regional lymph nodes

21. All of the following are true regarding the etiology of melanoma, except:
    A. Ultraviolet exposure is related to the development of melanoma.
    B. Carriers of the *CDKN2A* mutation have a 70 % chance of developing melanoma by age 80.
    C. Half of those with melanoma possess the *CDKN2A* mutation.
    D. An increasing number of nevi also increase the risk for melanoma.

22. Which of the following is incorrect regarding the ABCD's of melanoma?
    A. A refers to asymmetry of a lesion.
    B. B refers to border irregularity.
    C. C refers to color variation of a lesion.
    D. D refers to diameter of a lesion >5 mm.

23. Which is the most common variant of melanoma?
    A. Superficial spreading
    B. Nodular melanoma
    C. Lentigo malignant melanoma
    D. Acral lentiginous

24. Which variant of melanoma is most likely to be found under the nail of the thumb?
    A. Superficial spreading
    B. Nodular melanoma
    C. Lentigo maligna melanoma
    D. Acral lentiginous

25. A nodular melanoma is found on a 60-year-old woman's right cheek. It is ulcerated and 2.0 mm thick. There are no regional lymph nodes. What is the correct 7th edition AJCC stage?
    A. T1aN0
    B. T1bN0
    C. T2aN0
    D. T2bN0

26. Melanoma that invades but does not fill the papillary dermis is Clark's level:
    A. II
    B. III
    C. IV
    D. V

27. Which one of the following patients is least likely to undergo sentinel lymph node biopsy?
    A. Ulcerated 1 mm thick melanoma
    B. 1 mm thick, Clark level IV melanoma
    C. 1 mm thick melanoma with satellitosis
    D. Non-ulcerated 1 mm thick melanoma

28. Which is true regarding the management of thin stage I primary cutaneous melanoma lesions?
    A. Radiation therapy does not typically play a role.
    B. Wide local excision of lesions <1 mm thick should include 5 mm of clear margins.
    C. Wide local excision of lesions >1 mm thick should include 1 cm of clear margins.
    D. Adjuvant radiation after wide local excision is important because local recurrence with excision alone is >20 %.

29. All are true regarding nodal treatment for melanoma, except:
    A. Randomized trials have not shown a survival benefit for elective nodal dissection at the time of initial surgery.
    B. Sentinel lymph node biopsy can identify those patients that will benefit from nodal dissection.
    C. Sentinel lymph node biopsy has been shown to improve overall survival.
    D. Elective regional irradiation of head and neck melanoma has been shown to yield almost 90 % regional control at 10 years.

30. Which one of the following scenarios is least likely to require adjuvant nodal irradiation?
    A. One 2.5 cm lymph node found on elective lymph node dissection
    B. Four lymph nodes found on elective dissection, largest measuring 2.5 cm
    C. One lymph node found on therapeutic lymph node dissection
    D. One 2.5 cm lymph node found on repeat axillary lymph node dissection

31. Regarding the ECOG 1684 trial of high-dose interferon therapy, all of the following are true, except:
    A. Patients with melanoma >4 mm thick were included.
    B. Patients with positive lymph nodes were excluded.
    C. Relapse-free survival and overall survival were improved with IFN therapy.
    D. IFN therapy was given for a total of 52 weeks.

32. Regarding the ECOG 1690 trial evaluating interferon therapy duration, which of the following is false?
    A. Two years versus 1 year of IFN were compared to observation.
    B. There was an improvement in relapse-free survival with the longer duration of IFN compared to observation.
    C. There was an improvement in relapse-free survival with the shorter duration of IFN compared to observation.
    D. There was no improvement in overall survival with the longer duration of IFN.

33. Regarding the ECOG 1694 trial comparing interferon with a ganglioside GM_2 melanoma vaccine, which is true?
    A. Contrary to the prior 2 ECOG interferon trials, this trial showed that node-negative patients derived the greatest benefit from adjuvant interferon.
    B. The vaccine improved both relapse-free and overall survival.
    C. The vaccine improved only relapse-free survival.
    D. The vaccine improved only overall survival.

34. All of the following are true regarding a randomized trial comparing dacarbazine +/− ipilimumab reported by Robert et al., except:
    A. The addition of ipilimumab improved overall survival.
    B. Median survival was improved 2 months with the addition of ipilimumab.
    C. The most common reason for ipilimumab discontinuation was gastrointestinal toxicity.
    D. Elevation of the liver enzymes was the most frequently observed bowel toxicity.

35. In a prospective single-arm study of the oral *BRAF* inhibitor, PLX4032, all of the following are true, except:
    A. PLX4032 is an inhibitor of the V600E *BRAF* mutation.
    B. Patients with all sites of metastases were included.

C. There was an >80 % response rate in those with the V600E mutation.

D. Median overall survival has not yet been reached in those with the V600E mutation.

36. What radiation fractionation was used in a prospective series from M.D. Anderson Cancer Center (Ang et al.) using hypofractionated postoperative radiotherapy for cutaneous melanoma of the head and neck region?

A. 30 Gy in 6 fractions

B. 24 Gy in 6 fractions

C. 30 Gy in 5 fractions

D. 24 Gy in 4 fractions

37. What is the approximate 5-year local-regional control rate according to a prospective series from M.D. Anderson Cancer Center (Ang et al.) using hypofractionated postoperative radiotherapy for cutaneous melanoma of the head and neck region?

A. 55 %

B. 65 %

C. 75 %

D. 85 %

38. The Tasman Radiation Oncology Group randomized trial of postoperative radiotherapy for melanoma at high risk for local relapse employed which radiotherapy dose fractionation:

A. 30 Gy in 5 fractions

B. 30 Gy in 6 fractions

C. 48 Gy in 12 fractions

D. 48 Gy in 20 fractions

39. Which of the following pathologic scenarios would not have been eligible for the Tasman Radiation Oncology Group randomized trial of postoperative radiotherapy for melanoma at high risk for local relapse?

A. One positive cervical lymph node

B. Two positive parotid lymph nodes

C. Three positive groin nodes

D. One positive groin node with extracapsular extension

40. Which of the following is correct regarding the outcome of the Tasman Radiation Oncology Group randomized trial of postoperative radiotherapy for melanoma at high risk for local relapse?

A. Improved local control and improved survival with post-op RT

B. No improved local control and no improved survival with post-op RT

C. Improved local control but no improved survival with post-op RT

D. No improved local control but improved survival with post-op RT

Answers and Rationales

1. The correct answer is C. Basal cell and squamous cell carcinomas together constitute the most common malignancy in the United States. Basal cell carcinomas are four times more common than squamous cell carcinomas and have a more indolent growth pattern. They rarely metastasize. Cure rates are high, and surgical resection is the primary modality of treatment, except for BCCs of the nose, ear, and lower eyelids, in which radiation may have better functional and cosmetic results. Jemal A et al. Cancer statistics 2005. CA Cancer J Clin. 2005;55:10–30.

2. The correct answer is A. All of the listed syndromes are associated with increased incidence of skin carcinomas except ataxia-telangiectasia. Cleaver JE. Defective repair replication of DNA in xeroderma pigmentosum. Nature. 1968;218:652–6. Anderson DE et al. The nevoid basal cell carcinoma syndrome. Am J Hum Genet. 1967;19:12–22. Lutzner MA. Epidermodysplasia verruciformis: an autosomal recessive disease characterized by viral warts and skin cancer. A model for viral oncogenesis. Bull Cancer (Paris). 1978;65:169–82.

3. The correct answer is C. Basal cell nevus syndrome (Gorlin's syndrome) is inherited in an autosomal dominant pattern and comprises a group of defects involving the skin, nervous system, eyes, endocrine glands, and bone. Physical symptoms of the syndrome involve multiple nevoid basal cell carcinomas, a broad nose, cleft palate, protruding brow, protruding jaw with odontogenic keratocysts (jaw cysts), plantar/palmar pits, and hypertelorism (wide-set eyes). There is also an association with medulloblastoma. Gorlin RJ, Goltz RW. Multiple nevoid basal-cell epithelioma, jaw cysts and bifid rib: a syndrome. N Engl J Med. 1960;262:908–12. Morelli JG. Tumors of the skin. In: Kliegman RM, Behrman RE, Jenson HB, Stanton BF, editors. Nelson textbook of pediatrics. 19th ed. Philadelphia: Saunders Elsevier; 2011 chap 662.

4. The correct answer is A. The most common variant of basal cell carcinoma is the nodular-ulcerative (rodent ulcer) variant. It presents as a papule with a central umbilication that grows into a central ulceration and can be confused with melanoma. Superficial basal cell carcinoma presents as red, scaly macules with indistinct margins and can be confused with psoriasis. Morpheaform basal cell carcinoma presents as flat, indurated, ill-defined macules with a shiny surface that depresses as it grows into a plaque. Infiltrative basal cell carcinoma appears yellowish and blends into adjacent skin. Patterson JAK et al. Cancers of the skin. In: DeVita VT, Hellman S, Rosenberg SA, editors. Cancer principles and practice of oncology. 3rd ed. Philadelphia: JB Lippincott; 1989. p. 1469–98.

5. The correct answer is B. The 5th and 7th cranial nerves are most likely to be affected by a locally aggressive BCC. Veness MJ, Ang KK. Cutaneous Carcinoma. In: Gunderson LL, Tepper JE, editors. Clinical radiation oncology. 3rd ed. Philadelphia: Elsevier Saunders; 2012. p.757–69.

6. The correct answer is B. Merkel cell carcinoma is a neoplasm that arises from neural crest cells. It manifests as a firm, painless, pink nodule or plaque in the head/neck or extremities. Lymph nodes are involved at presentation in 20 % of cases. Morrison WH et al. The essential role of radiation therapy in securing locoregional control of Merkel cell carcinoma. Int J Radiat Oncol Biol Phys. 1990;19:583–591. Merkel F. Tastzellen und Tastkoerperchen bei den haushieren und beim Menschen. Arch Mikr Anat. 1875;11:636–52.

7. The correct answer is D. Morrison et al. reported on 54 patients with Merkel cell carcinoma treated with excision then postoperative radiotherapy of 60 Gy to the primary, 51 Gy to the primary echelon nodes, and 50 Gy to the supraclavicular nodes, at M.D. Anderson Cancer Center. Overall local failure was 35 %; overall regional failure was 67 %. Ninety-one percent of patients relapsed during the first year, with the median time to relapse—4.9 months. The predominant pattern of failure was distant metastasis. In those with lymph node metastases, median survival was 13 months versus 40 months in those without lymph node metastases. Morrison WH et al. The essential role of radiation therapy in securing locoregional control of Merkel cell carcinoma. Int J Radiat Oncol Biol Phys. 1990;19:583–391.

8. The correct answer is A. Sebaceous carcinoma arises most commonly in the upper eyelid and is the second most common eyelid neoplasm (most common—BCC) and second most lethal neoplasm (most lethal—melanoma). While they present as slow-growing, non-tender nodules, they behave more aggressively than squamous cell carcinoma. Civatte J et al. Adnexal skin carcinomas. In: Andrade R, Gumport SL, Popkin GL, et al. editors.: Cancer of the skin, vol 2. Philadephia: WB Saunders; 1976. p. 1045–68. Rulon DB et al. Cutaneous sebaceous neoplasms. Cancer. 1974;33:82–102. Batsakis JG et al. Sebaceous cell lesions of the head and neck. Arch Otolaryngol. 1972;95:151–7. Rao NA et al. Sebaceous carcinomas of the ocular adnexa: a clinicopathologic study of 104 cases, with five-year follow-up data. Hum Pathol. 1982;13:113–22.

9. The correct answer is D. A Marjolin's ulcer refers to an aggressive, ulcerating squamous cell carcinoma that arises in an area of prior trauma, chronic inflammation, and, most commonly, a burn. Chong AJ et al. Images in clinical medicine. Marjolin's ulcer. N Engl J Med. 2005;352:e9.

10. The correct answer is C. Nevus of Ota (congenital melanosis bulbi, oculodermal melanocytosis) is a blue hyperpigmentation of the face usually noted unilaterally. It results from entrapment of melanocytes in the upper third of the dermis and involves the first two branches of the trigeminal nerves. The sclera is involved in 2/3 of cases. Women are 5× more likely to develop Nevus of Ota than men, and it is more common in Asians (rare in whites). Rapini RP et al. Dermatology: 2-volume set. St. Louis: Mosby. p. 1720–2. Chan HH, Kono T. Nevus of Ota: clinical aspects and management. Skinmed. 2(2):89–96.

11. The correct answer is B. A 4.5 cm squamous cell carcinoma of the cheek is staged as T2, which includes tumors >2 cm but ≤ 5 cm. Edge SB, Byrd DR, Compton CC, et al., editors. Cutaneous squamous cell carcinoma and other cutaneous carcinomas. AJCC cancer staging handbook. 7th ed. New York: Springer; 2010.

12. The correct answer is B. When there are multiple tumors present, this is denoted by putting the number of tumors in parenthesis, with the T stage denoting the largest lesion. T2 (4) Edge SB, Byrd DR, Compton CC, et al., editors. Cutaneous squamous cell carcinoma and other cutaneous carcinomas. AJCC cancer staging handbook. 7th ed. New York: Springer; 2010..

13. The correct answer is C. Skin carcinomas of the H zone (medial canthus, glabella, nasolabial folds, and periauricular region) are well treated with definitive radiotherapy. A series of 1,000 patients treated with radiotherapy alone showed 5-year local control of >90 %. The size of the primary lesion is the major determinant of local control, and for tumors of the same size, basal cell carcinomas have higher control rates. Late complications of radiation include fibrosis and atrophy. Fitzpatrick PJ et al. Basal and squamous cell carcinoma of the eyelids and their treatment by radiotherapy. Int J Radiat Oncol Biol Phys. 1984;10:449–54. Petrovich Z et al. Carcinoma of the lip and selected sites of head and neck skin. A clinical study of 896 patients. Radiother Oncol. 1987;8:11–7.

14. The correct answer is D. Elective nodal irradiation is not a component of therapy for squamous or basal cell carcinomas, given their low incidence of nodal involvement, except in cases of recurrent carcinoma after previous surgery. In those patients who have lymph node metastases >3 cm, or + extracapsular extension on lymph node dissection, adjuvant nodal radiation is indicated. Veness MJ, Ang KK. Cutaneous carcinoma. In: Gunderson LL, Tepper JE, editors. Clinical radiation oncology. 3rd ed. Philadelphia: Elsevier Saunders; 2012. p. 757–69.

15. The correct answer is D. In previously untreated T4 skin carcinomas treated with 60–75 Gy over 6–8 weeks, 5-year local control was 67 %. Those with bony invasion or perineural spread had reduced local control. Lee WR et al. Radical radiotherapy for T4 carcinoma of the skin of the head and neck: a multivariate analysis. Head Neck. 1993;15:32–324.

16. The correct answer is C. After resection, a lymph node with extracapsular extension requires nodal irradiation. The larger treatment volume requires a lower dose per fraction; 1.8–2 Gy fractions are typically employed. For a lymph node with extracapsular extension, 63 Gy is recommended. Peters LJ et al. Evaluation of the dose for postoperative radiation therapy of head and neck cancer: first report of a prospective randomized trial. Int J Radiat Oncol Biol Phys. 1993;26(1):3–11.

17. The correct answer is A. Of the listed subtypes, superficial type is not a subtype of Merkel cell carcinoma. The trabecular subtype is the most common subtype. Veness MJ, Ang KK. Cutaneous carcinoma. In: Gunderson LL, Tepper JE, editors. Clinical radiation oncology. 3rd ed. Philadelphia: Elsevier Saunders; 2012. p. 757–69.

18. The correct answer is D. Merkel cell tumors are neuroendocrine tumors, and those stain positive for neuron-specific enolase. They are S-100 negative (melanoma is S-100 positive). They are leukocyte antigen negative (positive in lymphoma). Veness MJ, Ang KK. Cutaneous carcinoma. In: Gunderson LL, Tepper JE, editors. Clinical radiation oncology. 3rd ed. Philadelphia: Elsevier Saunders; 2012. p. 757–69.

19. The correct answer is A. Melanoma stains positive for both S-100 and HMB-45. Nonaka D et al. Differential expression of S100 protein subtypes in malignant melanoma, and benign and malignant peripheral nerve sheath tumors. J Cutan Pathol. 2008;35(11);1014–19. Gown AM et al. Monoclonal antibodies specific for melanocytic tumors distinguishes subpopulations of melanocytes. Am J Pathol. 1986;123(2):195–203.

20. The correct answer is B. All of the listed choices are primary determinants of survival from melanoma except maximum diameter of the primary. In addition, the site of distant disease (if present) is also a determinant. Ballo MT, Ang KK. Malignant melanoma. In: Gunderson LL, Tepper JE, editors. Clinical radiation oncology. 3rd ed. Philadelphia: Elsevier Saunders; 2012. p. 771–82.

21. The correct answer is C. Ultraviolet exposure has been linked to melanoma development, and higher numbers of melanoma are seen in those with a history of sun exposure and those who live in high-ambient sunlight areas. While those with the *CDKN2A* mutation will have a 70 % chance of developing melanoma by age 80, few people with melanoma actually have this mutation. There is an increasing risk of melanoma development in those with an increasing number of nevi. Beral V et al. Cutaneous factors related to the risk of malignant melanoma. Br J Dermatol. 1983;109:165–72. Gellin GA et al. Malignant melanoma. A controlled study of possibly associated factors. Arch Dermatol. 1969;99:43–48. English DR et al. Sunlight and cancer. Cancer Causes Control. 1997;8:271–83. Hussussian CJ et al. Germline p16 mutations in familial melanoma. Nat Genet. 1994;8:15–21. Aitken J et al. CDKN2a variants in a population-based sample of Queensland families with melanoma. J Natl Cancer Inst. 1999;3:446–52. Bishop DT et al. Geographical variation in the penetrance of CDKN2a mutation in melanoma. J Natl Cancer Inst. 2002;94:894–903. Bliss JM et al. Risk of cutaneous melanoma associated with pigmentation characteristics and freckling: systematic overview of 10 case controlled studies. The International Melanoma Analysis Group (IMAGE). Int J Cancer. 1995;62:367–76.

22. The correct answer is D. The ABCD's of melanoma are recognized signs for early diagnosis. A refers to asymmetry of a lesion. B refers to border irregularity. C refers to color variation of a lesion. D refers to diameter of a lesion >6 mm, not 5 mm. Ballo MT, Ang KK. Malignant melanoma. In: Gunderson LL, Tepper JE, editors. Clinical radiation oncology. 3rd ed. Philadelphia: Elsevier Saunders; 2012. p. 771–82.

23. The correct answer is A. Superficial spreading is the most common variant, accounting for 70 % of cases. It is more common in women and often arises in a junctional nevus. As the malignant cells resemble the cells of Paget's disease, this is also called pagetoid melanoma. Enlargement of the lesion entails invasion of the dermis and subcutaneous tissues by clusters of malignant cells. Nodular melanoma is the second most common variant (15–25 %) and is more common in men, arising on the trunk, head, or neck of middle-aged persons. These manifest as raised blue-black lesions. Lentigo maligna melanoma is less common (10 %) and occurs mostly on the face or neck of white women >50 years, arising from a lentigo maligna (precursor lesion). These are typically tan, flat lesions that have been present for many years. Acral lentiginous melanoma occurs on the palms, soles, or under the nail beds. It is much more common in dark-skinned persons. Clark WH et al. The developmental biology of primary human malignant melanoma. Semin Oncol. 1975;2:83–103. McCovern VJ, Murad TM. Pathology of melanoma: an overview. In: Balch CM, Milton GW, editors. Cutaneous melanoma: clinical management and treatment results worldwide. Philadelphia: JB Lippincott; 1985. p. 29–53. Clark WH, Mihm MC. Lentigo maligna and lentigo-maligna melanoma. Am J Pathol. 1969;55:39–67. Arrington JH et al. Plantar lentiginous melanoma: a distinctive variant of human cutaneous malignant melanoma. Am J Surg Pathol. 1977;1:131–143. Seiji M, Takahashi M. Acral melanoma in Japan. Hum Pathol. 1982;13:607–45.

24. The correct answer is D. Acral lentiginous melanoma is the most likely variant to be found under the nail of the thumbs or great toes. Ballo MT, Ang KK. Malignant melanoma. In: Gunderson LL, Tepper JE, editors. Clinical radiation oncology. 3rd ed. Philadelphia: Elsevier Saunders; 2012. p. 771–82.

25. The correct answer is D. Melanoma staging has used two microstaging systems. The Breslow system classifies lesions by thickness, whereas the Clark level classifies lesions by level of invasion. The Breslow system has been found to be more accurate in predicting outcome. In this system, ulceration is denoted with a "b." T1 refers to lesions ≤1.0 mm; T1a is lesions level II or III; T1b is lesions level IV or V or with ulceration. T2 lesions are 1.01–2.0 mm thick.

26. The correct answer is A. Invasion but not filling the papillary dermis is consistent with Clark's level II. Filling of the papillary dermis, with compression of the reticular dermis is Clark's level III. Clark's level staging is used only to describe thin T1 tumors. Ballo MT, Ang KK. Malignant melanoma. In: Gunderson LL, Tepper JE, editors. Clinical radiation oncology. 3rd ed. Philadelphia: Elsevier Saunders; 2012. p. 771–82.

27. The correct answer is D. Sentinel lymph node biopsy is generally recommended for any melanoma >1.0 mm thick. For lesions <1.0 mm thick, sentinel lymph node biopsy is still employed for ulcerated lesions, lesions with associated satellitosis, or lesions that are Clark levels IV or V. Ballo MT, Ang KK. Malignant melanoma. In: Gunderson LL, Tepper JE, editors. Clinical radiation oncology. 3rd ed. Philadelphia: Elsevier Saunders; 2012. p. 771–82.

28. The correct answer is A. Surgery is the primary management of melanoma. For stage I and II lesions, wide local excision is performed, with sentinel lymph node biopsy additionally in lesions >1 mm. Wide margins are important for decreasing the risk of local recurrence. Lesions <1 mm thick should have 1 cm of clear margins; lesions >1 mm thick should have 2 cm of clear margins. Adjuvant radiotherapy is not frequently employed as recurrence is usually <10 %. High-risk features (thickness >4 mm, head or neck site, ulceration, satellitosis increase this risk to ~15 %. Veronesi U, et al. Thin stage I primary cutaneous malignant melanoma. Comparison of excision with margins of 1 or 3 cm [Erratum: N Engl J Med. 1991;325:292] N Engl J Med. 1991;318:1159–62. Thomas JM et al. Excision margins in high-risk malignant melanoma. N Engl J Med. 2004;350:757–66. Heaton KM et al. Surgical margins and prognostic factors in patients with thick (>4 mm) primary melanoma. Ann Surg Oncol. 1998;5:322–28.

29. The correct answer is C. There is no randomized data that shows a survival benefit for elective nodal dissection at the time of initial surgery. There is a nonrandomized study from the Sydney Melanoma unit, which showed a survival benefit from elective nodal dissection in patients with intermediate thickness (0.76–4 mm). A retrospective review of 157 patients with head and neck melanoma from M.D. Anderson Cancer Center who underwent elective nodal irradiation instead of dissection however showed excellent regional control, 89 % at 10 years, despite the fact that almost 40 patients had occult regional metastases. Sentinel lymph node biopsy has largely replaced upfront elective nodal dissection as the sentinel lymph node generally is able to predict which patients will benefit from nodal dissection, though this hasn't been shown to improve survival. Milton GW et al. Prophylactic lymph node dissection in clinical stage I cutaneous malignant melanoma: results of surgical treatment in 1319 patients. Br J Surg. 1982; 49: 2420–30. Doubrovsky A et al. Sentinel node biopsy provides more accurate staging than elective lymph node dissection in patients with cutaneous melanoma. Ann Surg Oncol. 2004;11:829–36. Ang KK et al. Postoperative radiotherapy for cutaneous melanoma of the head and neck region. Int J Radiat Oncol Biol Phys. 1994;30:795–98.

30. The correct answer is A. Of the listed scenarios, a single 2.5 cm lymph node found on elective lymph node dissection is least likely to undergo adjuvant nodal irradiation. Factors that increase the risk for regional recurrence, thus necessitating regional irradiation, include the following: size of lymph node >3.0 cm, four or more involved lymph nodes, extracapsular extension of lymph node (strongest predictor), need for therapeutic dissection, need for repeat

dissection, and location of lymph node in cervical basin. Calabro A, et al., Patterns of relapse in 1,001 consecutive patients with melanoma nodal metastases. Arch Surg. 1989;124:1051–5. Monsour PD et al. Local control following therapeutic nodal dissection for melanoma. J Surg Oncol. 1993;54:18–22. Miller EJ et al. Loco-regional nodal relapse in melanoma. Surg Oncol. 1992;1:333–40. Bowsher WG et al. Morbidity, mortality and local recurrence following regional node dissection for melanoma. Br J Surg. 1986;73:906–8.

31. The correct answer is B. The ECOG 1684 trial sought to determine the benefit of high-dose interferon therapy. Eligible patients had either a primary melanoma >4 mm thick, or lymph nodes detected at LND, or palpable LNs at any stage, or recurrent regional lymph node disease. IFN was given IV five times per week for 48 weeks, then SQ three times per week for an additional 4 weeks. IFN was found to improve both relapse-free and overall survival (46 % vs. 37 %, $p=0.02$) at 5 years, with the greatest benefit in those with palpable or recurrent nodal disease. Kirkwood JM et al. Interferon- alfa-2b adjuvant therapy of high-risk resected cutaneous melanoma: the Eastern Cooperative Oncology Group Trial EST 1684. J Clin Oncol. 1996;14:7–17.

32. The correct answer is C. The ECOG 1690 trial sought to determine the benefit of longer duration (2 years) interferon therapy versus 1 year of observation. The longer duration of IFN was found to improve relapse-free compared to observation, though there was no difference between the 1-year arm and observation. Those patients with 2–3 nodes appeared to benefit most. There was no overall survival benefit seen with IFN. Kirkwood JM et al. High- and low-dose interferon alpha-2b in high-risk melanoma: first analysis of intergroup trial E1690/s9111/c9190. J Clin Oncol. 2000;18:2444–58.

33. The correct answer is A. The ECOG 1694 trial compared high-dose interferon with a ganglioside GM_2 melanoma vaccine in 880 patients. Interim analysis showed inferiority of the vaccine. Interestingly, contrary to the prior 2 ECOG trials, which showed a benefit in lymph-node-positive patients, this trial showed that lymph-node-negative patients, specifically T4N0 patients benefited from interferon. Kirkwood JM et al., High-dose interferon alpha-2b significantly prolongs relapse-free and overall survival compared with the GM2-kLH/QA-21 vaccine in patients with resected stage IIB-III melanoma: results of intergroup trial E1694/S9512/C509801. J Clin Oncol. 2001;19:2370–80.

34. The correct answer is C. In a randomized trial, 500 patients with previously untreated metastatic melanoma were randomized to one of two arms: dacarbazine +/− ipilimumab for a total of 22 weeks. Those without progression at week 24 were eligible to continue maintenance ipilimumab. The addition of ipilimumab improved overall survival and median survival (11.2 m vs. 9.1 m). The most common reason for ipilimumab discontinuation was disease progression. Of the study drug-related toxicities, liver enzyme elevation was the most common. Robert C et al. Ipilimumab plus Dacarbazine for previously untreated metastatic melanoma. N Engl J Med. 2011;364:2517–26.

35. The correct answer is B. PLX4032 is an oral BRAF inhibitor with activity against the V600E mutation specifically. A single-arm prospective study was carried out which showed good response of V600E mutated melanomas to this drug. The study consisted of 2 phases: a dose-escalation phase ($n = 55$), which found the maximally tolerated dose to be 960 mg BID, and the extension phase ($n = 32$). Eligible patients could have metastatic disease, except in the brain. Patients were monitored with CT every 8 weeks with results classified by RECIST criteria. In the dose-escalation phase, mutation testing was not required, and there was a 69 % overall response rate. Patients without the V600E mutation exhibited no tumor regression. In the extension phase, all patients had the V600E mutation, and there was an 81 % overall response rate. In these patients, the median progression-free survival is 7 months, and median overall survival has not yet been reached. Flaherty KT et al. Inhibition of mutated, activated BRAF in metastatic melanoma. N Engl J Med. 2010;363:809–19.

36. The correct answer is C. A prospective series from M.D. Anderson Cancer Center enrolled 174 patients with resected melanoma to one of three arms: (1) elective irradiation after wide local excision (WLE) alone of lesions ≥1.5 mm or Clark's levels IV–V, (2) elective irradiation after WLE of the primary lesion and limited neck dissection, and (3) irradiation after neck dissection for nodal relapse. Radiotherapy consisted of 30 Gy delivered in twice-weekly fractions of 6 Gy. Ang KK et al. Postoperative radiotherapy for cutaneous melanoma of the head and neck region. Int J Radiat Oncol Biol Phys. 1994;30(4):795–8.

37. The correct answer is D. A prospective series from M.D. Anderson Cancer Center enrolled 174 patients with resected melanoma to one of three groups: (1) elective irradiation after wide local excision (WLE) alone of lesions ≥1.5 mm or Clark's levels IV–V, (2) elective irradiation after WLE of the primary lesion and limited neck dissection, and (3) irradiation after neck dissection for nodal relapse. Radiotherapy consisted of 30 Gy delivered in twice-weekly fractions of 6 Gy. With a median of 35 months, actuarial 5-year local-regional control was 88 %, significantly higher than the projected 50 % expected after surgery alone. Actuarial 5-year survival for the whole group was 47 %. In group 1 patients, primary lesion thickness strongly affected the 5-year survival. Ang KK et al. Postoperative radiotherapy for cutaneous melanoma of the head and neck region. Int J Radiat Oncol Biol Phys. 1994;30(4):795–8.

38. The correct answer is D. The Tasman Radiation Oncology Group phase III study randomized 250 patients at high risk for regional relapse (≥1 parotid lymph node, ≥2 cervical or axillary lymph nodes, ≥3 groin lymph nodes; + extracapsular extension; or a minimum diameter of 3 cm in the neck or axilla or 4 cm in the groin to undergo either observation or radiotherapy after lymphadenectomy). Radiation consisted of 48 Gy/20 fractions. Burmeister B, et al. Adjuvant radiotherapy improves regional (lymph node field) control in melanoma patients after lymphadenectomy: results of an intergroup randomised trial (TROG 02.01/ANZMTG 01.02). ASTRO Abstract #3, 2009.

39. The correct answer is A. The Tasman Radiation Oncology Group phase III study randomized 250 patients at high risk for regional relapse (≥1 parotid lymph node, ≥2 cervical or axillary lymph nodes, ≥3 groin lymph nodes; + extracapsular extension; or a minimum diameter of 3 cm in the neck or axilla or 4 cm in the groin to undergo either observation or radiotherapy after lymphadenectomy). Radiation consisted of 48 Gy/20 fractions. With a median follow-up of 27 months, the addition of radiation was found to improve local control, though there was no improvement in survival. Burmeister B et al. Adjuvant radiotherapy improves regional (lymph node field) control in melanoma patients after lymphadenectomy: results of an intergroup randomised trial (TROG 02.01/ANZMTG 01.02). ASTRO Abstract #3, 2009.

40. The correct answer is C. The Tasman Radiation Oncology Group phase III study randomized 250 patients at high risk for regional relapse (≥1 parotid lymph node, ≥2 cervical or axillary lymph nodes, ≥3 groin lymph nodes; + extracapsular extension; or a minimum diameter of 3 cm in the neck or axilla or 4 cm in the groin to undergo either observation or radiotherapy after lymphadenectomy). Radiation consisted of 48 Gy/20 fractions. With a median follow-up of 27 months, the addition of radiation was found to improve local control, though there was no improvement in survival. Burmeister B et al. Adjuvant radiotherapy improves regional (lymph node field) control in melanoma patients after lymphadenectomy: results of an intergroup randomised trial (TROG 02.01/ANZMTG 01.02). ASTRO Abstract #3, 2009.

Chapter 3
Head and Neck Cancer

Kristina H. Young, Celine Bicquart Ord, and John M. Holland

Questions

1. The incidence of head and neck cancer in the United States is approximately
   _____ cases per year.
   - A. 100,000
   - B. 50,000
   - C. 30,000
   - D. 15,000

2. Which of the following is associated with an improved outcome in oropharyngeal
   cancer?
   - A. p16 mutation
   - B. Lack of EBV viral load
   - C. p53 mutation
   - D. HPV infection

K.H. Young, MD, PhD (✉)
Department of Radiation Medicine, Oregon Health & Sciences University,
3181 S.W. Sam Jackson Park Rd, KPV4, Portland, OR 97239, USA
e-mail: youngkri@ohsu.edu

C.B. Ord, MD
Department of Radiation Oncology, Scott & White Memorial Hospital,
Temple, TX 76508, USA
e-mail: cord@sw.org

J.M. Holland
Department of Radiation Oncology, Oregon Health and Science University,
3181 SW Sam Jackson Park Rd, KPV4, Portland, OR 97239-3098, USA
e-mail: hollanjo@ohsu.edu

C.B. Ord et al. (eds.), *Radiation Oncology Study Guide*,
DOI 10.1007/978-1-4614-6400-6_3, © Springer Science+Business Media New York 2013

3. How does the human papillomavirus promote carcinogenesis?
   A. E7 protein binds p53; E6 protein binds Rb.
   B. E6 protein binds p53; E7 protein binds Rb.
   C. E6 protein promotes p16 expression.
   D. None of the above.

4. All of the following are subsites of the larynx except:
   A. True vocal cord
   B. Pyriform sinus
   C. Aryepiglottic fold
   D. Suprahyoid epiglottis

5. The most commonly involved subsite of the oropharynx is:
   A. Soft palate
   B. Tonsil
   C. Base of tongue
   D. Pharyngeal wall

6. Which of the following nerves is not associated with otalgia related to a mass in
   the oral tongue, base of tongue, larynx, or hypopharynx?
   A. Auriculotemporal branch of CN V
   B. Jacobson nerve of CN IX
   C. Posterior auricular nerve of CN VII
   D. Arnold nerve of CN X

7. What is the approximate risk of lymph node metastases for a T1a true vocal
   cord cancer?
   A. 2 %
   B. 7 %
   C. 10 %
   D. 15 %

8. Which of the following lymph node levels contains the Delphian node?
   A. Level III
   B. Level IV
   C. Level V
   D. Level VI

9. What is the primary lymph node drainage for the supraglottic larynx?
   A. Level II
   B. Level V
   C. Level VI
   D. Level I

10. Of the listed tumor sites, which is least likely to demonstrate bilateral nodal involvement?
    A. Soft palate
    B. Base of tongue
    C. Pharyngeal wall
    D. Tonsil

11. Which of the following skull base structures is matched properly with the CN that traverses it?
    A. Cavernous sinus: CN II
    B. Foramen ovale: CN V2
    C. Jugular foramen: CN IX
    D. Foramen lacerum: CN V3

12. Which of the following is not a subsite of the hypopharynx?
    A. Pyriform sinus
    B. Postcricoid area
    C. Posterior pharyngeal wall
    D. Palatine tonsil

13. The inferior border of the hypopharynx is:
    A. C2
    B. Hyoid
    C. Cricoid
    D. Sternal notch

14. What structure anatomically divides the superficial and deep parotid?
    A. CN V2
    B. Zygomatic branch of CN VII
    C. Buccal branch of CN VII
    D. Mandibular branch of CN VII

15. A patient presents with a 3.5 cm tumor located in the right base of tongue, with three right level III LNs, the largest measuring 5 cm, with no distant metastases. What is the correct AJCC 7th edition TNM grouping and stage for this patient?
    A. Stage III: T3N1
    B. Stage IVA: T3N1
    C. Stage III: T2N2b
    D. Stage IVA: T2N2b

16. Which of the following is not an indication for postoperative radiation in the head and neck?
    A. Tumor >3cm
    B. ≥2 involved lymph nodes
    C. Perineural invasion
    D. Extracapsular extension

17. In the postoperative setting, what is the most appropriate dose in a nodal region associated with extracapsular spread?
    A. 54 Gy
    B. 57.6 Gy
    C. 63 Gy
    D. 68.4 Gy

18. GORTEC 94-01 demonstrated a benefit to concurrent chemoradiation over radiation alone in advanced oropharynx cancer in terms of:
    A. Local control but not overall survival benefit.
    B. Local control and overall survival benefit.
    C. Local control and distant-metastasis-free benefit.
    D. There was no benefit.

19. Based on the combined analysis of EORTC 22931 and RTOG 9501, which two pathologic findings are associated with a chemotherapy benefit?
    A. Perineural invasion, positive margins
    B. Angiolymphatic invasion, positive margins
    C. ≥2 involved lymph nodes, perineural invasion
    D. Extracapsular extension, positive margins

20. Which of the following is a correct pairing for anatomic boundaries of lymph node stations in the neck?
    A. Level II – caudal edge of medial pterygoid to platysma
    B. Level III – bottom edge of cricoid to clavicle
    C. Level V – skull base to clavicle
    D. Level VI – bottom edge of cricoid to clavicle

21. What were the reported 3-year overall survivals with and without concurrent cisplatin, respectively, in patients with unresectable head and neck squamous cell carcinoma, based on the Intergroup study reported by Adelstein et al.?
    A. 61 % versus 42 %
    B. 57 % versus 44 %
    C. 37 % versus 23 %
    D. 27 % versus 14 %

22. The addition of concurrent cetuximab to radiation offers which of the following benefits, based on the Bonner NEJM 2006 data:
    A. Local control but not overall survival benefit.
    B. Local control and progression-free survival but not overall survival benefit.
    C. Local control, progression-free, and overall survival benefit.
    D. There was no benefit.

23. What is the approximate 3-year OS for patients receiving the Posner induction regimen of TPF (docetaxel, cisplatin, 5-FU) followed by concurrent carboplatin and radiation for unresectable H&N cancer?
    A. 70 %
    B. 60 %
    C. 50 %
    D. 40 %

24. Based on the MACH-NC meta-analysis, what are the hazard ratios (HR) for death compared to RT alone with concurrent chemoradiation and induction chemotherapy, then radiation, respectively?
    A. Concurrent HR 1.0; induction HR 1.0
    B. Concurrent HR 0.8; induction HR 0.6
    C. Concurrent HR 0.8; induction HR 1.0
    D. Concurrent HR 0.6; induction HR 0.8

25. Hyperfractionated radiation for H&N cancers has demonstrated a benefit in:
    A. Local control
    B. Overall survival
    C. Disease-free survival
    D. A and B only

26. To what dose should you limit the mandible to minimize the risk of osteoradionecrosis?
    A. 50 Gy
    B. 60 Gy
    C. 70 Gy
    D. 80 Gy

27. Which of the following is effective for reducing toxicity associated with H&N radiation?
    A. Viscous lidocaine
    B. Limiting the parotid mean dose to <35 Gy
    C. Amifostine
    D. Hyperfractionation

28. Of the following sites of primary tumors, which location would be most likely to have a positive retropharyngeal lymph node?
    A. Nasopharynx
    B. Tonsil
    C. Base of tongue
    D. Suprahyoid epiglottis

29. Approximately what percentage of local control is lost per week of interruptions or break in radiation for head and neck cancer?
    A. 2 %
    B. 5 %
    C. 10 %
    D. 15 %

30. A patient presents with a mass in the nasopharynx extending into the sphenoid bone with bilateral 3 cm retropharyngeal LNs, without evidence of distant metastases. What is the correct 7th edition AJCC tumor staging for this patient?
    A. Stage IVa: T4N2
    B. Stage IVa: T3N2
    C. Stage III: T4N1
    D. Stage III: T3N1

31. What is the most common site for a nasopharynx primary?
    A. Torus tubarius
    B. Fossa of Rosenmuller
    C. Parapharyngeal space
    D. Posterior pharyngeal wall

32. Which of the following is not a risk factor for developing nasopharyngeal cancer?
    A. Tobacco
    B. Alcohol
    C. EBV infection
    D. Preserved meat consumption

33. Which WHO grade is most associated with EBV exposure?
    A. WHO grade I (1) – keratinizing
    B. WHO grade IIa (2) – keratinizing
    C. WHO grade IIa (2) – nonkeratinizing
    D. WHO grade IIb (3) – undifferentiated

34. According to Intergroup 0099 data, the 3-year OS for patients undergoing concurrent chemoradiation followed by chemotherapy alone was:
    A. 50 %
    B. 60 %
    C. 70 %
    D. 80 %

35. At which plasma EBV DNA concentration was overall survival and relapse-free survival found to be statistically decreased, as reported by Lin et al. in the New England Journal of Medicine?
    A. 1,000 copies per milliliter
    B. 1,500 copies per milliliter
    C. 2,000 copies per milliliter
    D. 2,500 copies per milliliter

36. What is the estimated percent of 2-year larynx preservation reported in the VA Larynx Trial?
    A. 45 %
    B. 55 %
    C. 65 %
    D. 75 %

37. What is the estimated locoregional control for preoperative versus postoperative radiation for supraglottic primaries based on RTOG 73-03?
    A. 30 % versus 60 %
    B. 40 % versus 60 %
    C. 50 % versus 80 %
    D. 60 % versus 80 %

38. For a left true vocal cord lesion involving 75 % of the TVC alone, what is the recommended treatment?
    A. Laryngectomy
    B. Concurrent chemoRT to 70 Gy in 35 fractions
    C. RT alone to the primary and at risk nodes to 70 Gy in 35 fractions
    D. RT alone to the primary to 63 Gy in 28 fractions

39. Based on RTOG 91-11, concurrent chemoRT was superior to induction chemotherapy followed by radiation and radiation alone due to:
    A. Overall survival benefit
    B. Local control benefit
    C. Larynx preservation rate
    D. Both B and C

40. What was the 2-year larynx preservation rate in the concurrent chemoRT arm of RTOG 91-11?
    A. 95 %
    B. 88 %
    C. 70 %
    D. 65 %

41. What was the 5-year larynx preservation rate in the concurrent chemoRT arm of 91-11?
    A. 92 %
    B. 84 %
    C. 76 %
    D. 64 %

42. What is the median overall survival in recurrent or metastatic H&N cancer treated with combination platinum, 5-FU, and cetuximab?
    A. 6 months
    B. 10 months
    C. 12 months
    D. 15 months

43. A suggested larynx constraint to minimize the risk of long-term side effects is:
    A. V30<30 %
    B. V40<30 %
    C. V50<30 %
    D. V60<30 %

44. Which of the following is a common side effect of amifostine?
    A. Anaphylaxis
    B. Fever
    C. Hypotension
    D. Headache

45. What is the name of the most lateral retropharyngeal lymph node?
    A. Delphian node
    B. Virchow's node
    C. The node of Rouviere
    D. Cloquet's node

46. A woman presents with a tumor of the infrahyoid epiglottis that invades the inner cortex of the right side of the thyroid cartilage with three enlarged lymph nodes in the right neck, the largest measuring 5 cm. What is the correct AJCC TNM grouping?
    A. T3N2a
    B. T3N2b
    C. T4aN2a
    D. T4aN2b

47. A man presents with a tumor of the left true vocal cord resulting in fixation of the cord. There are also two enlarged lymph nodes in the right neck, the largest measuring 4 cm. What is the correct AJCC TNM grouping?
    A. T3N2b
    B. T3N2c
    C. T2N2b
    D. T2N2c

48. A man presents with a 3 cm tumor of the left pyriform sinus, extending to the esophagus with two enlarged lymph nodes in the right neck, the largest measuring 6.5 cm. What is the correct AJCC TNM grouping?
    A. T3N2c
    B. T3N3
    C. T4N2c
    D. T4N3

49. A patient presents with a shock-like sensation in the extremities with neck flexion 4 months after receiving head and neck radiation. What is the most likely cause of his symptoms?
    A. Brachial plexopathy
    B. Lhermitte's syndrome
    C. Sciatica
    D. Guillain-Barre syndrome

50. On physical exam, the tongue is found to deviate the left; what CN is involved?
    A. R CN XII
    B. R CN IX
    C. L CN XII
    D. L CN IX

51. What is the maximum dose constraint for the optic chiasm/optic nerves per QUANTEC?
    A. 40 Gy
    B. 45 Gy
    C. 50 Gy
    D. 55 Gy

52. All of the following make up the anatomic boundaries of the tonsillar fossa except:
    A. Palatoglossus muscle
    B. Palatopharyngeal muscle
    C. Inferior glossotonsillar sulcus
    D. Posterior pharyngeal wall

53. What structure lies within Meckel's cave?
    A. CN VII
    B. Carotid artery
    C. CN V1
    D. Trigeminal ganglion

54. Which nerve exits the skull via the supraorbital notch?
    A. CN V1
    B. CN V2
    C. CN V3
    D. CN VII

55. Which of these foramina is the most lateral?
    A. Foramen ovale
    B. Foramen rotundum
    C. Foramen spinosum
    D. Foramen lacerum

56. What passes through the foramen spinosum?
    A. CN V1
    B. CN V2
    C. Middle meningeal artery and vein
    D. Carotid artery

57. What is the approximate rate of PEG tube dependence following chemoradiation for head and neck cancer?
    A. 5 %
    B. 15 %
    C. 25 %
    D. 30 %

58. Which of the following foramina is most anterior?
    A. Foramen ovale
    B. Foramen rotundum
    C. Foramen spinosum
    D. Foramen lacerum

59. Which of the following does not pass through the superior orbital fissure?
    A. CN III
    B. CN IV
    C. CN V1
    D. CN V2

60. All of the following nerves innervate the tongue except:
    A. Vagus
    B. Glossopharyngeal
    C. Mandibular branch of the trigeminal
    D. Maxillary branch of the trigeminal

61. After head and neck radiation, all of the following studies are appropriate for follow-up except:
    A. TSH.
    B. CXR.
    C. Head and neck CT.
    D. All of the above are acceptable.

62. The cavernous sinus houses all of the following except:
    A. CN II
    B. CN III
    C. CN IV
    D. CN VI

63. What cervical spine level corresponds to the hyoid?
    A. C2
    B. C3
    C. C4
    D. C5

64. What cervical spine level corresponds to the true vocal cords?
    A. C2-3
    B. C3-4
    C. C4-5
    D. C5-6

65. Pain in the thyroid cartilage upon palpation is indicative of:
    A. Postcricoid extension
    B. Tumor invasion into the thyroid cartilage
    C. Level IV LN involvement
    D. Delphian node involvement

66. Which is the most common site of sinonasal cancers?
    A. Nasal cavity
    B. Ethmoid sinus
    C. Maxillary sinus
    D. Sphenoid sinus

67. In which profession is adenocarcinoma of the nasal cavity most often reported?
    A. Nickel workers
    B. Steel workers
    C. Coal miners
    D. Carpenters

68. What is the posterior boundary of the nasal cavity proper?
    A. Limen nasi
    B. Choana
    C. Hard palate
    D. Base of skull

69. A tumor arising in the upper nasal cavity would extend to the orbit by traversing what structure?
    A. Fovea ethmoidalis
    B. Lamina papyracea
    C. Inferior turbinate
    D. Gingivolabial sulcus

70. Which of the following is histologically dissimilar to the other listed diseases?
    A. Small-cell lung cancer
    B. Ewing's sarcoma
    C. Esthesioneuroblastoma
    D. Melanoma

71. Ohngren's line divides the maxillary sinus and is comprised of a line drawn from the medial canthus to what structure?
    A. Angle of the mandible
    B. Tragus
    C. Antihelix
    D. Helix

72. What is the correct 7th edition AJCC stage for a left maxillary sinus tumor that invades the pterygoid plates and presents with a single ipsilateral 3.0 cm lymph node?
    A. T4aN1
    B. T3N1
    C. T4aN2
    D. T3N2

73. What is the correct 7th edition AJCC stage for a right ethmoid sinus tumor that invades the pterygoid plates and presents with two ipsilateral lymph nodes, largest measuring 5.4 cm?
    A. T3N2b
    B. T4aN2b
    C. T3N2c
    D. T4aN2c

74. According to the AJCC 7th edition staging manual, what is the T stage when tumors invade the cribriform plate for carcinomas of the maxillary sinus and ethmoid sinus, respectively?
    A. T3, T3
    B. T3, T4a
    C. T4a, T3
    D. T4a, T4a

75. What is the correct Kadish stage for an esthesioneuroblastoma that invades the maxillary sinus?
    A. Kadish stage A
    B. Kadish stage B
    C. Kadish stage C
    D. Kadish stage D

76. Which of the following statements is false regarding primary therapy of nasal vestibule tumors?
    A. Radiation is preferred due to better cosmesis.
    B. Over 90 % of lesions <2 cm are cured with radiation alone.
    C. External beam radiation is preferable to brachytherapy for local control.
    D. Late complications can be mitigated with proper fractionation.

77. Which of the following is false regarding esthesioneuroblastoma?
    A. Distant progression is the predominant cause of death in Kadish stage C patients.
    B. Ultimate local control of Kadish stage A patients is >90%.
    C. Locoregional failure is the predominant mode of failure of stage A and B patients.
    D. Elective nodal radiation is not indicated.

78. All of the following are in the major salivary gland group except:
    A. Parotid gland
    B. Submandibular gland
    C. Sublingual gland
    D. Submucosal gland in the hard palate

79. All of the following are true regarding parotid tumors except:
    A. This is the most common site of salivary gland tumors.
    B. The majority of adult parotid tumors are benign.
    C. Most arise in the deep lobe of the parotid.
    D. Parotid tumors in children are more likely to be malignant than tumors in adults.

80. Which of the following is not true regarding *carcinoma ex pleomorphic adenoma*?
    A. These arise from preexistent benign mixed tumors.
    B. The most common site of distant metastasis is the lung.
    C. Regional failure is rare, but distant failure is common.
    D. Adenocarcinoma is one of the most common histologies of *carcinoma ex pleomorphic adenoma*.

81. All of the following are true regarding adenoid cystic carcinoma except:
    A. These have frequent regional nodal involvement.
    B. The lung is the most frequent site of distant metastasis.
    C. Perineural invasion is not rare.
    D. These are more commonly seen in submandibular and minor salivary glands.

82. All of the following statements about molecular factors of salivary gland tumors are true except:
    A. Proliferating cell nuclear antigen (PCNA) has been shown to correlate with poorer outcomes in mucoepidermoid carcinoma.
    B. Proliferating cell nuclear antigen (PCNA) has not been shown to correlate with poorer outcomes in adenoid cystic carcinoma.
    C. Ki-67 overexpression has been shown to correlate with poorer outcomes in mucoepidermoid carcinoma.
    D. p53 expression has been detected in the majority of salivary gland tumors.

83. A 60-year- old man presents with a growing painless submandibular mass. It has been growing for the last 9 months. What is the next best step in management?
    A. Continued observation
    B. Fine-needle aspiration of the mass
    C. Incisional biopsy of the mass
    D. Excisional biopsy of the mass

84. A man undergoes resection of a right parotid tumor that was causing paralysis of the facial nerve. Surprisingly, a 3 cm left cervical lymph node was also found at the time of surgery. What is the correct 7th edition AJCC stage?
    A. T4aN2b
    B. T4aN2c
    C. T4bN2b
    D. T4bN2c

85. All of the following are true regarding resection for parotid cancers except:
    A. The facial nerve is always resected in an oncologic resection.
    B. Frey's syndrome can occur after resection.
    C. Tarsorrhaphy may be needed to protect the eye after resection.
    D. Nerve grafting can aid in recovery of facial strength.

86. Which of the following is false regarding thyroid cancers?
    A. Papillary and follicular carcinomas are more common in women than men.
    B. Patients with papillary thyroid carcinoma tend to be older than those with follicular carcinoma.
    C. Medullary carcinoma is associated with the MEN-2 syndrome.
    D. Papillary thyroid carcinoma is associated with Cowden's syndrome.

87. Which proto-oncogene is found in more than 90 % of familial medullary thyroid cancers?
    A. *ras*
    B. *myc*
    C. *kit*
    D. *RET*

88. Which type of thyroid carcinoma arises from the parafollicular cell?
    A. Medullary
    B. Papillary
    C. Follicular
    D. Anaplastic

89. Comparing papillary and follicular thyroid cancers, which of the following is false?
    A. Papillary thyroid cancers present more frequently with clinically evident lymphadenopathy.
    B. Follicular thyroid cancers present more frequently with distant metastatic disease.
    C. Papillary thyroid cancers present more frequently with larger- and higher-grade tumors.
    D. Follicular carcinomas present in older patients.

90. Which of the following statements regarding medullary thyroid cancers is not true?
    A. These arise from the C cell of the thyroid.
    B. These secrete calcitonin.
    C. The familial variant appears at a younger age than the sporadic form.
    D. The familial variant has a worse prognosis than the sporadic form.

91. All of the following stages of thyroid cancer are classified as AJCC stage IV except:
    A. T3N1a
    B. T4aN0
    C. T4bN0
    D. T1N1M1

92. What percentage of Hurthle cell features must be exhibited in follicular cells to classify it as a Hurthle cell carcinoma?
    A. 50 %
    B. 75 %
    C. 95 %
    D. 100 %

93. Which type of thyroid cancer requires the demonstration of angioinvasion or thyroid capsule invasion for definitive diagnosis?
    A. Papillary
    B. Follicular
    C. Medullary
    D. Anaplastic

94. Which type of thyroid cancer can be diagnosed preoperatively by amyloid staining by Congo red?
    A. Papillary
    B. Follicular
    C. Medullary
    D. Anaplastic

95. Which of the following is false regarding radioactive iodine therapy?
    A. Radioactive remnant ablation is used for completely resected follicular cell-derived carcinoma.
    B. Radioactive remnant ablation may improve the value of follow-up thyroglobulin measurement during follow-up.
    C. Patients with papillary thyroid carcinoma concentrate radioactive iodine ablation better than those with follicular thyroid carcinoma.
    D. Radioactive remnant ablation employs lower doses than radioactive iodine ablation.

96. Approximately what percentage of head and neck squamous cell carcinomas presents as an unknown primary?
    A. <5 %
    B. 10 %
    C. 15 %
    D. 20 %

97. What subtype of thyroid cancer is associated with the characteristic pathological feature of "Orphan Annie" nuclei?
    A. Follicular
    B. Medullary
    C. Papillary
    D. Anaplastic

98. What is the most common site where a primary cancer is ultimately found in head and neck cancer of unknown primary?
    A. Oral cavity
    B. Oropharynx
    C. Larynx
    D. Nasopharynx

99. Which of the following sites is least likely to be included in radiation treatment for head and neck cancer of unknown primary?
    A. Contralateral neck
    B. Oropharynx
    C. Larynx
    D. Nasopharynx

100. Which one of the following scenarios will not likely require subsequent neck dissection after radiation for head and neck unknown primary?
    A. N2 or N3 at presentation
    B. Gross neck disease after open biopsy
    C. Persistent neck mass 3 months after completion of therapy
    D. N1 at presentation

101. In a primary cancer, in which of the following sites is not likely to metastasize to level Ia in the neck?
    A. Floor of mouth
    B. Anterior oral tongue
    C. Cheek
    D. Anterior mandibular alveolar ridge

102. What are the cranial, caudal, and posterior borders of level IIa in the neck?
    A. Caudal edge of lateral process of C2, caudal edge of hyoid bone, posterior border of the internal jugular vein
    B. Cranial edge of lateral process of C2, cranial edge of hyoid bone, anterior border of the internal jugular vein
    C. Caudal edge of lateral process of C1, caudal edge of hyoid bone, posterior border of the internal jugular vein
    D. Cranial edge of lateral process of C1, cranial edge of hyoid bone, posterior border of the internal jugular vein

103. What are the anterior and posterior borders of level V in the neck?
    A. Posterior border of sternocleidomastoid muscle, anterior border of the trapezius muscle
    B. Posterior border of sternocleidomastoid muscle, posterior border of the trapezius muscle
    C. Anterior border of sternocleidomastoid muscle, anterior border of the trapezius muscle
    D. Anterior border of sternocleidomastoid muscle, posterior border of the trapezius muscle

104. Which primary tumor site is associated with the highest propensity for lymph node involvement?
    A. Supraglottic larynx
    B. Nasopharynx
    C. Piriform sinus
    D. Tonsillar fossa

105. Which primary tumor site is associated with the highest propensity for lymph node involvement of level V?
    A. Oral cavity
    B. Nasopharynx
    C. Hypopharynx
    D. Oropharynx

106. In a retrospective series of tonsillar carcinoma treated with radiation to the primary tumor and ipsilateral neck alone reported by O'Sullivan et al., which of the following is false?
    A. The incidence of contralateral neck recurrence was <5 %.
    B. No recurrences were seen in N0 patients.
    C. T stage predicted for contralateral neck recurrence.
    D. The majority of patients that failed in the contralateral neck also failed at the primary site.

107. All of the following were found to be "moderate" risk factors for locoregional relapse as described by Peters et al. in the trial for postoperative radiotherapy in head and neck cancer except:
    A. Extracapsular extension
    B. Positive margin at the primary
    C. Two or more invaded lymph nodes
    D. Two or more involved node levels

108. Which is true regarding the postoperative chemoradiation trials reported by the EORTC and RTOG?
    A. Both showed a survival benefit with the addition of chemotherapy to postoperative radiation.
    B. The majority of patients in the EORTC study received all the planned cycles of chemotherapy.
    C. Acute toxicity did not increase with the addition of chemotherapy.
    D. The incidence of distant metastases did not decrease with the addition of chemotherapy.

109. What is the most common oral cavity cancer subsite?
    A. Lower lip
    B. Tongue
    C. Floor of mouth
    D. Buccal mucosa

110. All of the following are true regarding squamous cell carcinomas of the lip except:
    A. They are more common on the lower than upper lip.
    B. Perineural invasion is common.
    C. Lymph node involvement is approximately 20 % when the commissure is involved.
    D. Leukoplakia commonly precedes the development of carcinoma.

111. What is the most appropriate treatment for a 1.9 cm squamous cell carcinoma of the lower lip that involves the left commissure?
    A. Surgery alone
    B. Surgery and postoperative radiotherapy
    C. Neoadjuvant radiation then surgery
    D. Radiation alone

112. What structure constitutes the floor of the mouth?
    A. Anterior belly of the digastric muscle
    B. Mylohyoid muscle
    C. Submandibular glands
    D. Posterior surface of the tongue

113. Which of the following lymph node groups is considered "first echelon" for floor of mouth cancers?
    A. Retropharyngeal
    B. Submandibular
    C. Upper jugular
    D. Lower jugular

114. Which one of the structure/sensory innervation pairings is incorrect?
    A. Lower lip-mental nerve
    B. Upper lip-infraorbital nerve
    C. Floor of mouth-lingual nerve
    D. Oral tongue-hypoglossal nerve

115. Based on a review by Mohit-Tabatabai et al. who found that the probability of subclinical neck metastases is related to thickness of the primary floor of mouth lesion, they recommend elective neck treatment for any lesion greater than _____ mm.
    A. 0.5
    B. 1.0
    C. 1.5
    D. 5.0

116. Deviation of the tongue to the affected side of a hypoglossal nerve injury is a result of:
    A. Unopposed action of the unaffected contralateral genioglossus muscle
    B. Unopposed action of the unaffected contralateral hyoglossus muscle
    C. Unopposed action of the unaffected contralateral styloglossus muscle
    D. Unopposed action of the unaffected contralateral palatoglossus muscle

117. What is the incidence of "skip metastases" in squamous cell carcinoma of the oral tongue?
    A. 5 %
    B. 10 %
    C. 15 %
    D. 20 %

118. Lower gingival squamous cell carcinomas drain most commonly to which lymph node group?
    A. Submental
    B. Submandibular
    C. Upper jugular
    D. Posterior cervical

119. Which one of the following lymph node groups is considered "first echelon" for retromolar trigone tumors?
    A. Submental
    B. Submandibular
    C. Subdigastric
    D. Upper jugular

120. What is the risk of clinically positive ipsilateral nodes and subclinically involved lymph nodes at presentation, respectively, for retromolar trigone tumors?
    A. 40 %, 40 %
    B. 40 %, 25 %
    C. 25 %, 40 %
    D. 25 %, 25 %

121. All of the following are true regarding carcinoma of the hard palate except:
    A. Squamous cell carcinoma is the most common histology.
    B. The incidence of osteoradionecrosis is less than in the mandible.
    C. Surgery is the mainstay of therapy.
    D. The risk of developing a subsequent metachronous primary carcinoma is >25 %.

122. What is the annual rate of development of a second head and neck squamous cell carcinoma?
    A. 1–3 %
    B. 4–7 %
    C. 8–10 %
    D. 11–15 %

123. What structures are the origin and termination of the base of tongue region, respectively?
    A. Lingual sulcus terminalis, base of the pharyngeal epiglottis
    B. Lingual sulcus terminalis, base of the lingual epiglottis
    C. Lingual sulcus terminalis, glossopharyngeal sulcus
    D. Lingual sulcus terminalis, epiglottis tip

124. All of the muscles of the soft palate are innervated by the vagus nerve except:
    A. Tensor veli palatini
    B. Palatoglossus
    C. Palatopharyngeus
    D. Levator veli palatini

125. A 3 cm left tonsil tumor is found to invade the left medial pterygoid. There is
     one ipsilateral 3.0 cm lymph node. What is the correct 7th edition AJCC stage?
     A. T2N1
     B. T2N2a
     C. T4aN1
     D. T4aN2a

126. All of the following are true regarding the findings of various fractionation
     schemes in the treatment of tonsil carcinoma with radiation alone from Withers
     et al. except:
     A. For every day of treatment prolongation for a constant total dose, local
        control is decreased 1 %.
     B. For every 1Gy increment in total dose in a constant treatment duration,
        local control increased 2 %.
     C. Larger fraction size is correlated with a higher incidence of mucosal late
        complications.
     D. Field size directly correlated with the incidence of mandibular
        complications.

127. All of the following are true regarding the findings of the Overgaard phase III
     trial of treatment duration except:
     A. The majority of patients had larynx cancer.
     B. Patients were randomized to 6 versus 5 fractions weekly.
     C. Local control was improved with the accelerated fractionated group.
     D. Late toxicity was worse in the accelerated fractionated group.

128. Which is not true regarding the RTOG 90-03 trial of altered fractionation?
     A. The majority of patients had oropharyngeal cancer.
     B. This was a three-arm trial: standard versus split-course accelerated versus
        hyperfractionation.
     C. There was no overall survival difference between any of the arms.
     D. Acute toxicity was worse in the altered fractionation arms.

129. What was the overall survival benefit seen with the addition of concurrent
     chemotherapy to radiation in the Meta-Analysis of Chemotherapy in Head and
     Neck Cancer (MACH-NC)?
     A. 5 %
     B. 6 %
     C. 7 %
     D. 8 %

130. All of the following are true regarding the GORTEC 94-01 trial of radiation +/– chemotherapy for tonsillar carcinoma except:
    A. Total radiation dose was 70 Gy.
    B. Chemotherapy consisted of 3 cycles of cisplatin on days 1, 22, and 43.
    C. The incidence of distant metastasis was unchanged with the addition of chemotherapy.
    D. Late effects were similar between the arms.

131. Which of the following statements is false regarding RTOG 05-22?
    A. All oropharynx cancers were eligible.
    B. Radiation was delivered using an accelerated radiation technique.
    C. All patients received concurrent cisplatin.
    D. The experimental arm also received concurrent C225.

132. Which of the following statements regarding RTOG 05-22 is false?
    A. The majority of patients completed the planned cycles of cisplatin in both arms.
    B. C225 improved progression-free but not overall survival.
    C. C225 increased grades 3–4 mucositis.
    D. Late reactions were not different between the arms.

133. All of the following are true regarding a phase III trial evaluating the benefit of adding cetuximab to radiation for locally advanced head and neck carcinoma as reported by Bonner et al. except:
    A. The majority of patients had oropharynx cancer.
    B. Acute mucositis was not increased with the addition of cetuximab.
    C. All radiation was delivered by standard fractionation.
    D. The skin reaction noted with cetuximab is a "maculopapular rash."

134. What is true regarding the addition of cetuximab to radiation for advanced head and neck cancer as reported by Bonner et al.?
    A. Five-year overall survival with cetuximab is 36 % versus 26 % without.
    B. Those patients with grade 2 or higher rash had improved survival compared to those with grade 1 rash.
    C. Cetuximab is administered starting day 1 of radiation.
    D. If the patient was postoperative, the dose of cetuximab was halved.

135. All are true of Hong's chemoprevention trial for patients with head and neck cancer s/p definitive treatment except:
    A. The chemoprevention agent was 13-cis-retinoic acid.
    B. Chemoprevention initially decreased the incidence of second primary tumors, as well as the rate of relapse from treatment of the first primary tumor.
    C. Chemoprevention initially decreased the incidence of second primary tumors, but not the rate of relapse from treatment of the first primary tumor.
    D. After 3 years, the chemopreventive effect abated, and the incidence of second primary tumors was similar with or without the agent.

136. What is the most frequently involved cranial nerve in nasopharyngeal carcinoma?
    A. V
    B. VI
    C. VII
    D. VIII

137. A woman presents to her doctor with dysphagia and altered taste sensation. On physical exam, she is found to have atrophy of the left tongue and a tumor in the left fossa of Rosenmuller. Which syndrome accounts for these symptoms?
    A. Jacod's syndrome
    B. Villaret's syndrome
    C. Frey's syndrome
    D. Horner's syndrome

138. What is the mechanism of Jacod's syndrome?
    A. Extension of tumor through foramen lacerum into the cavernous sinus
    B. Compression of the structures in the retropharyngeal space
    C. Obstruction of the Eustachian tube opening
    D. None of the above

139. All of the following are true regarding Intergroup 0099 assessing the addition of chemotherapy to radiation for nasopharyngeal cancer except:
    A. Concurrent chemotherapy consisted of cisplatin on days 1, 22, and 43.
    B. Concurrent chemotherapy consisted of cisplatin on days 1, 22, and 43 and 5-FU on days 1–4, every 3 weeks.
    C. The trial closed at interim analysis.
    D. Total radiation dose was 70 Gy.

140. Which one of the following statements regarding re-irradiation of nasopharyngeal carcinoma is incorrect?
    A. Re-irradiation can be accomplished with stereotactic radiosurgery, offering 2-year local control rates of approximately 50 %.
    B. The duration of the disease-free interval prior to re-irradiation does not influence survival after re-irradiation.
    C. Total deliverable dose above 60 Gy improves actuarial survival.
    D. Five-year overall survival after re-irradiation is approximately 50 %.

141. All of the following are included in the radiation treatment volume of locally advanced T4 nasopharynx carcinoma except:
    A. Posterior two thirds of the maxillary sinus
    B. Sphenoid sinus
    C. Base of skull
    D. Posterior one third of the nasal cavity

142. Which one of the following statements is true regarding the use of IMRT for nasopharynx cancer in the single-institution experience reported by Lee et al.?
    A. Four-year local control was 80 %.
    B. Four-year locoregional control was 85 %.
    C. The majority of patients experienced only grade 1 xerostomia.
    D. There was no grade 2 or higher xerostomia.

143. All of the following are true regarding the phase II RTOG 0225 trial of IMRT +/− chemotherapy for nasopharynx cancer except:
    A. The majority of patients had WHO type 1 nasopharynx cancer.
    B. Chemotherapy was given as per the Intergroup 0099 trial.
    C. There were no reports of grade 4 xerostomia.
    D. Two-year local control was >90 %.

144. Which of the following risk factors is least common in larynx cancer?
    A. Gastroesophageal reflux disease
    B. Tobacco
    C. Human papillomavirus
    D. Alcohol use

145. Larynx cancers most commonly present in which subsite of the larynx?
    A. Glottic
    B. Supraglottic larynx
    C. Subglottic larynx
    D. They present equally in all sites.

146. Regarding the nodal metastatic pattern of hypopharyngeal cancers, which of the following is false?
    A. Bilateral nodes at presentation occur in 15 % of patients.
    B. Levels II and III are the most frequently involved.
    C. Three-quarters of hypopharyngeal cancers present with nodal metastases.
    D. Hypopharyngeal cancers do not metastasize to the retropharyngeal nodes.

147. What is the least common subsite of hypopharyngeal cancer?
    A. Pharyngeal wall.
    B. Postcricoid pharynx.
    C. Pyriform sinus.
    D. They present equally in all sites.

148. Regarding the patterns of spread of larynx cancers, which of the following is not true?
    A. Glottic larynx tumors rarely spread to lymph nodes or distantly.
    B. Most subglottic tumors actually originate in the glottic larynx.
    C. The most common site of distant metastasis is the bone.
    D. Regional spread from supraglottic tumors is primarily to level II.

149. All of the following are indications for postoperative radiation after laryngectomy for larynx cancer except:
    A. Thyroid/cricoid cartilage invasion
    B. Emergency tracheotomy performed before radiation
    C. Extensive subglottic disease presence
    D. Difficult and prolonged surgery

150. What was the initially reported 5-year voice preservation rate in the Lefebvre EORTC phase III trial for pyriform sinus cancer?
    A. 35 %
    B. 45 %
    C. 55 %
    D. 65 %

151. What are the superior and posterior borders of an anterior T1 glottic larynx field, respectively?
    A. Top of the thyroid notch, bottom of the cricoid cartilage
    B. Bottom of the thyroid cartilage, bottom of the cricoid cartilage
    C. Top of the thyroid notch, anterior margin of the vertebral bodies
    D. Bottom of the thyroid notch, posterior margin of the vertebral bodies

152. All of the following are removed in a supraglottic laryngectomy except:
    A. Pre-epiglottic space
    B. False vocal cords
    C. True vocal cords
    D. Epiglottis

153. Which of the following is not a contraindication to supraglottic laryngectomy?
    A. Subglottic extension.
    B. Bilateral arytenoid involvement.
    C. Extension to the anterior commissure.
    D. These are all contraindications to supraglottic laryngectomy.

154. Which of the following is not a contraindication to hemilaryngectomy?
    A. Bilateral true vocal cord involvement
    B. Partial fixation of one true vocal cord
    C. Bilateral arytenoid involvement
    D. Epiglottic invasion

Answers and Rationales

1. The correct answer is B. Approximately 52,000 new cases per year of head and neck cancer are diagnosed in the United States with an estimated 11,000 deaths per year. There is a male predominance of about 2:1. Siegel R, et al. Cancer statistics, 2012. CA-A Cancer J Clin. 2012;62(1):10–29.

2. The correct answer is D. HPV infection is associated with p16 expression and portends a better outcome. Three-year overall survival rate among patients with HPV-positive oropharyngeal cancers in RTOG 0129 was 82.4 % versus 57.1 % in HPV-negative tumors. High EBV viral load is associated with poor outcome in nasopharyngeal cancer. p53 mutation is associated with tobacco use and worse outcome. Ang KK et al. Human papillomavirus and survival of patients with oropharyngeal cancer. N Engl J Med. 2010;363(1):24–35. Lin J-C et al. Quantification of plasma Epstein-Barr virus DNA in patients with advanced nasopharyngeal carcinoma. N Engl J Med. 2004;350(24):2461–70. Twu C-W et al. Comparison of the prognostic impact of serum anti-EBV antibody and plasma EBV DNA assays in nasopharyngeal carcinoma. Int J Radiat Oncol Biol Phys. 2007;67(1):130–7. Westra WH et al. Inverse relationship between human papillomavirus-16 infection and disruptive p53 gene mutations in squamous cell carcinoma of the head and neck. Clin Cancer Res. 2008;14(2):366–9. Field JK et al. p53 expression and mutations in squamous cell carcinoma of the head and neck: expression correlates with the patients' use of tobacco and alcohol. Cancer Detect Prev. 1994;18(3):197–208.

3. The correct answer is B. HPV promotes carcinogenesis via two mechanisms: E6 protein stimulates ubiquitin-mediated degradation of p53 inhibiting apoptosis while E7 protein binds to Rb and disrupts its ability to stall cells at the G1/S restriction point. p16 expression is upregulated as a result of Rb inactivation. Munger K et al. Mechanisms of human papillomavirus-induced oncogenesis. J Virol. 2004;78:11451–60.

4. The correct answer is B. The larynx can be subdivided into three subsites: the supraglottic, glottic, and subglottic. The supraglottic larynx consists of the AE folds, arytenoids, false cords, suprahyoid epiglottis, and infrahyoid epiglottis. The glottic larynx consists of the true vocal cords and anterior and posterior commissures. The subglottic larynx extends inferiorly from the glottis to the lower margin of the cricoid cartilage. The pyriform sinus is considered part of the hypopharynx. Edge SB, Byrd DR, Compton CC, et al., editors. Larynx. AJCC cancer staging handbook. 7th ed. New York: Springer; 2010.

5. The correct answer is B. The most common primary subsite within the oropharynx is the tonsil. Halperin EC, Perez CA, Brady LW, editors. Perez and Brady's principles and practice of radiation oncology. 5th ed. Philadelphia: Lippincott Williams & Wilkins; 2008.

6. The correct answer is C. Otalgia is a common presenting symptom of H&N cancer. The three major nerves responsible for otalgia are the auriculotemporal branch of CN V felt in the preauricular area, referred from the oral tongue; the Jacobsen nerve of CN IX felt in the tympanic cavity, referred from the base of tongue; and the Arnold nerve of CN X felt in the postauricular area, referred from the larynx and hypopharynx. The posterior auricular nerve is an efferent branch of CN VII. Netter FH. In: Kelly P, editor. Atlas of human anatomy. 3rd ed. Teterboro: Icon Learning Systems; 2003.

7. The correct answer is A. The glottic larynx has little to no lymphatic drainage; therefore, lymph node metastasis is rare. For a T1a true vocal cord cancer, this risk is ~2 %. Netter FH. In: Kelly P, editor. Atlas of human anatomy. 3rd ed. Teterboro: Icon Learning Systems; 2003. Garden AS, Morrison WH, Ang KK. Larynx and hypopharynx cancer. In: Gunderson LL, Tepper JE, editors. Clinical radiation oncology. 3rd ed. Philadelphia: Elsevier Saunders; 2012. p. 639–64.

8. The correct answer is D. The Delphian node is found in level VI. Netter FH. In: Kelly P, editor. Atlas of human anatomy. 3rd ed. Teterboro: Icon Learning Systems; 2003. Garden AS, Morrison WH, Ang KK. Larynx and hypopharynx cancer. In: Gunderson LL, Tepper JE, editors. Clinical radiation oncology, 3rd ed. Philadelphia: Elsevier Saunders; 2012. p. 639–64.

9. The correct answer is A. The primary lymphatic drainage of the supraglottic larynx is level II. Netter FH. In: Kelly P, editor. Atlas of human anatomy. 3rd ed. Teterboro: Icon Learning Systems; 2003. Lindberg R. Distribution of cervical lymph node metastases from squamous cell carcinoma of the upper respiratory and digestive tracts. Cancer. 1972;29(6):1446–49. Byers RM et al. Rationale for elective modified neck dissection. Head Neck Surg. 1988;10(3):160–7.

10. The correct answer is D. The frequency and distribution of LN involvement depends in large part on the primary tumor site. Nasopharyngeal and hypopharyngeal tumors have the highest nodal involvement, approximately 70–80 % of cases. Contralateral nodes are reported for midline tumors or tumors with bilateral lymphatic drainage such as the soft palate, base of tongue, and pharyngeal wall. Recent reports have suggested that well-lateralized tonsillar tumors may be adequately treated with ipsilateral LN management only (5-year freedom from contralateral nodal recurrence rate 96 %). Grégoire V et al. Selection and delineation of lymph node target volumes in head and neck conformal radiotherapy. Proposal for standardizing terminology and procedure based on the surgical experience. Radiother Oncol. 2000;56(2):135–50. Chronowski GM et al. Unilateral radiotherapy for the treatment of tonsil cancer. Int J Radiat Oncol Biol Phys. 2012;83(1):204–9.

11. The correct answer is C. The contents of the cavernous sinus are CN III, CN IV, CN V1, CN V2, and CN VI. CN V2 travels through foramen rotundum. CN V3 travels through foramen ovale. The jugular foramen contains CNs IX, X, and XI. CN XII travels through the hypoglossal canal. Netter FH. In: Kelly P, editor. Atlas of human anatomy. 3rd ed. Teterboro: Icon Learning Systems; 2003.

12. The correct answer is D. The hypopharynx extends superiorly from the hyoid to the cricoids inferiorly. Netter FH. In: Kelly P, editor. Atlas of human anatomy. 3rd ed. Teterboro: Icon Learning Systems; 2003. Garden AS, Morrison WH, Ang KK. Larynx and hypopharynx cancer. In: Gunderson LL, Tepper JE, editors. Clinical radiation oncology, 3rd ed. Philadelphia: Elsevier Saunders; 2012. p. 639–64.

13. The correct answer is C. The inferior border of the hypopharynx is the lower level of the cricoid cartilage, with the superior border being at the level of the hyoid bone. Garden AS, Morrison WH, Ang KK. Larynx and hypopharynx cancer. In: Gunderson LL, Tepper JE, editors. Clinical radiation oncology, 3rd ed. Philadelphia: Elsevier Saunders; 2012. p. 639–64.

14. The correct answer is C. The parotid gland is divided by CN VII. CN VII has five major divisions: temporal, zygomatic, buccal, marginal mandibular, and cervical. The buccal branch divides the parotid into deep and superficial lobes. Netter FH. In: Kelly P, editor. Atlas of human anatomy. 3rd ed. Teterboro: Icon Learning Systems; 2003.

15. The correct answer is D. Based on 7th edition AJCC staging, the patient has a T2 (tumor 3.5 cm), N2b (ipsilateral nodes <6 cm), M0, and therefore stage IVA cancer. Edge SB, Byrd DR, Compton CC, et al., editors. Pharynx. AJCC cancer staging handbook. 7th ed. New York: Springer; 2010.

16. The correct answer is A. In a subgroup analysis within Lester Peters' study of dose escalation in postoperative stage III/IV H&N cancer, a benefit was seen with radiation in patients with ECE alone or with two or more of the following risk factors: oral cavity primary, close/positive margins, perineural invasion, ≥ 2 LNs involved, largest LN>3 cm, treatment delay >6 months, or poor performance status. Peters LJ et al. Evaluation of the dose for postoperative radiation therapy of head and neck cancer: first report of a prospective randomized trial. Int J Radiat Oncol Biol Phys. 1993;26(1):3–11.

17. The correct answer is C. According to the Lester Peters' study of dose escalation in the post-operative setting, the minimal effective dose was 57.6 Gy giving a primary LRC 63 % versus 92 % versus 89 % for doses of <54 Gy, 57.6 Gy, and 63 Gy, respectively. The regions at risk for microscopic disease due to +ECE benefited from a minimum dose of 63 Gy with 2-year LRC of 52 % versus 74 % versus 72 % for doses of 57.6 Gy, 63 Gy, and 68.4 Gy, respectively.

Peters LJ et al. Evaluation of the dose for postoperative radiation therapy of head and neck cancer: first report of a prospective randomized trial. Int J Radiat Oncol Biol Phys. 1993;26(1):3–11.

18. The correct answer is B. GORTEC 94-01 randomized 222 patients with stage III or IV oropharyngeal carcinoma to radiation +/− concurrent chemotherapy. This trial demonstrated that concurrent chemoradiation with 3 cycles of carboplatin and 5-FU (weeks 1, 4, 7) compared to RT alone (70Gy in 35 fractions) resulted in improved 5-year OS 22 % versus 16 % ($p = 0.05$), 5-year DFS 27 % versus 15 % ($p = 0.01$), and 5-year local control 48 % versus 25 % ($p = 0.002$). There was no difference in the incidence of distant metastases. There was increased incidence of grades 3–4 mucositis. Denis F et al. Final results of the 94-01 French head and neck oncology and radiotherapy group randomized trial comparing radiotherapy alone with concomitant radiochemotherapy in advanced-stage oropharynx carcinoma. J Clin Oncol. 2004;22(1):69–76.

19. The correct answer is D. Independently, the RTOG 9501 study found ≥2LNs involved, +margins, and ECE as groups benefiting from chemoradiotherapy. EORTC 22391 found stage III–IV cancers, oropharynx and oral cavity with level 4 or 5 LNs, perineural disease, vascular embolisms, positive margins, and ECE benefitted chemoradiotherapy. The combined analysis of both studies found that patients with positive margins and/or ECE benefited from chemoradiation over radiation alone HR 0.524. Bernier J et al. Postoperative irradiation with or without concomitant chemotherapy for locally advanced head and neck cancer. N Engl J Med. 2004;350:1945–52. Cooper JS et al. Postoperative concurrent radiotherapy and chemotherapy for high-risk squamous-cell carcinoma of the head and neck. N Engl J Med. 2004;350:1937–44. Bernier J et al. Defining risk levels in locally advanced head and neck cancers: a comparative analysis of concurrent postoperative radiation plus chemotherapy trials of the EORTC (#22931) and RTOG (#9501). Head Neck. 2005;27:843–50.

20. The correct answer is C. According to the guidelines for boundaries of neck node levels, as reported by Grégoire et al., the only correct pairing is that level V extends from the skull base posterolaterally to the clavicle. Grégoire V et al. Selection and delineation of lymph node target volumes in head and neck conformal radiotherapy. Proposal for standardizing terminology and procedure based on the surgical experience. Radiother Oncol. 2000;56(2):135–50.

21. The correct answer is C. The Intergroup study by Adelstein et al. randomized unresectable H&N squamous cell carcinomas to one of three arms; arm A included radiation alone to 70 Gy in 35 fractions, arm B included the same radiation plus concurrent cisplatin q 3 weeks, and arm C included split-course radiation with cisplatin q 3 weeks plus 5-FU with a break after 30 Gy to evaluate for conversion to resectability and possible surgery. About 55–60 % of patients in each arm had an oropharynx primary. Patients in arm B (RT + concurrent

cisplatin) demonstrated a 3-year OS benefit of 37 % compared to 23 % in the RT alone group. Three-year DFS was 51 % versus 33 %. No benefit was seen in the split-course arm. Adelstein DJ et al. An intergroup phase III comparison of standard radiation therapy and two schedules of concurrent chemoradiotherapy in patients with unresectable squamous cell head and neck cancer. J Clin Oncol. 2003;21(1):92–8.

22. The correct answer is C. Patients with locoregionally advanced H&N squamous cell carcinoma were randomized to RT alone versus RT with concurrent weekly cetuximab (400 mg/m² loading 1 week prior followed by 250 mg/m² weekly). Concurrent RT and cetuximab demonstrated a benefit with LR progression HR 0.68 ($p=0.005$), OS HR 0.74 ($p=0.03$), and PFS HR 0.70 ($p=0.006$). Median OS was 49.0 months with concurrent treatment versus 29.3 months with RT alone. About 80 % of patients had detectable EGFR. Bonner JA et al. Radiotherapy plus cetuximab for squamous-cell carcinoma of the head and neck. N Engl J Med. 2006;354(6):567–78. Bonner JA et al. Radiotherapy plus cetuximab for locoregionally advanced head and neck cancer: 5-year survival data from a phase 3 randomized trial, and relation between cetuximab-induced rash and survival. Lancet Oncol. 2010;11(1):21–8.

23. The correct answer is B. The TAX 324 study randomized 501 patients to induction of docetaxel, cisplatin, and 5-FU (TPF) versus cisplatin and 5-FU (PF); patients in both arms subsequently underwent concurrent chemoradiation with weekly carboplatin to 70 Gy in 35 fractions. The OS HR 0.70 ($p=0.006$) favored TPF, with 3-year OS of 62 % versus 48 % for TPF and PF induction, respectively. There was no difference in DM. There was an LRC benefit with LRF in 30 % versus 38 % for TPF and PF induction, respectively. Posner MR et al. Cisplatin and fluorouracil alone or with docetaxel in head and neck cancer. N Engl J Med. 2007;357(17):1705–15.

24. The correct answer is C. The MACH-NC meta-analysis evaluated 93 trials comparing concurrent, induction, or adjuvant chemotherapy with radiation. The oropharynx was the most common primary site (37 %). The addition of concurrent chemotherapy yielded an 8 % 5-year actuarial survival benefit. Overall survival at 5 years was 27 % in the radiation alone group versus 35 % in the chemoradiation arm. The HR for death was 0.8 for concurrent chemoRT compared to RT alone and 0.96 for induction chemotherapy followed by radiation compared to RT alone. Adjuvant chemotherapy following RT had an HR of 1.06. Pignon J-P, le Maître A, Maillard E, Bourhis J. Meta-analysis of chemotherapy in head and neck cancer (MACH-NC): an update on 93 randomized trials and 17,346 patients. Radiother Oncol. 2009;92(1):4–14.

25. The correct answer is A. RTOG 90-03 and EORTC 22791 demonstrated improved LC, but no benefit in OS or DFS. In RTOG 90-03, there was a trend towards DFS, but this was not statistically significant. Similarly, EORTC 22791

demonstrated a trend towards OS benefit but was not statistically significant. Fu KK et al. A Radiation Therapy Oncology Group (RTOG) phase III randomized study to compare hyperfractionation and two variants of accelerated fractionation to standard fractionation radiotherapy for head and neck squamous cell carcinomas: first report of RTOG 9003. Int J Radiat Oncol Biol Phys. 2000;48(1):7–16. Horiot JC et al. Hyperfractionation versus conventional fractionation in oropharyngeal carcinoma: final analysis of a randomized trial of the EORTC cooperative group of radiotherapy. Radiother Oncol. 1992; 25(4): 231–41.

26. The correct answer is C. Osteoradionecrosis is more common with doses >70 Gy. Mendenhall WM, Foote RL, Sandow PL, Fernandes RP. Oral cavity cancer. In: Gunderson LL, Tepper JE, editors. Clinical radiation oncology. 3rd ed. Philadelphia: Elsevier Saunders; 2012. p. 553–84.

27. The correct answer is C. Amifostine has been shown to reduce acute and late xerostomia and dysphagia resulting from H&N chemoradiation. In the Antonadou study, the control group underwent a prolonged treatment time due to interruptions resulting from grade 4 mucositis. Viscous lidocaine can help reduce painful mucositis but does not reduce the incidence of toxicities. The mean dose to the parotid should be <26 Gy to avoid xerostomia. Hyperfractionation demonstrated increased acute toxicity, not decreased. Antonadou D et al. Prophylactic use of amifostine to minimize radiochemotherapy-induced mucositis and xerostomia in head-and-neck cancer. Int J Radiat Oncol Biol Phys. 2002;52(3):739–47. Fu KK et al. A Radiation Therapy Oncology Group (RTOG) phase III randomized study to compare hyperfractionation and two variants of accelerated fractionation to standard fractionation radiotherapy for head and neck squamous cell carcinomas: first report of RTOG 9003. Int J Radiat Oncol Biol Phys. 2000;48(1):7–16. Horiot JC et al. Hyperfractionation versus conventional fractionation in oropharyngeal carcinoma: final analysis of a randomized trial of the EORTC cooperative group of radiotherapy. Radiother Oncol. 1992;25(4):231–41.

28. The correct answer is A. An analysis of LN positivity in H&N primaries in various locations revealed tumors within the nasopharynx, hypopharynx, oropharynx, and posterior soft palate had a propensity for retropharyngeal LN involvement. Grégoire V et al. Selection and delineation of lymph node target volumes in head and neck conformal radiotherapy. Proposal for standardizing terminology and procedure based on the surgical experience. Radiother Oncol. 2000;56(2):135–50. Grégoire V et al. CT-based delineation of lymph node levels and related CTVs in the node-negative neck: DAHANCA, EORTC, GORTEC, NCIC,RTOG consensus guidelines. Radiother Oncol. 2003;69(3):227–36.

29. The correct answer is C. H&N cancer treatment prolongation is associated with a higher level of local recurrence and treatment failure attributed, in part, to

accelerated repopulation. One study estimated that each day of treatment prolongation was associated with 1.4 % loss of local control and each week prolongation was associated with 10–12 % loss of local control. Increasing the dose by 0.5 Gy per day may compensate for the treatment prolongation using BED-T modeling. Bese NS et al. Effects of prolongation of overall treatment time due to unplanned interruptions during radiotherapy of different tumor sites and practical methods for compensation. Int J Radiat Oncol Biol Phys. 2007;68(3):654–61.

30. The correct answer is D. Per the 7th edition AJCC staging system for nasopharynx, invasion into the sphenoid sinus constitutes T3 disease. The nodal staging of nasopharynx cancer is unlike other sites of H&N cancer. Bilateral retropharyngeal lymph node involvement is still N1. Edge SB, Byrd DR, Compton CC, et al., editors. Larynx. AJCC cancer staging handbook. 7th ed. New York: Springer; 2010.

31. The correct answer is B. The most common anatomic location from which nasopharyngeal cancer arises is the fossa of Rosenmuller. The anatomic borders of the nasopharynx are the sphenoid bone (superior), soft palate (inferior), clivus/C1-2 (posterior), and posterior edge of the choanae (anterior). Netter FH. In: Kelly P, editor. Atlas of human anatomy. 3rd ed. Teterboro: Icon Learning Systems; 2003. Lee N, Laufer M, Ove R, Foote RL, Bonner JA. Nasopharyngeal carcinoma. In: Gunderson LL, Tepper JE, editors. Clinical radiation oncology. 3rd ed. Philadelphia: Elsevier Saunders; 2012. p. 619–38.

32. The correct answer is B. Unlike many H&N cancers, nasopharyngeal cancer is not associated with alcohol consumption. EBV infection is very common, and many studies have demonstrated that EBV copy number is associated with patient outcome. Lin J-C et al. Quantification of plasma Epstein-Barr virus DNA in patients with advanced nasopharyngeal carcinoma. N Engl J Med. 2004;350(24):2461–70.

33. The correct answer is D. Nasopharyngeal cancer has three histologic subtypes classified as WHO grade I (keratinizing representing 20 % of cases), WHO grade IIa (nonkeratinizing representing 30–40 % of cases), and WHO grade IIb (undifferentiated or lymphoepithelial representing 40–50 % of cases). EBV is classically associated with WHO grade IIb and is endemic in Asia. WHO grade I disease is keratinizing, which is a poor prognostic feature, and is associated with smoking. Lee N, Laufer M, Ove R, Foote RL, Bonner JA. Nasopharyngeal carcinoma. In: Gunderson LL, Tepper JE, editors. Clinical radiation oncology. 3rd ed. Philadelphia: Elsevier Saunders; 2012. p. 619–38.

34. The correct answer is D. The Intergroup 0099 study randomized patients with what would now be T2 and N+ nasopharyngeal cancer to RT alone (70 Gy) versus concurrent chemoradiation with cisplatin q 3 weeks to 70 Gy followed by reduced dose cisplatin and 5-FU × 3 cycles. There was a benefit of chemoradiation in 3-year PFS 24 % versus 69 % and 3-year OS 47 % versus 78 %.

Al-Sarraf M et al. Chemoradiotherapy versus radiotherapy in patients with advanced nasopharyngeal cancer: phase III randomized Intergroup study 0099. J Clin Oncol. 1998;16(4):1310–7.

35. The correct answer is B. Plasma concentrations of EBV DNA were detected by real-time quantitative polymerase-chain-reaction assay in 94 of 99 patients with stage III/IV nasopharyngeal carcinoma and no evidence of metastasis (M0). Patients with relapse had higher pretreatment plasma EBV DNA concentrations than those that did not have relapse, $p = 0.02$. In those with complete remission, plasma EBV DNA concentration was persistently low or undetectable. In those with pretreatment plasma EBV DNA concentrations of >1,500 copies per milliliter, overall and relapse-free survival were significantly lower than those with concentrations <1,500 copies per milliliter. Lin J-C et al. Quantification of plasma Epstein-Barr Virus DNA in patients with advanced nasopharyngeal carcinoma. N Engl J Med. 2004;350:2461–70.

36. The correct answer is C. The VA Larynx Trial randomized patients with stage III/IV laryngeal SCC to induction chemotherapy with cisplatin and 5-FU followed by definitive RT (66–76 Gy) versus total laryngectomy followed by adjuvant RT (50.4 Gy + 10–23 Gy boost). Patients who failed definitive RT could undergo salvage laryngectomy. Two-year OS was equivalent at 68 % for both groups. Larynx preservation rate was 64 %. Wolf et al. Induction chemotherapy plus radiation compared with surgery plus radiation in patients with advanced laryngeal cancer. The Department of Veterans Affairs Laryngeal Cancer Study Group. N Engl J Med. 1991;324(24):1685–90.

37. The correct answer is C. RTOG 73-03 randomized 277 patients with supraglottic larynx and hypopharynx primaries to 50 Gy pre-op RT versus 60 Gy postoperative RT. LRC significantly favored post-op radiation at 58 % versus 70 %, and in a subset analysis, the supraglottic larynx group benefitted the most with LRC 50 % versus 80 % and death related to local recurrence measured at 10 % versus 30 %. Tupchong L et al. Randomized study of preoperative versus postoperative radiation therapy in advanced head and neck carcinoma: long-term follow-up of RTOG study 73-03. Int J Radiat Oncol Biol Phys. 1991;20(1):21–8.

38. The correct answer is D. Yamazaki et al. randomized 180 patients with T1N0 glottic carcinomas to two treatment arms: arm A (2 Gy per fraction) and arm B (2.25 Gy per fraction). The groups were further stratified to dose based on TVC involvement, <2/3 of the TVC versus ≥2/3 of the TVC. Arm A was subdivided to 60 Gy versus 66 Gy, and arm B was subdivided to 56 Gy versus 63 Gy. The 5-year LC was superior in the 2.25 Gy/fraction arm: 77 % versus 92 %. There was no difference in overall survival. Yamazaki H, et al. Radiotherapy for early glottic carcinoma (T1N0M0): results of prospective randomized study of radiation fraction size and overall treatment time. Int J Radiat Oncol Biol Phys. 2006;64(1):77–82.

39. The correct answer is D. RTOG 91-11 randomized 547 patients with locally advanced laryngeal cancer to one of 3 arms: (1) cisplatin + 5-FU induction chemotherapy followed by RT to 70 Gy in 35 fractions, (2) concurrent cisplatin + RT to 70 Gy, and (3) RT alone to 70 Gy. Patients with large-volume T4 disease were not eligible. Two-year LRC was 61 % versus 78 % versus 56 %, favoring concurrent chemoradiation. Two-year laryngeal preservation rate was 75 % versus 88 % versus 70 %. There was no difference in overall survival (all about 75 % at 2 years and 55 % at 5 years). The 5-year results presented in 2006 show a persistent LRC and larynx preservation benefit in the concurrent chemoRT arm. Larynx preservation for the concurrent chemoRT arm at 5 years was 83.6 % versus 70.5 % with induction chemotherapy versus 65.7 % with RT alone. The most updated results with a median of 10.8 years of follow-up still show a persistent locoregional control and larynx preservation benefit. Forastiere AA, et al. Concurrent chemotherapy and radiotherapy for organ preservation in locally advanced laryngeal cancer. N Engl J Med. 2003;349(22):2091–98. Forastiere AA, et al. Long-term results of Intergroup RTOG 91-11: a phase III trial to preserve the larynx-induction cisplatin/5-FU and radiation therapy versus concurrent cisplatin and radiation therapy versus radiation therapy. J Clin Oncol. 2006 ASCO Meeting Proceedings. Part I. Vol. 24, No 18S (20 June Supplement):5517. Forastiere, AA et al. Long-term results of RTOG 91-11: a comparison of three nonsurgical treatment strategies to preserve the larynx in patients with locally advanced larynx cancer. J Clin Oncol. 2013;31(7):845–852.

40. The correct answer is B. RTOG 91-11 randomized 547 patients with locally advanced laryngeal cancer to one of three arms: (1) cisplatin + 5-FU induction chemotherapy followed by RT to 70 Gy in 35 fractions, (2) concurrent cisplatin + RT to 70 Gy, and (3) RT alone to 70 Gy. Two-year laryngeal preservation rate was 75 % versus 88 % versus 70 %. There was no difference in overall survival (all about 75 % at 2 years). Forastiere AA et al. Concurrent chemotherapy and radiotherapy for organ preservation in locally advanced laryngeal cancer. N Engl J Med. 2003;349(22):2091–8.

41. The correct answer is B. RTOG 91-11 randomized 547 patients with locally advanced laryngeal cancer to one of three arms: (1) cisplatin + 5-FU induction chemotherapy followed by RT to 70 Gy in 35 fractions, (2) concurrent cisplatin + RT to 70 Gy, and (3) RT alone to 70 Gy. Two-year laryngeal preservation rate was 75 % versus 88 % versus 70 %. The 5-year results presented in 2006 show a persistent LRC and larynx preservation benefit in the concurrent chemoRT arm. Larynx preservation for the concurrent chemoRT arm at 5 years was 83.6 % versus 70.5 % with induction chemotherapy versus 65.7 % with RT alone. There is still no overall survival benefit (5-year OS: 55 %). Forastiere AA, et al. Long-term results of Intergroup RTOG 91-11: a phase III trial to preserve the larynx-induction cisplatin/5-FU and radiation therapy versus concurrent cisplatin and radiation therapy versus radiation therapy. J Clin Oncol. 2006 ASCO Meeting Proceedings. Part I. Vol. 24, No 18S (20 June Supplement):5517.

42. The correct answer is B. According to the EXTREME trial (Vermorken et al.), which randomized patients with recurrent or metastatic HNSCC to platinum+ 5-FU versus platinum+5-FU+cetuximab, median OS was 7.4 months versus 10.1 months, respectively. PFS was 3.3 months versus 5.6 months favoring the addition of cetuximab. The overall response rate was 20 % versus 36 % favoring the addition of cetuximab. Vermorken JB et al. Platinum-based chemotherapy plus cetuximab in head and neck cancer. N Engl J Med. 2008; 359(11): 1116–27.

43. The correct answer is C. A typical dose constraint for the larynx is V50<30%. Garden AS, Morrison WH, Ang KK. Larynx and hypopharynx cancer. In: Gunderson LL, Tepper JE, editors. Clinical radiation oncology. 3rd ed. Philadelphia: Elsevier Saunders; 2012. p. 639–64.

44. The correct answer is C. Hypotension and nausea are frequent side effects of amifostine. Antonadou D et al. Prophylactic use of amifostine to prevent radiochemotherapy-induced mucositis and xerostomia in head-and-neck cancer. Int J Radiat Oncol Biol Phys. 2002;52(3):739–47.

45. The correct answer is C. The superior most lateral retropharyngeal lymph node is called the node of Rouviere, named for French Anatomy Professor Henri Rouviere (1876–1952). Virchow's node is an enlarged left supraclavicular lymph node, often signifying gastrointestinal malignancy. The Delphian node is a prelaryngeal lymph node involved in subglottic and thyroid malignancies. Cloquet's node is the superior most deep inguinal lymph node. Netter FH. In: Kelly P, editor. Atlas of human anatomy. 3rd ed. Teterboro: Icon Learning Systems; 2003.

46. The correct answer is B. The larynx staging is divided by anatomic location/ subsite into supraglottic, glottic, and subglottic larynx. An infrahyoid epiglottic tumor is a tumor of the supraglottic subsite. Invasion of the inner cortex of the thyroid cartilage constitutes T3 disease. Multiple lymph nodes ipsilaterally, all less than 6 cm, constitutes N2b nodal disease. Edge SB, Byrd DR, Compton CC, et al., editors. Larynx. AJCC cancer staging handbook. 7th ed. New York: Springer; 2010.

47. The correct answer is B. The larynx staging is divided by anatomic location/ subsite into supraglottic, glottic, and subglottic larynx. Tumors of the vocal cord are located in the true glottis. A tumor that causes fixation of the vocal cord is T3. As the lymph nodes are in the contralateral neck, the nodal stage is N2c. Edge SB, Byrd DR, Compton CC, et al., editors. Larynx. AJCC cancer staging handbook. 7th ed. New York: Springer; 2010.

48. The correct answer is B. A tumor in the pyriform sinus is located in the hypopharyngeal subsite. This patient has T3N3 disease. Tumors in the hypopharynx that extend to the esophagus are T3. Any lymph node larger than 6 cm is N3. Edge SB, Byrd DR, Compton CC, et al., editors. Larynx. AJCC cancer staging handbook. 7th ed. New York: Springer; 2010.

49. The correct answer is B. Lhermitte's syndrome is a demyelinating condition of the cervical spine that results in shock-like sensation in the extremities with neck flexion occurring 2–6 months after radiation to the region. Brachial plexopathy is characterized by numbness and pain of the shoulder, arm, or hand with associated weakness related to damage to the brachial plexus. Sciatica is likely unrelated to the H&N radiation but can present as shock-like sensations down the legs with straight leg raise. Guillain-Barre syndrome is a progressive demyelinating disease that spreads inferior to superior and is associated with autoantibodies following an illness. Leung WM et al. Lhermitte's sign among nasopharyngeal cancer patients after radiotherapy. Head Neck. 2005;27(3):187–94.

50. The correct answer is C. The tongue deviates to the side of the lesion, in this case, L CN XII. Netter FH. In: Kelly P, editor. Atlas of human anatomy. 3rd ed. Teterboro: Icon Learning Systems; 2003.

51. The correct answer is D. QUANTEC recommends keeping the Dmax of the optic nerves/chiasm to 55 Gy. Dmax <55 Gy is associated with a <3 % risk of optic neuropathy. Many clinicians employ an optic nerve/chiasm Dmax of 54 Gy. QUANTEC (Quantitative Analyses of Normal Tissue Effects in the Clinic. Int J Radiat Oncol Biol Phys. 2010;76(2):Suppl, 1 Mar. Mayo C et al. Radiation dose-volume effects of optic nerves and chiasm. Int J Radiat Oncol Biol Phys. 2010;76(3):S28–35.

52. The correct answer is D. The tonsillar fossa is defined by the palatoglossus muscle, palatopharyngeal muscle, and inferior glossotonsillar sulcus. The posterior pharyngeal wall is not a border of the tonsillar fossa. Netter FH. In: Kelly P, editor. Atlas of human anatomy. 3rd ed. Teterboro: Icon Learning Systems; 2003.

53. The correct answer is D. The trigeminal ganglion lies within Meckel's cave. Netter FH. In: Kelly P, editor. Atlas of human anatomy. 3rd ed. Teterboro: Icon Learning Systems; 2003.

54. The correct answer is A. CN V1 exits the supraorbital notch. Netter FH. In: Kelly P, editor. Atlas of human anatomy. 3rd ed. Teterboro: Icon Learning Systems; 2003.

55. The correct answer is C. Traversing anterior to posterior: foramen rotundum, ovale, spinosum, and lacerum. Traversing medial to lateral: lacerum, rotundum, ovale, and spinosum. Netter FH. In: Kelly P, editor. Atlas of human anatomy. 3rd ed. Teterboro: Icon Learning Systems; 2003.

56. The correct answer is C. The middle meningeal artery and vein traverse the foramen spinosum. CN V1 passes through the superior orbital fissure. CN V2 passes through the foramen rotundum. The carotid artery passes through the carotid canal. Netter FH. In: Kelly P, editor. Atlas of human anatomy. 3rd ed. Teterboro: Icon Learning Systems; 2003.

57. The correct answer is B. PEG-dependency rates are estimated at 15–20 % following chemoradiation for oropharynx cancer. Cannon GM, Harari PM, Gentry LR, Avey GD, Siu LL. Oropharyngeal cancer. In: Gunderson LL, Tepper JE, editors. Clinical radiation oncology, 3rd ed. Philadelphia: Elsevier Saunders; 2012. p. 585–618

58. The correct answer is B. Traversing ant to post: foramen rotundum, ovale, spinosum, and lacerum. Traversing medial to lateral: lacerum, rotundum, ovale, and spinosum. Netter FH. In: Kelly P, editor. Atlas of human anatomy. 3rd ed. Teterboro: Icon Learning Systems; 2003.

59. The correct answer is D. The superior orbital fissure contains CNs III, IV, V1, and VI as well as the superior ophthalmic vein. CN V2 passes through the foramen rotundum. Netter FH. In: Kelly P, editor. Atlas of human anatomy. 3rd ed. Teterboro: Icon Learning Systems; 2003.

60. The correct answer is D. Regarding its sensory innervation, the tongue is innervated posteriorly by the superior laryngeal branch of the vagus nerve, posterolaterally by the glossopharyngeal nerve, anteriorly by the lingual nerve of the mandibular branch of the trigeminal nerve, and anterolaterally by the chorda tympani and lingual nerve branches of the facial nerve. Netter FH. In: Kelly P, editor. Atlas of human anatomy. 3rd ed. Teterboro: Icon Learning Systems; 2003.

61. The correct answer is D. Follow-up should include TSH if the thyroid is irradiated, CXR to evaluate for metastases, surveillance CT of the head and neck, and visual inspection with laryngoscopy.

62. The correct answer is A. The cavernous sinus includes CNs III, IV, VI, V1, V2, and the internal carotids. Netter FH. In: Kelly P, editor. Atlas of human anatomy. 3rd ed. Teterboro: Icon Learning Systems; 2003.

63. The correct answer is B. The hyoid resides at approximately the same level as C3. Netter FH. In: Kelly P, editor. Atlas of human anatomy. 3rd ed. Teterboro: Icon Learning Systems; 2003.

64. The correct answer is D. The TVCs lie at approximately C5–C6. Netter FH. In: Kelly P, editor. Atlas of human anatomy. 3rd ed. Teterboro: Icon Learning Systems; 2003.

65. The correct answer is B. The sensation of pain elicited upon palpation of the thyroid cartilage is indicative of thyroid invasion. Loss of the laryngeal click is associated with postcricoid extension. Garden AS, Morrison WH, Ang KK. Larynx and hypopharynx cancer. In: Gunderson LL, Tepper JE, editors. Clinical radiation oncology, 3rd ed. Philadelphia: Elsevier Saunders; 2012. p. 639–64.

66. The correct answer is C. The maxillary sinus is by far the most common site of sinonasal cancer (55 %). The nasal cavity and ethmoid sinus have almost equal incidence, 23 % and 20 %, respectively. The sphenoid and frontal sinuses are rare sites of sinonasal cancer. Fletcher GH. Nasal and paranasal sinus carcinoma. In: Fletcher GH, editor. Textbook of radiotherapy. Philadelphia: Lea & Febiger; 1980. p. 408–25.

67. The correct answer is D. Carpenters exposed to dust of hardwoods and exotic woods have been observed to have a higher incidence of adenocarcinoma of the nasal cavity. Nickel workers develop squamous cell carcinomas more commonly. Torjussen W et al. Histopathological changes of nasal mucosa in nickel workers: a pilot study. Cancer. 1979;44:963–74. Schwaab G et al. Epidemiology of cancer of the nasal cavities and paranasal sinuses. Neurochirurgie. 1997;43:963–74. Zheng W et al. Risk factors for cancers of the nasal cavity and paranasal sinuses among white men in the United States. Am J Epidemiol. 1993;138:965–72. Acheson ED et al. Nasal cancer in woodworkers in the furniture industry. Br Med J. 1968;2:587–96.

68. The correct answer is B. The listed anatomic structures detail the anterior, posterior, inferior, and superior boundaries of the nasal cavity proper, respectively. Beitler JJ, Wadsworth JT, Hudgins PA, Ang KK. Sinonasal cancer. In: Gunderson LL, Tepper JE, editors. Clinical radiation oncology, 3rd ed. Philadelphia: Elsevier Saunders; 2012. p. 665–90.

69. The correct answer is B. A tumor arising in the upper nasal cavity would extend to the orbit by traversing the lamina papyracea, a thin porous bone that makes up the medial orbital wall. The fovea ethmoidalis is the "roof of the ethmoid sinus," made up of a portion of the frontal bone. Beitler JJ, Wadsworth JT, Hudgins PA, Ang KK. Sinonasal cancer. In: Gunderson LL, Tepper JE, editors. Clinical radiation oncology. 3rd ed. Philadelphia: Elsevier Saunders; 2012. p. 665–90.

70. The correct answer is D. All listed diseases are "small round-cell" tumors except melanoma. Esthesioneuroblastoma is a tumor of neural crest origin arising in the olfactory portion of the nasal cavity. Beitler JJ, Wadsworth JT, Hudgins PA, Ang KK. Sinonasal cancer. In: Gunderson LL, Tepper JE, editors. Clinical radiation oncology. 3rd ed. Philadelphia: Elsevier Saunders; 2012. p. 665–90.

71. The correct answer is A. Ohngren's line is drawn from the medial canthus to the angle of the mandible and divides the maxillary sinus into a super and substructure. Tumors arising in the superstructure have a poorer prognosis. Beitler JJ, Wadsworth JT, Hudgins PA, Ang KK. Sinonasal cancer. In: Gunderson LL, Tepper JE, editors. Clinical radiation oncology. 3rd ed. Philadelphia: Elsevier Saunders; 2012. p. 665–90.

72. The correct answer is A. A maxillary sinus tumor that invades into the pterygoid plates is T4a. Invasion of the pterygoid fossa is T3. A single 3.0 cm ipsilateral lymph node is N1. A 3.1 cm lymph node would be N2. Edge SB, Byrd DR, Compton CC, et al., editors. Nasal cavity and paranasal sinuses. AJCC cancer staging handbook. 7th ed. New York: Springer; 2010.

73. The correct answer is B. An ethmoid sinus tumor that invades into the pterygoid plates is T4a. Multiple ipsilateral lymph nodes ≤6 cm are N2b. N2c describes bilateral or contralateral lymph node involvement ≤6 cm. Edge SB, Byrd DR, Compton CC, et al., editors. Nasal cavity and paranasal sinuses. AJCC cancer staging handbook. 7th ed. New York: Springer; 2010.

74. The correct answer is C. Whereas invasion of the cribriform plates constitutes T4a disease in maxillary sinus cancer, it is T3 in ethmoid sinus cancer. Edge SB, Byrd DR, Compton CC, et al., editors. Nasal cavity and paranasal sinuses. AJCC cancer staging handbook. 7th edition. New York: Springer; 2010.

75. The correct answer is B. Invasion of one paranasal sinus is Kadish stage B. Stage C refers to an esthesioneuroblastoma that extends beyond the nasal cavity and paranasal sinuses or distant metastasis. Beitler JJ, Wadsworth JT, Hudgins PA, Ang KK. Sinonasal cancer. In: Gunderson LL, Tepper JE, editors. Clinical radiation oncology. 3rd ed. Philadelphia: Elsevier Saunders; 2012. p. 665–90.

76. The correct answer is C. Nasal vestibule tumors are preferentially treated with radiation due to excellent outcomes and cosmesis. Excellent local control has been obtained with both external beam and brachytherapy approaches. In small (<2 cm) lesions, local control exceeds 90 %. With proper fractionation, late complications are minimized. Wong CS et al. External irradiation for squamous cell carcinoma of the nasal vestibule. Int J Radiat Oncol Biol Phys. 1986;12:1943–46. Chobe R et al. Radiation therapy for carcinoma of the nasal vestibule. Otolaryngol Head Neck Surg. 1988;98:67–71. Langendjk JA et al. Radiotherapy of squamous cell carcinoma of the nasal vestibule. Int J Radiat Oncol Biol Phys. 2004;59:1319–25. McCollough WM et al. Radiotherapy alone for squamous cell carcinoma of the nasal vestibule: management of the primary site and regional lymphatics. Int J Radiat Oncol Biol Phys. 1993;26:73–9. Mak ACA et al. Radiation therapy of carcinoma of the nasal vestibule. Eur J Cancer. 1980;16:81–5.

77. The correct answer is A. Esthesioneuroblastoma is a disease characterized by locoregional failure, even in stage C patients. Elkon et al. reported on 78 patients and found that local control of stage A patients is >90 %. Sixty percent of stage C patients died of their disease, with the majority dying of local tumor progression, not distant progression. As isolated nodal failure is < 15 %, elective nodal irradiation is not routinely recommended. Elkon D et al. Esthesioneuroblastoma. Cancer. 1979;44:1087–94.

78. The correct answer is D. All of the listed glands are part of the major salivary group except the submucosal glands in the hard palate. These glands comprise 50 % of the minor salivary gland group. Other sites of submucosal glands are in the buccal mucosa, nasal cavity, oropharynx, and paranasal sinuses. Quon J, Lin A, Weiss J, Alonso-Basanta M, Dutta P, Newman JG. Salivary gland cancer. In: Gunderson LL, Tepper JE, editors. Clinical radiation oncology. 3rd ed. Philadelphia: Elsevier Saunders; 2012. p. (691–706).

79. The correct answer is C. Parotid tumors are the most common type of salivary gland tumor. The majority (>80 %) are benign in adults; parotid tumors are more commonly malignant in children. The majority of parotid tumors arise from the superficial lobe of the parotid. Quon J, Lin A, Weiss J, Alonso-Basanta M, Dutta P, Newman JG. Salivary gland cancer. In: Gunderson LL, Tepper JE, editors. Clinical radiation oncology. 3rd ed. Philadelphia: Elsevier Saunders; 2012. p. (691–706).

80. The correct answer is C. Carcinoma *ex pleomorphic adenoma* is a malignant tumor that arises from preexistent benign mixed tumors. Adenocarcinoma and salivary duct carcinoma are the two most common histologies. These tumors can be aggressive locally, with frequent recurrence after surgery and frequent (>50 %) metastasis to regional lymph nodes. They produce distant metastases, most commonly to the lung. Quon J, Lin A, Weiss J, Alonso-Basanta M, Dutta P, Newman JG. Salivary gland cancer. In: Gunderson LL, Tepper JE, editors. Clinical radiation oncology. 3rd ed. Philadelphia: Elsevier Saunders; 2012. p. 691–706.

81. The correct answer is A. Adenoid cystic carcinomas are tumors more commonly seen in the submandibular and minor salivary glands. While regional lymph node metastasis is rare, distant metastasis is common, with the lung being the most common site. These can behave aggressively locally, with frequent perineural invasion (>50 %) at diagnosis, and grow intracranially along nerves. Quon J, Lin A, Weiss J, Alonso-Basanta M, Dutta P, Newman JG. Salivary gland cancer. In: Gunderson LL, Tepper JE, editors. Clinical radiation oncology. 3rd ed. Philadelphia: Elsevier Saunders; 2012. p. 691–706.

82. The correct answer is B. p53 expression has been detected in the majority of salivary gland tumors, with poorer prognosis noted with increasing expression. Proliferating cell nuclear antigen (PCNA) has also been found to correlate with poorer outcomes in both mucoepidermoid and adenoid cystic carcinoma. Ki-67 overexpression, an indicator of proliferation, has similarly been shown to correlate with poor outcomes in mucoepidermoid tumors. Albeck H et al. Familial clusters of nasopharyngeal carcinoma and salivary gland carcinomas in Greenland natives. Cancer. 1993;72:196–200. Cho K et al. Proliferating cell nuclear antigen and c-erb B-2 oncoprotein expression in adenoid cystic carcinoma of the salivary glands. Head Neck. 1999;21:414–9. Frankenthaler RA et al.

High correlation with survival of proliferating cell nuclear antigen expression in mucoepidermoid carcinoma of the parotid gland. Otolaryngol Head Neck Surg. 1994;111:460–6. Pires FR et al. Prognostic factors in head and neck mucoepidermoid carcinoma. Arch Otolaryngol Head Neck Surg. 2004;130:174–80. Gallo O et al. p53 oncoprotein expression in parotid gland carcinoma is associated with clinical outcome. Cancer. 1995;75:2037–44.

83. The correct answer is B. A growing, painless mass suggests malignancy. Most submandibular and parotid tumors present as painless masses. Fine-needle aspiration to provide a histological diagnosis is the next best step in management. Excisional and incisional biopsies are discouraged because they are associated with higher rates of local recurrence, can harm adjacent critical structures, and require subsequent wide local excision of the scar. Quon J, Lin A, Weiss J, Alonso-Basanta M, Dutta P, Newman JG. Salivary gland cancer. In: Gunderson LL, Tepper JE, editors. Clinical radiation oncology. 3rd ed. Philadelphia: Elsevier Saunders; 2012. p. 691–706.

84. The correct answer is B. Involvement of the facial nerve is T4a. Though only 3 cm, the contralateral lymph node is N2c. Edge SB, Byrd DR, Compton CC, et al., editors. (Major) salivary glands. AJCC cancer staging handbook. 7th ed. New York: Springer; 2010.

85. The correct answer is A. Resection of parotid tumors is guided by the extent of tumor. In cases where the facial nerve is clearly involved, it is removed; otherwise, it is generally preserved. Adverse effects of facial nerve sacrifice are Frey's syndrome (gustatory sweating and loss of earlobe sensation), as well as need for gold weight placement in the upper eyelid to close and protect the eye. If the facial nerve is sacrificed, nerve grafting can help to recover facial function. Quon J, Lin A, Weiss J, Alonso-Basanta M, Dutta P, Newman JG. Salivary gland cancer. In: Gunderson LL, Tepper JE, editors. Clinical radiation oncology. 3rd ed. Philadelphia: Elsevier Saunders; 2012. p. 691–706.

86. The correct answer is B. Papillary and follicular carcinomas are more common in women than men, with papillary carcinomas tending to present at a younger age. Papillary carcinoma is associated with Cowden's syndrome, while medullary carcinoma is associated with MEN-2. Ain KB. Papillary thyroid carcinoma. Endocrinol Metab Clin North Am. 1995;24:711–60. Grebe SKG et al. Follicular thyroid cancer. Endocrinol Metab Clin North Am. 1995;24:761–801. Farid NR et al. Molecular basis of thyroid cancer. Endocr Rev. 1994;15:202–32.

87. The correct answer is D. The *RET* proto-oncogene is found in 90 % of familial medullary thyroid cancers. Those who are found to have the mutation in infancy typically undergo total thyroidectomy at ages 5–7 to prevent the development of medullary thyroid cancer. Ledger GA et al. Genetic testing in the diagnosis and management of multiple endocrine neoplasia type II. Ann Intern Med.

1995;122:118–26. Wells SA et al. Predictive DNA testing and prophylactic therapy in patients at risk for multiple endocrine neoplasia type 2A. Ann Surg. 1994;120:1377–81. Wohlik N et al. Application of genetic screening to the management of medullary thyroid carcinoma and multiple endocrine neoplasia type 2. Endocrinol Metab Clin North Am. 1996;25:1–15.

88. The correct answer is A. All of the listed thyroid cancers are derived from the follicular cell except medullary thyroid carcinoma, which derives from the parafollicular (C cell). Papillary thyroid carcinoma is the most common subtype. Anaplastic thyroid carcinoma is the least common subtype. Nel CJ et al. Anaplastic carcinoma of the thyroid: a clinicopathologic study of 82 cases. Mayo Clin Proc. 1985;60:51–8.

89. The correct answer is C. Papillary carcinoma presents in patients 30–50 years, while follicular carcinoma presents 10 years later. While papillary thyroid tumors tend to present with 2–3 cm primary tumors, follicular tumors tend to be larger and higher grade at presentation. Both present with primarily local disease, but papillary tumors present with clinically evidence lymphadenopathy in one third of cases, compared to 4–6 % in follicular carcinoma. Distant metastases at presentation are much less common in papillary thyroid cancers. Hay ID. Papillary thyroid carcinoma. Endocrinol Metab Clin North Am. 1990;19:545–76. McConahey WM et al. Papillary thyroid cancer treated at Mayo Clinic, 1946 through 1970: initial manifestations, pathologic findings, therapy, and outcome. Mayo Clin Proc. 1986;61:978–96. Dinneen SF et al. Distant metastases in thyroid carcinoma: 100 cases observed at one institution during 5 decades. J Clin Endocrinol Metab. 1995;80:2041–5. Brennan MD et al. Follicular thyroid cancer treated at the Mayo Clinic, 1946 through 1970: initial manifestations, pathologic findings, therapy, and outcome. Mayo Clin Proc. 1991;66:11–9. Grebe SKG et al. Follicular thyroid cancer. Endocrinol Metab Clin North Am. 1995;24:761–801. Ruegemer JJ et al. Distant metastases in differentiated thyroid carcinoma: a multivariate analysis of Prognostic Variables. J Clin Endocrinol Metab. 1998;67(3):501–8.

90. The correct answer is D. Medullary thyroid cancer arises from the parafollicular (C cell) cell and secretes calcitonin. It is associated with MEN-2, though these cases are less common than the sporadic variants. The familial variant presents earlier, tends to involve both sides of the thyroid, and has a better prognosis, as it is curable with total thyroidectomy. Moley JF. Medullary thyroid cancer. Surg Clin N Am. 1995;75:405–20. Lips CJM et al. Clinical screenings as compared with DNA analysis in families with multiple endocrine neoplasia type 2A. N Engl J Med. 1994;331:828–35.

91. The correct answer is A. Any N1b, T4a, or T4b thyroid cancer is classified as stage IV cancer, though T4a denotes stage IVA, T4b denotes stage IVB, and M1 denotes stage IVC. The only N1a that is classified as stage IV occurs in

conjunction with a T4a primary. Edge SB, Byrd DR, Compton CC, et al., editors. Thyroid. AJCC cancer staging handbook. 7th ed. New York: Springer; 2010.

92. The correct answer is B. Seventy-five percent of the follicular cells must exhibit Hurthle cell features to classify it as a Hurthle cell carcinoma. Grebe SKG, Hay ID. Follicular thyroid cancer. Endocrinol Metab Clin North Am. 1995;24:761–801.

93. The correct answer is B. The definitive diagnosis of follicular or Hurthle cell carcinoma requires the demonstration of thyroid capsule invasion or angioinvasion. Grebe SKG, Hay ID. Follicular thyroid cancer. Endocrinol Metab Clin North Am. 1995;24:761–801.

94. The correct answer is C. Medullary carcinoma can be definitely diagnosed preoperatively by Congo red staining of amyloid or immunoperoxidase labeling of intracytoplasmic calcitonin of an FNA biopsy specimen. Moley JF. Medullary thyroid cancer. Surg Clin N Am. 1995;75:405–20.

95. The correct answer is C. Radioactive iodine ablation (RAI) and radioactive remnant ablation (RRA) are two means of adjuvant therapy to destroy residual thyroid tissue. RAI is used for patients with distant metastatic disease or gross residual disease and thus employs higher doses. RRA is used for patients that have undergone surgery and is intended to destroy residual macroscopically normal thyroid tissue in an effort to improve outcomes. Two benefits of this therapy are as follows: (1) later detection of possible recurrent disease by scanning is facilitated as there is no longer any functional thyroid tissue, and (2) serum thyroglobulin as a disease marker in follow-up may be more useful as there is no longer any functional thyroid tissue. Those with follicular thyroid carcinoma have been found to concentrate RAI better than those with papillary thyroid cancer. American Association of Clinical Endocrinologists. AACE/AAES medical/surgical guidelines for clinical practice: management of thyroid carcinoma. Endocr Pract. 2001;7:202–30. Grebe SKG, Hay ID. Follicular thyroid cancer. Endocrinol Metab Clin North Am. 1995;24:761–801. Sweeney DC, Johnston GS. Radioiodine therapy for thyroid cancer. Endocrinol Metab Clin North Am. 1995;24:803–39. Sawka AM et al. Clinical review 170. A systemic review and metaanalysis of the effectiveness of radioactive iodine remnant ablation for well-differentiated thyroid cancer. J Clin Endocrinol. 2004;89:3668–76. Simpson WJ et al. Papillary and follicular thyroid cancer: impact of treatment in 1578 patients. Int J Radiat Oncol Biol Phys. 1998;14:1063–71.

96. The correct answer is A. Less than 5 % of patients have neck metastases from an unknown primary head and neck squamous cell carcinoma. Mendenhall WM, Mancuso, AA, Werning JW. Unknown head and neck primary site cancer. In:Gunderson, LL, Tepper JE. editors. Clinical radiation oncology. 3rd ed. Philadelphia: Elsevier Saunders; 2012. p. 723–30.

97. The correct answer is C. "Orphan Annie" nuclei (nuclei that seem uniformly light blue staining, thus appearing empty) are associated with papillary thyroid cancer. KS, Kumar V, Robbins SL. Robbins pathologic basis of disease. 5th ed. Philadelphia: W.B. Saunders; 1994. p. 1137.

98. The correct answer is B. Upon evaluation of head and neck cancers of unknown primary, the oropharynx is the most common site of detected primaries. Martin H et al. Cervical lymph node metastasis as the first symptom of cancer. Surg Gynecol Obstet. 1944;76:133–59. Fletcher GH, et al. Oropharynx. In: MacComb WS, Fletcher GH, editors. Cancer of the head and neck. Baltimore: Williams & Wilkins. 1967, p. 179–212. Jones AS et al. Squamous carcinoma presenting as an enlarged cervical node. Cancer. 1993;72:1756–61.

99. The correct answer is C. When treating unknown primary of the head and neck, the volume includes the bilateral neck, entire oropharynx, and nasopharynx. The oral cavity is not treated unless the patient has submandibular lymph nodes. The larynx and hypopharynx are not routinely treated. Mendenhall WM et al. Squamous cell carcinoma metastatic to the neck from an unknown head and neck primary site. Am J Otolaryngol. 2001; 22:261–7. Reddy SP et al. Metastatic carcinoma in the cervical lymph nodes from an unknown primary site: results of bilateral neck plus mucosal irradiation vs. ipsilateral neck irradiation. Int J Radiat Oncol Biol Phys. 1997;37:797–802.

100. The correct answer is D. Of the listed scenario, those with N1 nodes at presentation are least likely to undergo subsequent neck dissection after radiation for unknown head and neck primary, as the node will likely resolve completely. Those with more advanced nodes at presentation, residual gross disease, or a persistent mass after therapy should undergo planned neck dissection. Peters LJ et al. Neck surgery in patients with primary oropharyngeal cancer treated by radiotherapy. Head Neck. 1996;18:552–9. Johnson CR et al. Radiotherapeutic management of bulky cervical lymphadenopathy in squamous cell carcinoma of the head and neck: is postradiotherapy neck dissection necessary? Radiat Oncol Investig. 1998;6:52–7. Mendenhall WM et al. Squamous cell carcinoma of the head and neck treated with radiation therapy: the role of neck dissection for clinically positive neck nodes. Int J Radiat Oncol Biol Phys. 1986;12:733–40. Brizel DM et al. Necessity for adjuvant neck dissection in setting of concurrent chemoradiation for advanced head-and-neck cancer. Int J Radiat Oncol Biol Phys. 2004;58:1418–23.

101. The correct answer is C. All of the listed sites would drain into level Ia (submental nodes) except a cheek primary, which is more likely to drain to level Ib. A lower lip primary would also drain into level Ia. Grégoire V, Duprez T, Lengelé B, Hamoir M. Management of the neck. In: Gunderson LL, Tepper JE, editors. Clinical radiation oncology. 3rd ed. Philadelphia: Elsevier Saunders; 2012. p. 731–56.

102. The correct answer is C. Level IIa extends cranially from the caudal edge of the lateral process of C1 to the caudal edge of the hyoid bone. The anterior border is the posterior edge of the submandibular bland, with the posterior border being the posterior border of the internal jugular vein. The internal jugular vein and spinal accessory nerve divide levels IIa and IIb. Grégoire V et al. Selection and delineation of lymph node target volumes in head and neck conformal radiotherapy. Proposal for standardizing terminology and procedure based on the surgical experience. Radiother Oncol. 2000;56(2):135–50.

103. The correct answer is A. Level V (posterior triangle lymph nodes) extends cranially from the convergence of the sternocleidomastoid and trapezius muscles down to the clavicle. The anterior border is the posterior edge of sternocleidomastoid muscle, with the posterior border being the anterolateral border of the trapezius muscle. Grégoire V et al. Selection and delineation of lymph node target volumes in head and neck conformal radiotherapy. Proposal for standardizing terminology and procedure based on the surgical experience. Radiother Oncol. 2000;56(2):135–50.

104. The correct answer is C. Hypopharynx primary tumors have the highest propensity for lymph node involvement (70 %). Grégoire V, Duprez T, Lengelé B, Hamoir M. Management of the neck. In: Gunderson LL, Tepper JE, editors. Clinical radiation oncology. 3rd ed. Philadelphia: Elsevier Saunders; 2012. p. 731–56.

105. The correct answer is B. Nasopharynx primary tumors have the highest propensity for lymph node metastasis to level V. Grégoire V, Duprez T, Lengelé B, Hamoir M. Management of the neck. In: Gunderson LL, Tepper JE, editors. Clinical radiation oncology. 3rd ed. Philadelphia: Elsevier Saunders; 2012. p. 731–56.

106. The correct answer is C. O'Sullivan et al. reported their retrospective experience of 228 patients with tonsil carcinoma, the majority of whom had T1-2 and N0-1 tumors, treated with radiation to the primary site and ipsilateral neck alone. Of the 228 patients, only eight failed (2 %) in the contralateral neck, with 5 also failing at the primary site. No failures occurred in the N0 patients ($n = 133$). Only involvement of midline structure was a prognostic factor for contralateral neck recurrence. O'Sullivan B et al. The benefits and pitfalls of ipsilateral radiotherapy in carcinoma of the tonsillar region. Int J Radiat Oncol Biol Phys. 2001;51:332–43.

107. The correct answer is A. Of the listed risk factors for locoregional recurrence, all are "moderate" except for extracapsular extension, which is "high risk." Additional "moderate" risk factors are primary tumor in the oral cavity, perineural invasion, involved node ≥3 cm, and more than 6 weeks between surgery and the start of radiation. A combination of two or more "moderate" risk factors

was also "high" risk. This trial demonstrated that those patients with "high" risk benefited from a postoperative dose of 63 Gy versus 57.6 Gy. In those with only one "moderate" risk factor, 57.6 Gy was sufficient. Peters LJ et al. Evaluation of the dose for postoperative radiation therapy of head and neck cancer: first report of a prospective randomized trial. Int J Radiat Oncol Biol Phys. 1993;26: 3–11.

108. The correct answer is D. The EORTC and RTOG both designed studies (EORTC 22931 and RTOG 9501) to assess the benefit of the addition of che-motherapy (cisplatin 100 mg/m^2) to postoperative radiotherapy (60–66 Gy). Cisplatin was planned for days 1, 22, and 43, but approximately half of patients in both studies were able to receive all 3 cycles due to increased acute local toxicity. While the EORTC trial showed a statistically significant benefit in terms of local control and overall survival for the addition of chemotherapy, only a locoregional control benefit was seen in the RTOG trial. No improve-ment in the rate of distant metastasis was seen in either study from the addition of chemotherapy. Subsequent meta-analysis of the combined studies found that two features were associated with a survival benefit from the addition of chemotherapy: (1) extracapsular extension and (2) positive margin. Bernier J et al. Postoperative irradiation with or without concomitant chemotherapy for locally advanced head and neck cancer. N Engl J Med. 2004;350:1945–52. Cooper JS et al. Postoperative concurrent radiotherapy and chemotherapy for high-risk squamous-cell carcinoma of the head and neck. N Engl J Med. 2004;350:1937–44. Bernier J et al. Defining risk levels in locally advanced head and neck cancers: a comparative analysis of concurrent postoperative radiation plus chemotherapy trials of the EORTC (#22931) and RTOG (#9501). Head Neck. 2005;27:843–50.

109. The correct answer is A. The lower lip is the most common involved subsite of oral cavity cancer (38 %). The tongue is the second most common (22 %), followed by the floor of mouth (17 %). The buccal mucosa is the least com-mon subsite (2 %). Krolls SO et al. Squamous cell carcinoma of the oral soft tissues: a statistical analysis of 14, 253 cases by age, sex, and race of patients. J Am Dent Assoc. 1976;92:571.

110. The correct answer is B. Squamous cell carcinoma of the lip typically starts on the vermillion border of the lower lip and can be preceded by leukoplakia. Lymph node involvement increases with depth of invasion, larger lesions, and commissure involvement (20 %). Overall, the incidence of lymph nodes at presentation is 5–10 %, and only 2 % have perineural involvement. Shklar G. The oral cavity, jaws, and salivary glands. In: Robbins S editor. Pathologic basis of disease. 3rd ed. Philadelphia: WB Saunders; 1984. p. 783–4. Byers RM et al. The therapeutic and prognostic implications of nerve invasion in cancer of the lower lip. Int J Radiat Oncol Biol Phys. 1978;4:215–7. Wurman LH et al. Carcinoma of the lip. Am J Surg. 1975;130:470–4. Cross JE et al. Carcinoma of the lip. A review of 563 case records of carcinoma of the lip at the Pondville hospital. Surg Gynecol Obstet. 1948;81:153–62.

111. The correct answer is D. Given the commissure involvement, despite the small size, radiation is the preferred treatment for optimal local control and cosmesis. If the lesion did not involve the commissure, surgery alone would be satisfactory (assuming no adverse pathological features). Stranc MF et al. Comparison of lip function: surgery vs. radiotherapy. Br J Plast Surg. 1987;40: 598–604. Harrison LB. Applications of brachytherapy in head and neck cancer. Semin Surg Oncol. 1997;13:177–84.

112. The correct answer is B. The mylohyoid muscle is the muscular floor of the floor of mouth. Mendenhall WM, Foote RL, Sandow PL, Fernandes RP. Oral cavity cancer. In: Gunderson LL, Tepper JE, editors. Clinical radiation oncology. 3rd ed. Philadelphia: Elsevier Saunders; 2012. p. 53–84.

113. The correct answer is B. The submandibular lymph nodes are first echelon for floor of mouth tumors, though drainage can also occur to the submental nodes. These lymph nodes then drain to the jugulo-omohyoid lymph node. Rouviére H. Anatomy of the human lymphatic system, Tobias MJ (trans). Ann Arbor: Edwards Brothers; 1938. p. 44–56. Mendenhall WM, Foote RL, Sandow, PL, Fernandes RP. Oral cavity cancer. In: Gunderson LL, Tepper JE, editors. Clinical radiation oncology. 3rd ed. Philadelphia: Elsevier Saunders; 2012. p. 553–84.

114. The correct answer is D. All pairings are correct except the sensory innervation of the oral tongue, which is provided by the lingual nerve, a branch of V3. The motor innervation of the oral tongue is provided by the hypoglossal nerve.

115. The correct answer is C. In a retrospective review of 84 patients with floor of mouth cancer, Mohit-Tabatabai et al. found that the probability of subclinical neck metastases increased with lesion thickness and recommend elective neck treatment for lesions >1.5 mm. Primary lesion size and grade did NOT significantly correlate with neck node development. Mohit-Tabatabai MA et al. Relation of thickness of floor of mouth stage I and II cancers to regional metastasis. Am J Surg. 1986;152:351–3.

116. The correct answer is A. The tongue deviates to the side of a hypoglossal nerve injury due to unopposed action of the unaffected contralateral genioglossus muscle. All listed muscles are the muscles that comprise the oral tongue. Mendenhall WM, Foote RL, Sandow PL, Fernandes RP. Oral cavity cancer. In: Gunderson LL, Tepper JE, editors. Clinical radiation oncology. 3rd ed. Philadelphia: Elsevier Saunders; 2012. p. 553–84.

117. The correct answer is C. Oral tongue cancer is associated with skip metastases 15.8 % of the time. Frequency and therapeutic implications of "skip metastases" in the neck from squamous carcinoma of the oral tongue. Head Neck. 1997;19(1):14–9.

118. The correct answer is B. Lower gingival squamous cell carcinomas drain most commonly to the submandibular nodes (60 %), with the upper jugular nodes

being the second most common site (40 %). Byers et al. reported the lymph node distribution after elective neck dissection for gingival tumors, and there was a 0 % incidence in the submental and posterior cervical lymph node groups. Byers RM et al. Rationale for elective modified neck dissection. Head Neck Surg. 1988;10:163.

119. The correct answer is C. The subdigastric lymph nodes are first echelon for retromolar trigone tumors. Mendenhall WM, Foote RL, Sandow PL, Fernandes RP. Oral cavity cancer. In: Gunderson LL, Tepper JE, editors. Clinical radiation oncology. 3rd ed. Philadelphia: Elsevier Saunders; 2012. p. 553–84.

120. The correct answer is B. Retromolar trigone tumors present with clinically positive ipsilateral neck nodes 40 % of the time of diagnosis, and 25 % have subclinical cervical lymph nodes. Byers RM et al. Rationale for elective modified neck dissection. Head Neck Surg. 1988;10:163.

121. The correct answer is A. Hard palate carcinomas are mostly of adenoid cystic or mucoepidermoid histology as they arise from minor salivary glands. Squamous cell carcinomas on the palate typically have secondarily spread from a gingival primary site. Surgery is the mainstay of therapy due to the frequent involvement of underlying bone, but radiation can be used postoperatively for close/positive margins, perineural invasion (especially with adenoid cystic), or bone invasion. Given the rich vascular supply of the palate from the greater palatine artery, the incidence of osteoradionecrosis is less than in the mandible. A University of Virginia report showed that of patients with hard palate carcinoma, 28 % will develop a metachronous primary, with the oral cavity as the most common site. Ratzer ER et al. Epidermoid carcinoma of the palate. Am J Surg. 1970;119:294–7. Barker GJ et al. Oral management of the cancer patient: a guide for the health care professional. Kansas City: The Curators of the University of Missouri; 1981. Chung CK et al. Squamous cell carcinoma of the hard palate. Int J Radiat Oncol Biol Phys. 1979;5:191–6.

122. The correct answer is B. The annual rate of developing a second squamous cell carcinoma is 4–7 %. Wynder EL. The epidemiology of cancers of the upper alimentary and upper respiratory tracts. Laryngoscope. 1978;88:50–1.

123. The correct answer is B. The base of tongue starts at the lingual sulcus terminalis (divides the oral and base of tongue) and then ends at the junction between the valleculae and base of the lingual epiglottis. Cannon GM, Harari PM, Gentry LR, Avey GD, Siu LL. Oropharyngeal cancer. In: Gunderson LL, Tepper JE, editors. Clinical radiation oncology. 3rd ed. Philadelphia: Elsevier Saunders; 2012. p. 585–618.

124. The correct answer is A. Of the five muscles of the soft palate (tensor veli palatini, palatoglossus, palatopharyngeus, levator veli palatini, and uvular), only the

tensor veli palatini is not innervated by the vagus nerve; it is innervated by the mandibular branch of the trigeminal nerve. Cannon GM, Harari PM, Gentry LR, Avey GD, Siu LL. Oropharyngeal cancer. In: Gunderson LL, Tepper JE, editors. Clinical radiation oncology. 3rd ed. Philadelphia: Elsevier Saunders; 2012. p. 585–618.

125. The correct answer is C. A 3.0 cm oropharynx tumor alone would be classified as T2, but the invasion of the medial pterygoid upstages it to T4a. Invasion of the lateral pterygoid would be T4b. A single ipsilateral 3 cm or less is N1. Edge SB, Byrd DR, Compton CC, et al., editors. Pharynx. AJCC cancer staging handbook. 7th ed. New York: Springer; 2010.

126. The correct answer is C. Withers et al. studied various fractionation schemes used to treat 676 patients with tonsil cancer treated with radiation alone at nine institutions in North America and England. Fractionation ranged from 51 Gy/16 fx to 75 Gy/37 fx, with a mean treatment duration of 37 days. They found that total treatment duration, total dose, and the presence of nodal disease significantly correlated with local control. For a constant total dose, every day of delay decreased local control by 1 %. For a constant treatment duration, every 1 Gy increased local control by 2 %. Local control was worse in those with nodal disease. Late complications were found to be worse in bone and muscle with increased fraction size, presumed because these are similar to late-responding tissues. Mucosal late toxicity (acute-responding) was not worse. Field size correlated with mandibular complications. Withers H et al. Local control of carcinoma of the tonsil by radiation therapy: an analysis of patterns of fractionation in nine institutions. Int J Radiat Oncol Biol Phys. 1995;33:549–62. Withers H et al. Late normal tissue sequelae from radiation therapy for carcinoma of the tonsil: patterns of fractionation study of radiobiology. Int J Radiat Oncol Biol Phys. 1995;33:563–8.

127. The correct answer is D. The Overgaard treatment duration phase III trial randomized patients with head and neck carcinoma (62 % larynx, 29 % pharyngeal) to receive either 5 of 6 fractions of 2 Gy daily to a total of 66–68 Gy. T1 glottic patients were treated to 62 Gy. Median treatment durations were 39 days (accelerated) and 46 days (standard). The accelerated group had improved local control (76 % vs. 64 %, $p = 0.00001$), though overall survival was not improved. While acute toxicity was worse in the accelerated arm, late toxicity was not different between the groups. Overgaard J et al. Five compared with six fractions per week of conventional radiotherapy of squamous-cell carcinoma of head and neck: DAHANCA 6 and 7 randomized controlled trial. Lancet. 2003;362:933–40.

128. The correct answer is B. RTOG 90-03 randomized 1,113 patients (60 % oropharynx) to one of four arms: (1) standard fractionation 70 Gy/35 fractions/7 weeks, (2) hyperfractionation 81.6 Gy/68 fractions/7 weeks, (3) split-course accelerated

fractionation 67.2 Gy/42 fractions/6 weeks with a split after 38.4 Gy, and (4) accelerated fractionation with concomitant boost 54 Gy/30 fractions/6 weeks with 18 Gy/12 BID fractions during last 2.5 weeks. The hyperfractionation and accelerated concomitant boost arms were found to have improved local control, though there was no survival difference between any of the arms. All three altered fractionation arms had increased acute, but not late, toxicity. Fu KK et al. A Radiation Therapy Oncology Group (RTOG) Phase II randomized study to compare hyperfractionation and two variants of accelerated fractionation to standard fractionation radiotherapy for head and neck squamous cell carcinoma: first report of RTOG 90-03. Int J Radiat Oncol Biol Phys. 2000;48:7–16.

129. The correct answer is D. The MACH-NC meta-analysis evaluated 87 trials comparing concurrent, induction, or adjuvant chemotherapy with radiation. The oropharynx was the most common primary site (37 %). The addition of concurrent chemotherapy yielded an 8 % 5-year actuarial survival benefit. Overall survival at 5 years was 27 % in the radiation alone group versus 35 % in the chemoradiation arm. The HR for death was 0.8 for concurrent chemoRT compared to RT alone and 0.96 for induction chemotherapy followed by radiation compared to RT alone. Adjuvant chemotherapy following RT had an HR of 1.06. Pignon J-P, le Maître A, Maillard E, Bourhis J. Meta-analysis of chemotherapy in head and neck cancer (MACH-NC): an update on 93 randomized trials and 17,346 patients. Radiother . 2009;92(1):4–14.

130. The correct answer is B. GORTEC 94-01 randomized 222 patients with stage III or IV oropharyngeal carcinoma to radiation +/− concurrent chemotherapy. This trial demonstrated that concurrent chemoradiation with 3 cycles of carboplatin and 5-FU (weeks 1, 4, 7) compared to RT alone (70 Gy in 35 fractions) resulted in improved 5-year OS 22 % versus 16 % ($p=0.05$), 5-year DFS 27 % versus 15 % ($p=0.01$), and 5-year local control 48 % versus 25 % ($p=0.002$). There was no difference in the incidence of distant metastases. There was increased incidence of grades 3–4 mucositis, but late effects were not different between the arms. Denis F, et al. Final results of the 94-01 French head and neck oncology and radiotherapy group randomized trial comparing radiotherapy alone with concomitant radiochemotherapy in advanced-stage oropharynx carcinoma. J Clin Oncol. 2004;22(1):69–76.

131. The correct answer is A. RTOG 0522 randomized 895 evaluable patients with stage III or IV head and neck cancer to receive accelerated radiation and 2 cycles of cisplatin +/− weekly cetuximab. Stage I and II patients were not eligible as these patients are suitable for radiation alone treatment. Over 90 % of patients in both arms received all planned cisplatin cycles. The addition of cetuximab did not improve progression-free survival or overall survival. While grades 3–4 mucositis and skin reaction were worse with the addition of cetuximab, grades 3–4 dysphagia was unchanged. Ang KK et al. J Clin Oncol. 2011;29:(suppl; abstr 5500).

132. The correct answer is B. RTOG 0522 randomized 895 evaluable patients with stage III or IV head and neck cancer to receive accelerated radiation and 2 cycles of cisplatin +/− weekly cetuximab. Stage I and II patients were not eligible as these patients are suitable for radiation alone treatment. Over 90 % of patients in both arms received all planned cisplatin cycles. The addition of cetuximab did not improve progression-free survival or overall survival. While grades 3–4 mucositis and skin reaction were worse with the addition of cetuximab, grades 3–4 dysphagia was unchanged. Ang KK et al. J Clin Oncol. 2011;29:(suppl; abstr 5500).

133. The correct answer is C. Patients with locoregionally advanced H&N squamous cell carcinoma (60 % oropharynx) were randomized to RT alone versus RT with concurrent weekly cetuximab (400 mg/m^2 loading 1 week prior followed by 250 mg/m^2 weekly). Radiation was delivered by standard fractionation and hyperfractionation or accelerated with concomitant boost technique. Concurrent RT and cetuximab demonstrated a benefit with LR progression HR 0.68 ($p = 0.005$), OS HR 0.74 ($p = 0.03$), and PFS HR 0.70 ($p = 0.006$). Median OS was 49.0 months with concurrent treatment versus 29.3 months with RT alone. About 80 % of patients had detectable EGFR. Cetuximab caused a maculopapular rash in 34 % of patients, though it resolved with the cessation of the drug. It did not cause an increase in acute mucositis. Bonner JA et al. Radiotherapy plus cetuximab for squamous-cell carcinoma of the head and neck. N Engl J Med. 2006;354(6):567–78. Bonner JA et al. Radiotherapy plus cetuximab for locoregionally advanced head and neck cancer: 5-year survival data from a phase 3 randomized trial, and relation between cetuximab-induced rash and survival. Lancet Oncol. 2010;11(1):21–8.

134. The correct answer is B. Patients with locoregionally advanced, previously untreated H&N SCC (60 % oropharynx) were randomized to RT alone versus RT with concurrent weekly cetuximab (400 mg/m^2 loading 1 week prior to start of radiation followed by 250 mg/m^2 weekly). Radiation was delivered by standard fractionation and hyperfractionation or accelerated with concomitant boost technique. Concurrent RT and cetuximab demonstrated a benefit with LR progression HR 0.68 ($p = 0.005$), OS HR 0.74 ($p = 0.03$), and PFS HR 0.70 ($p = 0.006$). Median OS was 49.0 months with concurrent treatment versus 29.3 months with RT alone. At 5 years, the overall survival benefit persisted: 46 % versus 36 %. About 80 % of patients had detectable EGFR. Cetuximab caused a maculopapular rash in 34 % of patients, though it resolved with the cessation of the drug. It did not cause an increase in acute mucositis. The update also showed that those experiencing grade 2 or higher rash had improved survival compared to those experiencing grade 1 rash. Bonner JA et al. Radiotherapy plus cetuximab for squamous-cell carcinoma of the head and neck. N Engl J Med. 2006;354(6):567–78. Bonner JA, et al. Radiotherapy plus cetuximab for locoregionally advanced head and neck cancer: 5-year survival data from a phase 3 randomized trial, and relation between cetuximab-induced rash and survival. Lancet Oncol. 2010;11(1):21–8.

135. The correct answer is B. In patients that had been definitively treated for a head and neck cancer with surgery and/or radiation, chemoprevention with 13-cis-retinoic acid was tested to assess for reduction in the incidence of second primary tumors. 13-cis-Retinoic acid was associated with a decrease in second primaries (4 % with vs. 24 % without, $p=0.005$), though this effect did not persist after 3 years, at which time the incidence was equal. 13-cis-Retinoic acid did not affect the rate of relapse from treatment of the first primary, nor did it improve overall survival. Khuri FR et al. Molecular epidemiology and retinoid chemoprevention of head and neck cancer. J Natl Cancer Inst. 1997;89:199–211. Hong WK et al. Prevention of second primary tumors with isotretinoin in squamous-cell carcinoma of the head and neck. N Engl J Med. 1990;323:795–801.

136. The correct answer is B. Cranial nerve VI is the most commonly involved nerve, followed by cranial nerve V. Perez CA et al. Carcinoma of the nasopharynx: factors affecting prognosis. Int J Radiat Oncol Biol Phys. 1992;23:271–80.

137. The correct answer is B. Villaret's syndrome (poststyloid parapharyngeal syndrome) is characterized by compression of the structures in the retropharyngeal space by enlarged retropharyngeal nodes. These structures include CNs IX–XII. Primary tumor may also invade this space. Compression of CN IX and CN X results in dysphagia; compression of CN XII results in tongue atrophy and paralysis. Unilateral Horner's due to compression of the cervical sympathetic chain can also be seen in conjunction with Villaret's. Jacod's syndrome (petrosphenoidal syndrome) results from superior extension of tumor through foramen lacerum and into the cavernous sinus. This can cause unilateral ptosis (CN III), complete ophthalmoplegia (CNs III, IV, VI), or supraorbital and superior maxillary pain or anesthesia (CN V1 and CN V2). Frey's syndrome is gustatory sweating and a loss of earlobe sensation due to facial nerve sacrifice. Lee N, Laufer M, Ove R, Foote RL, Bonner JA. Nasopharyngeal Carcinoma. In: Gunderson LL, Tepper JE, editors. Clinical radiation oncology. 3rd ed. Philadelphia: Elsevier Saunders; 2012. p. 619–38

138. The correct answer is A. Jacod's syndrome (petrosphenoidal syndrome) results from superior extension of tumor through foramen lacerum and into the cavernous sinus. This can cause unilateral ptosis (CN III), complete ophthalmoplegia (CNs III, IV, VI), or supraorbital and superior maxillary pain or anesthesia (CN V1 and CN V2). Lee N, Laufer M, Ove R, Foote RL, Bonner JA. Nasopharyngeal carcinoma. In: Gunderson LL, Tepper JE, editors. Clinical radiation oncology. 3rd ed. Philadelphia: Elsevier Saunders; 2012. p. 619–38.

139. The correct answer is B. The Intergroup 0099 study randomized 150 patients with what would now be T2 and N+ nasopharyngeal cancer to RT alone (70 Gy) versus concurrent chemoradiation to 70 Gy with concurrent cisplatin

(100 mg/m² on days 1, 22, 43) followed by adjuvant reduced dose cisplatin (80 mg/m²) and 5-FU on days 1–4 × 3 cycles. At interim analysis, given the overwhelming benefit of chemotherapy, the trial was closed. The addition of chemotherapy improved 3-year PFS 24 % versus 69 % ($p < 0.001$) and 3-year OS 47 % versus 78 %, ($p = 0.005$). Al-Sarraf M et al. Chemoradiotherapy versus radiotherapy in patients with advanced nasopharyngeal cancer: phase III randomized Intergroup study 0099. J Clin Oncol. 1998;16(4):1310–7.

140. The correct answer is B. There is meaningful salvage of nasopharyngeal recurrences. Wang et al. described their experience of re-irradiating 51 patients, with 5-year actuarial survival of those receiving >60 Gy being 45 % versus 0 % in those receiving less than 60 Gy. The duration of the disease-free interval prior to re-irradiation also correlated with 5-year actuarial survival of 66 % in those with a disease-free interval >24 months versus 13 % in those <24 months. Stereotactic radiosurgery (median dose 18 Gy) has been used to treat 12 patients at Stanford with recurrent nasopharynx cancer. At a median follow-up of 17 months, seven of 12 patients were locally controlled. Wang CC. Re-irradiation of recurrent nasopharyngeal carcinoma: treatment techniques and results. Int J Radiat Oncol Biol Phys. 1987;13:953–6. Cmelak AJ et al. Radiosurgery for skull base malignancies and nasopharyngeal carcinoma. Int J Radiat Oncol Biol Phys. 1997;37:997–1003.

141. The correct answer is A. All of the listed structures should be included in the radiation treatment volume for locally advanced T4 nasopharynx cancer except it is only the posterior one third of the maxillary sinus. Al-Sarraf M, LeBlanc M, Giri PG, et al. Chemoradiotherapy versus radiotherapy in patients with advanced nasopharyngeal cancer: phase III randomized Intergroup study 0099. J Clin Oncol. 1998;16(4):1310–7.

142. The correct answer is D. Lee et al. described their experience of treating 67 patients with nasopharyngeal carcinoma with IMRT. Four-year local and locoregional controls were 97 % and 98 %, respectively. The use of IMRT greatly improved rates of xerostomia, with the majority of patients (66 %) having grade 0 xerostomia and no patients having grade 2 or higher xerostomia. This report set the groundwork for RTOG 0225. Lee N et al. Intensity modulated radiotherapy in the treatment of nasopharyngeal carcinoma: an update of the UCSF experience. Int J Radiat Oncol Biol Phys. 2002;53(1): 12–22.

143. The correct answer is A. RTOG 0225 was a phase II trial looking at the feasibility and outcomes of IMRT for nasopharynx cancer. Chemotherapy was given for those with T2b or greater tumors. The majority (93.8 %) of patients ($n = 68$) had WHO grades 2 and 3 tumors. Chemotherapy was given as per the Intergroup 0099 trial with concurrent cisplatin (100 mg/m² on days 1, 22, 43) followed by adjuvant reduced dose cisplatin (80 mg/m²) and 5-FU on days 1–4

×3 cycles. Two-year local progression-free survival was 92.6 %. Two-year overall survival was 80.2 %. At 1 year from the start of IMRT, the rate of grade 2 xerostomia was 13.5 %, and there were no patients with grade 4 xerostomia. Lee N, et al. Intensity-modulated radiation therapy with or without chemotherapy for nasopharyngeal carcinoma: Radiation Therapy Oncology Group Phase II Trial 0225. J Clin Oncol. 2009;27(22):3684–90.

144. The correct answer is C. Of the listed risk factors, HPV is known to have an association with oropharynx, particularly tonsil cancers, but the association with larynx cancers is not as well established. Tobacco is strongly associated with the development of larynx cancer, and alcohol is felt to act synergistically with tobacco. GERD may predispose to cancer to due chronic irritation of the larynx. Wydner EL.Toward the prevention of laryngeal cancer. Laryngoscope. 1975;85:1190. Muscat JE, Wydner EL. Tobacco, alcohol, asbestos, and occupational risk factors for laryngeal cancer. Cancer. 1992;69:2244. Rothman et al. Epidemiology of laryngeal cancer. Epidemiol Rev. 1980;2:195. Frije et al. Carcinoma of the larynx in patients with gastroesophageal reflux. Am J Otolaryngol. 1996;17:386. Syrjanen S. Human papillomavirus (HPV) in head and neck cancer. J Clin Virol. 2005;32(Suppl 1):S59.

145. The correct answer is A. Larynx cancer presents significantly more commonly in the true glottic larynx and three times more common than in the supraglottic larynx. Subglottic cancers are the least common in incidence (2 %). Garden AS, Morrison WH, Ang KK. Larynx and hypopharynx cancer. In: Gunderson LL, Tepper JE, editors. Clinical radiation oncology. 3rd ed. Philadelphia: Elsevier Saunders; 2012. p. 639–64.

146. The correct answer is D. Hypopharyngeal cancers are the most common to present with lymph node metastases, occurring in 75 %, with levels II and III being the most frequently involved. Hypopharyngeal cancers can also metastasize to the retropharyngeal nodes and the deep jugular nodes. Bilateral nodes at presentation occur in 15 % of patients. Lindberg RD. Distribution of cervical lymph node metastases from squamous cell carcinoma of the upper respiratory and digestive tracts. Cancer. 1972;29:1446.

147. The correct answer is B. The most frequently involved subsite of the hypopharynx is the pyriform sinus, accounting for 70 % of hypopharyngeal tumors. The postcricoid pharynx is the least common site. Garden AS, Morrison WH, Ang KK. Larynx and hypopharynx cancer. In: Gunderson LL, Tepper JE, editors. Clinical radiation oncology. 3rd ed. Philadelphia: Elsevier Saunders; 2012. p. 639–64.

148. The correct answer is C. Due to the lack of lymphatic supply in the glottic larynx, tumors here rarely spread to lymph nodes or distantly. Conversely, hypopharyngeal tumors have the highest incidence of nodal and distant metastasis.

Head and neck cancer most commonly metastasizes to the lung, which is also the most common site of first metastasis. Merino OR et al. An analysis of distant metastases from squamous cell carcinoma of the upper respiratory and digestive tracts. Cancer. 1977;40:145.

149. The correct answer is D. All of the listed scenarios are indications for postoperative radiation after laryngectomy except for difficult and prolonged surgery. Klein et al. reported stomal recurrence in 13 of 54 patients with subglottic disease who did not receive adjuvant radiation. Goepfert et al. reported a 2-year local control of 63 % with radiation versus 37 % with laryngectomy alone for stage IV supraglottic cancer. Klein R, Fletcher GH. Evaluation of the clinical usefulness of radiological findings in squamous cell carcinoma of the larynx. AJR A J Roentgenol. 1964;92:43. Goepfert H et al. Optimal treatment for the technically resectable squamous cell carcinoma of the supraglottic larynx. Laryngoscope. 1975;85;14.

150. The correct answer is A. In the EORTC phase III trial for pyriform sinus cancers, 194 evaluable patients were randomized to one of two arms: (1) surgery + postoperative radiation (50–70 Gy) or (2) induction chemotherapy with bolus cisplatin 100 mg/m^2 on day 1 and 5-FU 1,000 mg/m^2 on days 1–5 × 2 cycles. After 2 cycles, partial and complete responders went on to receive radiation (70 Gy). Nonresponders underwent laryngectomy and postoperative radiation. Larynx preservation was 35 % at 5 years. Local and regional failures were equal in the two arms, but there were fewer distant failures in the induction chemotherapy arm. Median overall survival was improved with induction chemotherapy: 3.7 years versus 2.1 years. Lefebvre JL et al. Larynx preservation in pyriform sinus cancer: preliminary results of a European Organization for Research and Treatment of Cancer phase III trial. EORTC Head and Neck Cancer Cooperative Group. J Natl Cancer Inst. 1996;88(13):890–9.

151. The correct answer is C. A T1 glottic larynx field is an approximately 5×5 cm field that extends from the top of the thyroid notch superiorly to the bottom of the cricoid cartilage inferiorly. The posterior border is the anterior margin of the vertebral bodies; the anterior border is 1cm flash on the skin. Garden AS, Morrison WH, Ang KK. Larynx and hypopharynx cancer. In: Gunderson LL, Tepper JE, editors. Clinical radiation oncology. 3rd ed. Philadelphia: Elsevier Saunders; 2012. p. 639–64.

152. The correct answer is C. In a supraglottic laryngectomy, the pre-epiglottic space, false cords, a portion of the hyoid bone, epiglottis, aryepiglottic folds, and a portion of the thyroid cartilage are removed. The true vocal cords and the arytenoid cartilages are preserved. Garden AS, Morrison WH, Ang KK. Larynx and hypopharynx cancer. In: Gunderson LL, Tepper JE, editors. Clinical radiation oncology. 3rd ed. Philadelphia: Elsevier Saunders; 2012. p. 639–64.

153. The correct answer is D. Contraindications to supraglottic laryngectomy include subglottic extension, hypopharyngeal involvement, bilateral arytenoid involvement, extension to the true vocal cords, extension to the anterior commissure, and thyroid/cricoid cartilage invasion. Garden AS, Morrison WH, Ang KK. Larynx and hypopharynx cancer. In: Gunderson LL, Tepper JE, editors. Clinical radiation oncology. 3rd ed. Philadelphia: Elsevier Saunders; 2012. p. 639–64.

154. The correct answer is B. Contraindications to hemilaryngectomy include >5 mm subglottic extension, bilateral true vocal cord involvement, bilateral arytenoid involvement, epiglottic invasion, and extension to the false cords. Partial fixation of one true vocal cord is not a contraindication. Garden AS, Morrison WH, Ang KK. Larynx and hypopharynx cancer. In: Gunderson LL, Tepper JE, editors. Clinical radiation oncology. 3rd ed. Philadelphia: Elsevier Saunders; 2012. p. 639–64.

Chapter 4
Lung Cancer

Celine Bicquart Ord and Charles R. Thomas, Jr.

Questions

1. Historically, what percentage of newly diagnosed lung cancer is small-cell type?
   A. 20 %
   B. 30 %
   C. 40 %
   D. 50 %

2. Non-small-cell lung cancer most commonly presents at which stage?
   A. I
   B. II
   C. III
   D. IV

3. What molecular abnormality is NOT seen in small-cell lung cancer?
   A. *MYC* amplification
   B. *EGFR* expression
   C. *TP53* mutation
   D. *RB1* deletion

C.B. Ord, MD (✉)
Department of Radiation Oncology, Scott & White Memorial Hospital,
2401 S. 31st Street, Temple, TX 76508, USA
e-mail: cord@sw.org

C.R. Thomas Jr., MD (✉)
Department of Radiation Medicine, Oregon Health & Science University, Knight Cancer Institute,
3181 SW Sam Jackson Park Road, KPV4, Portland, OR 97239-3098, USA
e-mail: thomasch@ohsu.edu; thomas@gmail.com

C.B. Ord et al. (eds.), *Radiation Oncology Study Guide*,   107
DOI 10.1007/978-1-4614-6400-6_4, © Springer Science+Business Media New York 2013

4. Which of the following types of lung cancer is LEAST likely to metastasize to the brain?
   A. Adenocarcinoma
   B. Large-cell carcinoma
   C. Small-cell lung cancer
   D. Squamous cell carcinoma

5. Which of the following paraneoplastic syndromes associated with small-cell lung cancer is not correctable with therapy?
   A. SIADH
   B. Lambert-Eaton syndrome
   C. Atrial natriuretic peptide syndrome
   D. Cerebellar degeneration syndrome

6. All of the following are true regarding Lambert-Eaton syndrome except:
   A. Symptoms improve with repetition.
   B. It is a paraneoplastic syndrome associated with small-cell lung cancer.
   C. It results from anti-calcium channel antibodies of the presynaptic receptor.
   D. Symptoms are not improved with anti-myasthenia therapies.

7. Which of the following is a paraneoplastic syndrome most commonly associated with squamous cell carcinoma?
   A. Hypercalcemia
   B. Hyponatremia
   C. Hypertrophic pulmonary osteoarthropathy
   D. Gynecomastia

8. Which of the following is a paraneoplastic syndrome most commonly associated with adenocarcinoma?
   A. Hypercalcemia
   B. Hyponatremia
   C. Hypertrophic pulmonary osteoarthropathy
   D. Gynecomastia

9. Which of the following is a paraneoplastic syndrome most commonly associated with large-cell carcinoma?
   A. Hypercalcemia
   B. Hyponatremia
   C. Hypertrophic pulmonary osteoarthropathy
   D. Gynecomastia

10. All of the following statements regarding carcinoid tumors of the lung are true except:
    A. This is not the most common site of carcinoid tumors.
    B. The majority of these tumors are associated with carcinoid syndrome at presentation.
    C. The majority of these tumors are typical rather than atypical carcinoid tumors.
    D. In the lung, carcinoid tumors are primarily endobronchial, rather than parenchymal.

11. Which immunostain would most likely be negative in small-cell lung cancer?
    A. Chromogranin
    B. Synaptophysin
    C. CDX-2
    D. TTF-1

12. Which of the following statements regarding small-cell lung cancer is incorrect?
    A. Two-thirds of patients present with extensive-stage disease.
    B. Approximately 10 % present with superior vena cava syndrome.
    C. Approximately 10–20 % present with brain metastases at diagnosis.
    D. Median survival of limited-stage disease with chemotherapy with or without radiation is 7–11 months.

13. What percentage of patients with small-cell lung cancer with superior vena cava syndrome presents with a normal chest radiograph?
    A. 5 %
    B. 15 %
    C. 25 %
    D. 35 %

14. What was the overall survival benefit seen in both the Pignon and Warde meta-analyses regarding the addition of thoracic radiotherapy to chemotherapy for small-cell lung cancer?
    A. 5 %
    B. 7 %
    C. 10 %
    D. 12 %

15. Regarding the optimal timing of thoracic radiotherapy, reported by Murray et al. in the NCI Canada Study, all of the following are true except:
    A. Early radiotherapy started with the second cycle of chemotherapy.
    B. One component of chemotherapy included adriamycin.
    C. Total radiotherapy dose was 40 Gy.
    D. Early thoracic radiotherapy improved overall survival, but not local control.

16. According to a meta-analysis by Fried et al. regarding the timing of thoracic radiotherapy in addition to chemotherapy, which of the following constitutes "early" thoracic radiotherapy?
    A. Beginning within 7 weeks of starting chemotherapy
    B. Beginning within 8 weeks of starting chemotherapy
    C. Beginning within 9 weeks of starting chemotherapy
    D. Beginning within 10 weeks of starting chemotherapy

17. According to the Intergroup 0096 (Turrisi) trial comparing once daily versus twice daily radiotherapy for small-cell lung cancer, all of the following are true except:
    A. Grade 3 esophagitis was increased in the twice daily radiotherapy arm.
    B   Overall survival was improved in the twice daily radiotherapy arm.
    C. The 5-year overall survival in the once daily radiotherapy arm was 10 %.
    D. Dose per fraction in the once daily radiotherapy arm was 1.8 Gy.

18. What was the spinal cord tolerance in the BID fractionation arm of the Intergroup 0096 (Turrisi) trial?
    A. 36 Gy
    B. 45 Gy
    C. 50.4 Gy
    D. 54 Gy

19. What was the rate of grade three esophagitis in the BID fractionation arm of the Intergroup 0096 (Turrisi) trial?
    A. 11 %
    B. 20 %
    C. 27 %
    D. 33 %

20. Which of the following prophylactic cranial irradiation fractionation schemes has not been typically described for small-cell lung cancer?
    A. 8 Gy in 1 fraction
    B. 30 Gy in 10 fractions
    C. 36 Gy in 18 fractions
    D. 18 Gy in 10 fractions

21. What was the survival benefit seen in those with limited-stage small-cell lung cancer given prophylactic cranial irradiation after a complete response in the Auperin meta-analysis?
    A. 5 %
    B. 10 %
    C. 15 %
    D. 20 %

22. Regarding the published results from Lé Pechoux et al. regarding optimal prophylactic cranial irradiation dose, which of the following is not true?
   A. Patients had to be in complete remission prior to randomization for PCI.
   B. Both extensive and limited-stage responders were eligible to randomization.
   C. Patients were randomized to receive either 25 Gy or 36 Gy.
   D. There was no significant reduction in the total incidence of brain metastases with higher dose.

23. Regarding the addition of thoracic radiotherapy in extensive-stage small-cell lung cancer, which of the following observations from Jeremic et al. is not true?
   A. Patients with a complete response at distant sites were eligible.
   B. Patients randomized to receive radiotherapy were treated to 45 Gy with BID fractionation.
   C. Patients that received thoracic radiotherapy had significantly improved survival compared to those that did not receive thoracic radiotherapy.
   D. Concurrent carboplatin was given with thoracic radiotherapy.

24. Regarding prophylactic cranial irradiation (PCI) given for those with extensive-stage small-cell lung cancer as reported by Slotman et al., which of the following is true?
   A. There was a 5.4 % survival benefit associated with PCI at 3 years.
   B. A complete response was not required before PCI was given.
   C. Brain imaging to confirm the absence of brain metastases was required before PCI.
   D. Acceptable doses for PCI ranged from 20 Gy to 30 Gy.

25. Regarding the National Lung Screening Trial, all of the following are true except:
   A. Participants were randomized to undergo either low-dose CT or chest radiograph screening.
   B. Participants underwent a total of four screenings at 1-year intervals.
   C. Any nodule on low-dose CT ≥4 mm was classified as "suspicious for" lung cancer.
   D. Former smokers were required to have quit within 15 years of enrollment.

26. What level in the mediastinum are prevascular lymph nodes?
   A. 2
   B. 3
   C. 4
   D. 5

27. Mediastinal level 5 lymph nodes are best evaluated via which of the following?
   A. Endoscopic ultrasound with fine-needle aspiration
   B. Video-assisted thoracoscopy
   C. Chamberlain procedure
   D. CT-guided biopsy

28. From which lobe is there frequent nodal drainage to the contralateral paratracheal
    and anterior mediastinal lymph nodes?
    A. Right upper lobe
    B. Right middle lobe
    C. Left upper lobe
    D. Lingula

29. What 7th edition AJCC TNM stage is most appropriate for a 3.5-cm adenocar-
    cinoma of the left upper lobe of the lung with a separate 2.9-cm nodule in the
    left lower lobe without mediastinal or hilar lymph node metastases?
    A. T2aM1
    B. T4N0
    C. T4M1
    D. T2bM1

30. What 7th edition AJCC TNM stage is most appropriate for a 3.5-cm adenocar-
    cinoma of the right upper lobe of the lung with a 2.0-cm left supraclavicular
    lymph node metastasis?
    A. T2aN3
    B. T2bN3
    C. T2aM1
    D. T2bM1

31. What 7th edition AJCC TNM stage is most appropriate for a 7-cm squamous
    cell carcinoma of the right upper lobe of the lung with an ipsilateral pleural
    effusion and ipsilateral hilar lymph node involvement?
    A. T4N1M0
    B. T4N1M1a
    C. T3N1M1a
    D. T3N1M1b

32. All of the following are true regarding adenocarcinoma of the lung except:
    A. It can arise out of an old tuberculosis scar.
    B. It has the fastest doubling time of all subtypes of non-small-cell lung cancer.
    C. Stage-for-stage outcomes are worse compared to squamous cell lung cancer.
    D. It most commonly presents in a peripheral location.

33. Which of the following subtypes of lung cancer is least related to smoking?
    A. Bronchioalveolar carcinoma
    B. Squamous cell carcinoma
    C. Small-cell carcinoma
    D. Large-cell carcinoma

34. Which of the following was not found to be one of the three most important prognostic factors affecting survival in inoperable bronchogenic carcinoma of the lung, as reported in the Veterans Administration Lung Group Protocols?
    A. Karnofsky performance status
    B. Extent of disease
    C. Weight loss in the previous 6 months
    D. Response to treatment

35. Comparing lobectomy versus limited resection, which of the following statements regarding the Lung Cancer Study Group trial is incorrect?
    A. Participants with T1N0M0 lung cancer were randomized to lobectomy versus limited resection.
    B. There was no difference in local control between the two arms.
    C. Cancer-related mortality was worse in the limited resection arm.
    D. No participants in the limited resection group required postoperative ventilation for >24 h.

36. What is the best evidence-based treatment approach for an operable small T1a peripheral NSCLC?
    A. Lobectomy
    B. Wedge resection
    C. Stereotactic body radiation therapy
    D. Definitive chemoradiation

37. What is the 5-year overall survival of a cT1N0 lung cancer per the Mountain data?
    A. 90 %
    B. 80 %
    C. 70 %
    D. 60 %

38. What is the 5-year overall survival of a pT1N0 lung cancer per the Mountain data?
    A. 90 %
    B. 80 %
    C. 70 %
    D. 60 %

39. Regarding the published results of RTOG 0236 (JAMA 2010), a phase II study looking at stereotactic body radiation therapy in medically inoperable early-stage lung cancer, which of the following is true?
    A. T2 tumors were excluded from enrollment.
    B. The prescription dose was 18 Gy × 3 fractions.
    C. Three-year overall survival was 55 %.
    D. Three-year primary tumor control rate was 85 %.

40. Which of the following was found to be the treated BED equal to or over which there was a statistically significant improvement in both local control and overall survival, as described by Onishi et al.?
    A. ≥90 Gy
    B. ≥95 Gy
    C. ≥100 Gy
    D. ≥105 Gy

41. Regarding postoperative radiotherapy for lung cancer, all of the following are conclusions from the postoperative radiotherapy meta-analysis except:
    A. There was an absolute overall survival detriment of 7 % associated with postoperative radiotherapy in N0/N1 patients.
    B. Postoperative radiotherapy was associated with improved survival in patients with N2 disease.
    C. Both published and unpublished trials were included to avoid publication bias.
    D. Postoperative radiotherapy doses ranged from 30 to 60 Gy.

42. All are true regarding the Lung Cancer Study Group 773 Trial of postoperative radiotherapy for non-small-cell lung cancer as reported by Weisenberger et al. except:
    A. Adenocarcinoma was not included.
    B. Postoperative radiation dose was 50 Gy.
    C. Local control was improved only in patients with N2 disease.
    D. There was no overall survival benefit for the addition of radiation.

43. All are true regarding the Medical Research Council study of postoperative radiotherapy for non-small-cell lung cancer as reported by Stephens et al. except:
    A. Negative margins were required.
    B. Postoperative radiation dose was 40 Gy.
    C. Local recurrence was improved only in patients with N2 disease.
    D. Median survival was not improved with the addition of radiation in any subgroup.

44. Regarding adjuvant chemotherapy in lung cancer, which of the following statements about the International Adjuvant Lung Cancer Trial (IALT) is not true?
    A. Participants were not allowed to receive adjuvant radiotherapy.
    B. Participants were randomized to observation versus an adjuvant cisplatin doublet.
    C. Adjuvant chemotherapy was associated with a 4 % absolute survival benefit.
    D. The survival benefit seen with adjuvant chemotherapy was present for all stage groups.

45. All of the following are true statements about the CALGB 9633 trial which randomized resected T2N0M0 NSCLC to observation versus adjuvant carbo-platin/paclitaxel except:
   A. Adjuvant chemotherapy consisted of 4 cycles of carboplatin/paclitaxel.
   B. Neutropenia was the predominant toxicity seen with chemotherapy.
   C. There was a statistically significant survival benefit of chemotherapy only in those with tumors ≥4 cm.
   D. Only half of patients randomized to receive chemotherapy received all of the planned cycles.

46. In the randomized trial comparing preoperative chemotherapy plus surgery ver-sus surgery alone as reported by Rosell et. al., all of the following are true except:
   A. All patients received mediastinal radiotherapy after surgery.
   B. Preoperative chemotherapy consisted of 3 cycles of cisplatin/etoposide.
   C. Median survival was improved in those receiving preoperative chemotherapy.
   D. Local recurrence was greater in those that did not receive preoperative chemotherapy.

47. In the CALGB 8433 trial (Dillman et al.) comparing induction chemotherapy plus radiotherapy versus radiotherapy alone, all of the following are true except:
   A. Total radiotherapy dose in both arms was 60 Gy.
   B. Only patients with stage III NSCLC were eligible.
   C. Median survival was improved with the addition of induction chemotherapy.
   D. Induction chemotherapy consisted of cisplatin and etoposide.

48. The Intergroup 0139 trial randomized patients with NSCLC to undergo chemo-radiation alone versus chemoradiation + surgery. All of the following are true statements about 0139 except:
   A. N2 nodal status was required for eligibility.
   B. Chemotherapy consisted of cisplatin and etoposide for a total of 4 cycles.
   C. Total radiotherapy dose in the chemoradiation alone arm was 63 Gy.
   D. Total radiotherapy dose in the preoperative chemoradiation arm was 45 Gy.

49. All of the following are outcomes from the Intergroup 0139 trial which ran-domized patients with NSCLC to undergo chemoradiation alone versus chemo-radiation + surgery except:
   A. Esophagitis was the most common grade 3 or 4 toxicity.
   B. Overall survival was not improved with the addition of surgical resection.
   C. Progression-free survival was improved with the addition of surgery.
   D. Overall survival was improved in those who underwent lobectomy, but not pneumonectomy.

50. What trial initially established 60 Gy as the standard dose for unresectable, locally advanced NSCLC?
    A. RTOG 73-01
    B. RTOG 83-11
    C. RTOG 88-08
    D. RTOG 94-10

51. Which of the following is least likely to increase the risk of pneumonitis?
    A. Increased total radiation dose
    B. Increased volume of lung irradiated
    C. Poor pulmonary function from underlying COPD
    D. Treatment of upper lobe tumor

52. Regarding the use of amifostine as a radioprotectant during irradiation for NSCLC, all of the following are true except:
    A. Amifostine is a thioester that scavenges free radicals.
    B. Hypotension is a frequent side effect.
    C. It has been shown to significantly improve objective measures of esophagitis.
    D. Its trade name is Ethyol®.

53. What was the rate of esophagitis in the amifostine arm of RTOG 98-01, a phase III trial of non-small-cell lung cancer treated with chemoradiation with or without amifostine?
    A. 15 %
    B. 20 %
    C. 25 %
    D. 30 %

54. All of the following statements regarding the NSCLC dose escalation RTOG 0617 trial are true except:
    A. There was no survival benefit for treatment with 74 Gy versus 60 Gy.
    B. Toxicity rates were no different between the arms.
    C. Standard concurrent chemotherapy in all arms was carboplatin/paclitaxel.
    D. All arms of the trial were closed after the high-dose arms crossed the futility boundary.

55. All of the following regarding the NSCLC dose escalation RTOG 0617 trial are true except:
    A. All patients were planned to receive consolidation chemotherapy.
    B. IMRT was not allowed.
    C. One of the stratification features was use of PET staging.
    D. The total lung V20 was to be kept ≤37 %.

56. Which of the following was NOT an arm of the LAMP trial as reported by Belani et al.?
    A. Induction chemotherapy, followed by radiotherapy alone to 63 Gy
    B. Induction chemotherapy followed by concurrent chemoradiation
    C. Concurrent chemoradiation alone
    D. Concurrent chemoradiation followed by consolidative chemotherapy

57. Which of the following is not an observation from the LAMP trial as reported by Belani et al.?
    A. Neutropenia was the most common grade 3 or 4 toxicity.
    B. Esophagitis was worst in the concurrent chemoradiation arms.
    C. Median survival seemed to be improved with the addition of consolidative chemotherapy.
    D. Those patients in the consolidative chemotherapy arm had the lowest percentage of completion of the scheduled radiotherapy dose.

58. What was the elective nodal failure in those patients with NSCLC treated with involved nodal radiotherapy only as reported by Rosenzweig et al.?
    A. 4 %
    B. 6 %
    C. 8 %
    D. 10 %

59. All are true regarding the Hoosier Oncology Group consolidation docetaxel trial for inoperable stage III non-small-cell lung cancer as reported by Hanna et al. except:
    A. Total radiotherapy dose delivered was 59.4 Gy.
    B. Median survival was not improved with the addition of docetaxel.
    C. Concurrent chemotherapy consisted of carboplatin/paclitaxel.
    D. There was increased febrile neutropenia in the docetaxel group.

60. Which of the following statements correctly describes the methods of RTOG 94-10?
    A. Concurrent chemotherapy in the hyperfractionated arm consisted of cisplatin/vinblastine.
    B. Concurrent chemotherapy in the conventionally fractionated arms was cisplatin/etoposide.
    C. Total radiotherapy dose in conventionally fractionated arms was 60 Gy.
    D. Total radiotherapy dose in the hyperfractionated arm was 69.2 Gy.

61. Which of the following is not true regarding the RTOG 94-10 trial for inoperable, advanced non-small-cell lung cancer?
    A. Acute esophagitis was worst in the hyperfractionated arm.
    B. Late esophagitis was worst in the hyperfractionated arm.
    C. Median survival was 17 months in the concurrent chemotherapy, conventional RT arm.
    D. Stage II NSCLC was eligible for enrollment.

62. Which of the following was NOT an arm of RTOG 88-08 as reported by Sause et al.?
    A. 60Gy/30 fractions/6 weeks
    B. 60Gy/30 fractions/6 weeks with induction cisplatin/etoposide
    C. 60Gy/30 fractions/6 weeks with induction cisplatin/vinblastine
    D. 69.2 Gy in twice daily 1.2 Gy fractions

63. All of the following are treatment arms from the Schaake-Koning trial of unresectable non-small-cell lung cancer except:
    A. Split-course RT alone: 30 Gy then 25 Gy
    B. Split-course RT with weekly cisplatin
    C. Split-course RT with daily cisplatin
    D. Split-course RT with cisplatin on days 1, 22, and 43

64. All are true regarding the United Kingdom CHART regimen for lung cancer as reported by Saunders et al. except:
    A. CHART did not show a survival benefit compared to conventional radiotherapy.
    B. The CHART regimen consisted of 54 Gy delivered in TID fractions.
    C. Acute toxicity was increased in the CHART arm.
    D. There were no differences in late toxicities between the two arms.

65. All of the following are acceptable components of treatment for radiation-induced pneumonitis except:
    A. Prednisone prescribed at 1 mg/kg/day over a slow taper
    B. Prednisone 60 mg/day over a slow taper
    C. Trimethoprim-sulfamethoxazole
    D. Metronidazole

66. The symptom of sudden electric shocks extending down the spine with head flexion infrequently associated with treatment of non-small-cell lung cancer is known as:
    A. Nelson's syndrome
    B. Lhermitte's syndrome
    C. Garcin syndrome
    D. Lemierre's syndrome

67. Regarding the RTOG 0214 trial evaluation prophylactic cranial irradiation (PCI) for treated advanced-stage non-small-cell lung cancer, which of the following is true?
    A. PCI total dose was 25 Gy in 10 fractions.
    B. There was a small disease-free survival benefit with the addition of PCI.
    C. There was no overall survival benefit with the addition of PCI.
    D. The 1-year rate of brain metastases was not different between the arms.

68. Regarding the SWOG 0023 trial in which consolidation therapy after definitive chemoRT consisted of docetaxel × 3 cycles with or without gefitinib, all of the following are true except:
    A. Total radiotherapy dose delivered was 61 Gy.
    B. Cisplatin/etoposide was delivered concurrently.
    C. Median survival was improved with the addition of gefitinib.
    D. Stage IIIA and stage IIIB patients were eligible for enrollment.

69. What ipsilateral lung dosimetric constraint will reduce the risk of pneumonitis after chemoradiation for non-small-cell lung cancer to <10 %, as reported by Ramella et al.?
    A. V20 ipsilateral <52 %
    B. V20 ipsilateral <42 %
    C. V30 ipsilateral <30 %
    D. V30 ipsilateral <35 %

70. Which of the following is not a histologic subtype of malignant mesothelioma?
    A. Epithelioid
    B. Large cell
    C. Sarcomatoid
    D. Biphasic

71. Which histologic subtype of malignant mesothelioma has the best prognosis?
    A. Epithelioid
    B. Large cell
    C. Sarcomatoid
    D. Biphasic

72. Which biomarker as reported by Pass et al. can help identify early-stage pleural mesothelioma in patients with prior asbestos exposure?
    A. Chromogranin A
    B. Nuclear matrix protein 22
    C. Osteopontin
    D. Calcitonin

73. Which of the following chemotherapy doublets is not approved or recommended by the Food and Drug Administration nor the National Comprehensive Cancer Network?
    A. Cisplatin/pemetrexed
    B. Carboplatin/pemetrexed
    C. Cisplatin/gemcitabine
    D. Cisplatin/etoposide

74. Regarding the role of radiotherapy for malignant pleural mesothelioma, all of the following are true except:
    A. It can be used to prevent instrument-tract recurrence after pleural intervention.
    B. It can be used to palliate chest or bone pain.
    C. Definitive chemoradiation has been shown to yield equivalent overall survival compared to surgery.
    D. High-dose radiotherapy to the hemithorax yields significant toxicity.

75. What hypofractionated radiotherapy regimen yielded no local recurrences in the treated tract sites for malignant pleural mesothelioma as reported by Di Salvo et al.?
    A. 500 cGy × 3 fractions
    B. 600 cGy × 3 fractions
    C. 700 cGy × 3 fractions
    D. 800 cGy × 3 fractions

76. All of the following make malignant pleural mesothelioma unresectable except:
    A. Contralateral mediastinal involvement
    B. Multiple pleural plaques in ipsilateral lung
    C. Diaphragmatic invasion
    D. Distant spread to brain

Answers and Rationales

1. The correct answer is A. Historically, 20 % of newly diagnosed lung cancers were reported as small cell in histology. Of those that present with small-cell lung cancer, approximately 30 % present with limited-stage disease. A recent publication suggests that the incidence of small-cell lung cancer is declining and accounted for 10 and 11 % (male and female, respectively) of lung cancer cases ($n = 237,792$) in England between 1970 and 2007. Warde et al. Does thoracic irradiation improve survival and local control in limited-stage small cell carcinoma of the lung? A meta-analysis. J Clin Oncol. 1992;10:890–5. Riaz SP et al. Trends in incidence of small cell lung cancer and all lung cancer. Lung Cancer. 2012;75(3):280–4.

2. The correct answer is D. Non-small-cell lung cancer most commonly presents at stage IV. A rough estimate of the percentage of presentation of each stage: I (10 %), II (20 %), III (30 %), and IV (40 %). Wagner H. Non-small cell lung cancer. In: Gunderson LL, Tepper JE, editors. Clinical radiation oncology. 3rd ed. Philadelphia: Elsevier Saunders; 2012. p. 805–38.

3. The correct answer is B. Of the listed molecular abnormalities, *EGFR* expression has NOT been reported in small-cell lung cancers (SCLC). *TP53* mutation is seen in over 80 % SCLC, *RB1* deletion is seen in 90 %, and *MYC* amplification has been seen in 30 % of SCLC. *MYC* amplification has been associated with more recurrent, aggressive, and variant histologies of SCLC. Harbour JW et al. Abnormalities in structure and expression of the human retinoblastoma gene in SCLC. Science. 1988;241:353–7. Gazdar AF. Molecular markers for the diagnosis and prognosis of lung cancer. Cancer. 1992;69:1592–9. Gazdar A. The molecular and cellular basis of human lung cancer. Anticancer Res. 1994;13:261–8.

4. The correct answer is D. Of the listed histologies, squamous cell lung cancer is the least likely to metastasize to the brain. Adenocarcinoma, small cell, and large cell frequently metastasize to the brain. Wagner H. Non-small cell lung cancer. In: Gunderson LL, Tepper JE, editors. Clinical radiation oncology. 3rd ed. Philadelphia: Elsevier Saunders; 2012. p. 805–38.

5. The correct answer is D. Of all the listed paraneoplastic syndromes, cerebellar degeneration syndrome is not correctable with therapy. SIADH results from the excessive secretion of ADH, leading to hyponatremia and hypoosmolality. It improves with treatment of the underlying SCLC. Atrial natriuretic peptide (ANP) is a less common endocrinologic syndrome that can produce hyponatremia, natriuresis, and hypotension. It occurs in 15 % of SCLC and responds to therapy. Lambert-Eaton is a neurologic syndrome with symptoms similar to those of myasthenia gravis, though it improves with repetition (MG worsens

with repetition). This condition also improves with treatment of the underlying malignancy. Schild SE, Curran WJ. Small cell lung cancer. In: Gunderson LL, Tepper JE, editors. Clinical radiation oncology. 3rd ed. Philadelphia: Elsevier Saunders; 2012. p. 795–804.

6. The correct answer is D. Lambert-Eaton is a paraneoplastic syndrome of small-cell lung cancer with symptoms that resemble myasthenia gravis. Whereas *post*synaptic receptor anti-calcium channel antibodies are involved in myasthenia gravis, the *pre*synaptic receptor antibodies are involved in Lambert-Eaton. Another important difference is that symptoms improve with repetition in Lambert-Eaton, but worsen with repetition in myasthenia gravis. While treatment of the underlying disease is most effective in improving symptoms, these also do respond to anti-myasthenic therapies. Sellers T et al. Lung cancer histologic type and family history of cancer. Cancer. 1992;69:86–91.

7. The correct answer is A. Of the listed paraneoplastic syndromes, hypercalcemia is most commonly associated with squamous cell carcinoma. Hyponatremia is most commonly associated with small-cell carcinoma. Hypertrophic pulmonary osteoarthropathy is most commonly associated with adenocarcinoma. Gynecomastia is most commonly associated with large-cell carcinoma. Wagner H. Non-small cell lung cancer. In: Gunderson LL, Tepper JE, editors. Clinical radiation oncology. 3rd ed. Philadelphia: Elsevier Saunders; 2012. p. 805–38.

8. The correct answer is C. Of the listed paraneoplastic syndromes, hypertrophic pulmonary osteoarthropathy is most commonly associated with adenocarcinoma. Hypercalcemia is most commonly associated with squamous cell carcinoma. Hyponatremia is most commonly associated with small-cell carcinoma. Gynecomastia is most commonly associated with large-cell carcinoma. Wagner H. Non-small cell lung cancer. In: Gunderson LL, Tepper JE, editors. Clinical radiation oncology. 3rd ed. Philadelphia: Elsevier Saunders; 2012. p. 805–38.

9. The correct answer is D. Of the listed paraneoplastic syndromes, gynecomastia is most commonly associated with large-cell carcinoma. Hypertrophic pulmonary osteoarthropathy is most commonly associated with adenocarcinoma. Hypercalcemia is most commonly associated with squamous cell carcinoma. Hyponatremia is most commonly associated with small-cell carcinoma. Wagner H. Non-small cell lung cancer. In: Gunderson LL, Tepper JE, editors. Clinical radiation oncology. 3rd ed. Philadelphia: Elsevier Saunders; 2012. p. 805–38.

10. The correct answer is B. Carcinoid tumors are rare in the lung, with the most common site of presentation in the GI tract. Within the lung, carcinoid tumors tend to be typical in histology and endobronchial. While the minority (10–15 %) of typical carcinoid tumors present with carcinoid syndrome (flushing, diarrhea, wheezing), most eventually develop these symptoms. Wagner H. Non-small cell lung cancer. In: Gunderson LL, Tepper JE, editors. Clinical radiation oncology. 3rd ed. Philadelphia: Elsevier Saunders; 2012. p. 805–38.

11. The correct answer is C. Of the listed immunostains, CDX-2 would most likely be negative, as it is a stain for gastrointestinal malignancy. TTF-1 stains are common in lung neoplasms and in >90 % of SCLC. Chromogranin and synaptophysin are neuroendocrine stains frequently seen in small-cell lung cancer. Wagner H. Non-small cell lung cancer. In: Gunderson LL, Tepper JE, editors. Clinical radiation oncology. 3rd ed. Philadelphia: Elsevier Saunders; 2012. p. 805–38.

12. The correct answer is D. Small-cell lung cancer presents predominantly with extensive-stage disease (2/3). While this is the most common histology to present with superior vena cava syndrome, only ~10 % of patients present this way. Ten to twenty percent of patients present with brain metastases at diagnosis, but by 2 years, 50 % will have developed brain metastases. The median survival of extensive-stage disease with chemotherapy with or without radiation is 7–11 months. Median survival of limited-stage disease is 20–22 months. Schild SE, Curran WJ. Small cell lung cancer. In: Gunderson LL, Tepper JE, editors., Clinical radiation oncology. 3rd ed. Philadelphia: Elsevier Saunders; 2012. p. 795–804.

13. The correct answer is B. Fifteen percent of patients with superior vena cava syndrome from small-cell lung cancer have a normal chest radiograph. Armstrong BA et al. Role of irradiation in the management of superior vena cava syndrome. Int J Radiat Oncol Biol Phys. 1987;13(4):531–9. Wilson LD. Superior vena cava syndrome with malignant causes. N Engl J Med. 2007; 356:1862–9.

14. The correct answer is A. Both the Pignon and Warde meta-analyses comparing chemotherapy alone with chemotherapy plus thoracic radiotherapy showed a 5.4 % overall survival benefit. The Warde meta-analysis also showed a 25 % improvement in intrathoracic tumor control with the addition of radiotherapy. Warde et al. Does thoracic irradiation improve survival and local control in limited-stage small cell carcinoma of the lung? A meta-analysis. J Clin Oncol. 1992;10:890–5. Pignon JP et al. Meta-analysis of small-cell lung cancer. N Engl J Med. 1992; 327:1618–24.

15. The correct answer is C. In the NCI Canada study of the optimal timing of thoracic radiotherapy, 308 patients with limited-stage disease were randomized to early thoracic radiotherapy given with the second cycle of chemotherapy versus late thoracic radiotherapy given with the sixth cycle of chemotherapy. Chemotherapy consisted of cytoxan/adriamycin/vincristine alternating with cisplatin/etoposide for a total of 6 cycles; total radiotherapy dose was 40 Gy/15 fractions. At the end of chemoradiation, those without progression received prophylactic cranial irradiation (25 Gy/10 fractions). Early thoracic radiotherapy was found to improve progression-free survival and overall survival, but not local control (both 50 % at 3 years). Murray N et al. Importance of timing for thoracic irradiation in the combined modality treatment of limited-stage small-cell lung cancer. The National Cancer Institute of Canada Clinical Trials Group. J Clin Oncol. 1993;11(2):336–44.

16. The correct answer is C. In a meta-analysis of 7 trials ($n = 1,524$ patients) regarding the timing of thoracic radiotherapy in addition to chemotherapy for limited-stage SCLC, Fried et al. found that initiating radiotherapy within 9 weeks of starting chemotherapy conferred a 2-year overall survival benefit of 5.2 %, similar to the magnitude of adding thoracic radiotherapy to chemotherapy. Fried et al. Timing of thoracic irradiation in the combined-modality treatment of limited-stage small cell lung cancer: a meta-analysis [abstract O-70]. Lung Cancer. 2003; 41 (Suppl 2):23.

17. The correct answer is C. Intergroup 0096 compared daily radiotherapy 1.8–45 Gy to BID radiotherapy of 1.5–45 Gy, with concurrent cisplatin/etoposide, beginning on day 1. Twice daily radiotherapy yielded a survival advantage compared to daily radiotherapy, with 5-year OS (26 % vs. 16 %, $p = 0.04$), though the incidence of grade 3 esophagitis also increased (27 % vs. 11 %, $p < 0.001$). Starting with week 2, delivery of the afternoon fraction in the BID arm was delivered with off-cord obliques. Cord tolerance in this study was 36 Gy. Turrisi A et al. Twice-daily compared with once-daily thoracic radiotherapy in limited small cell lung cancer treated concurrently with cisplatin and etoposide. N Engl J Med. 1999; 340:265–71.

18. The correct answer is A. Intergroup 0096 compared daily radiotherapy 1.8–45 Gy, to BID radiotherapy of 1.5–45 Gy, with concurrent cisplatin/etoposide, beginning on day 1. Twice daily radiotherapy yielded a survival advantage compared to daily radiotherapy, with 5-year OS (26 % vs. 16 %, $p = 0.04$), though the incidence of grade 3 esophagitis also increased (27 % vs. 11 %, $p < 0.001$). Starting with week 2, delivery of the afternoon fraction in the BID arm was delivered with off-cord obliques. Cord tolerance in this study for the BID arm was 36 Gy. Turrisi A et al. Twice-daily compared with once-daily thoracic radiotherapy in limited small cell lung cancer treated concurrently with cisplatin and etoposide. N Engl J Med. 1999; 340:265–71.

19. The correct answer is C. Intergroup 0096 compared daily radiotherapy 1.8–45 Gy, to BID radiotherapy of 1.5–45 Gy, with concurrent cisplatin/etoposide, beginning on day 1. Twice daily radiotherapy yielded a survival advantage compared to daily radiotherapy, with 5-year OS (26 % vs. 16 %, $p = 0.04$), though the incidence of grade 3 esophagitis also increased (27 % vs. 11 %, $p < 0.001$). Starting with week two, delivery of the afternoon fraction in the BID arm was delivered with off-cord obliques. Cord tolerance in this study for the BID arm was 36 Gy. Turrisi A et al. Twice-daily compared with once-daily thoracic radiotherapy in limited small cell lung cancer treated concurrently with cisplatin and etoposide. N Engl J Med. 1999;340:265–71.

20. The correct answer is D. Of the listed prophylactic cranial irradiation (PCI) fractionation schemes, 18 Gy in 10 fractions has not been extensively studied in small-cell lung cancer, though it is used for PCI in acute lymphoblastic leukemia.

A multicenter trial in the United Kingdom reported by Gregor et al. described outcomes for patients with limited-stage SCLC +/− PCI. Reported fractionation delivered included 8 Gy in 1 fraction, 30 Gy in 10 fractions, and 36 Gy in 18 fractions. There was a reduction seen in brain relapse at 2 years in those that received PCI, from 59 % to 29 % ($p=0.0002$), though this did not translate into an overall survival benefit. Gregor A et al. Effects of prophylactic cranial irradiation for patients with small cell lung cancer in complete response [abstract]. Eur J Cancer. 1995;31A:S19.

21. The correct answer is A. The meta-analysis by Auperin et al. included seven randomized trials and found that PCI after a complete response in limited-stage SCLC conferred a 5.4 % survival benefit, similar to that of adding thoracic radiotherapy to chemotherapy. Auperin A et al. For the PCI overview collaborative group: prophylactic cranial irradiation for patients with small-cell lung cancer in complete remission. N Engl J Med. 1999;342:476–84.

22. The correct answer is B. Optimal PCI dose was studied in a randomized trial by Lé Pechoux et al. Patients with limited-stage small-cell lung cancer in complete remission were randomized to receive either 25 Gy in 10 fractions or 36 Gy. The 36 Gy could be delivered conventionally in 18 fractions or with an accelerated hyperfractionated approach of BID fractions of 1.5 Gy × 12 days of treatment. There was no difference in the 2-year incidence of brain metastases: 29 % standard versus 23 % high dose. The 2-year overall survival was 42 % in the standard-dose arm and 37 % in the high-dose arm, but this is felt to represent increased cancer-related death rather than treatment-related mortality. Twenty-five gray remains the standard dose for limited-stage small-cell PCI. Lé Pechoux C et al. Standard-dose versus higher-dose prophylactic cranial irradiation (PCI) in patients with limited-stage small-cell lung cancer in complete remission after chemotherapy and thoracic radiotherapy (PCI 99-01, EORTC 220003-08004, RTOG 0212, and IFCT 99-01): a randomised clinical trial. Lancet Oncol. 2009;10(5):467–74.

23. The correct answer is B. Jeremic et al. reported results from their prospective randomized trial in which patients with extensive-stage small-cell lung cancer that experienced a complete response at distant sites and complete/partial response of intrathoracic disease after 3 cycles of cisplatin/etoposide were randomized to either receive (1) BID thoracic radiotherapy to 54 Gy with concurrent carboplatin followed by 2 cycles cisplatin/etoposide or (2) 4 cycles of cisplatin/etoposide alone. Those that received thoracic radiotherapy experienced significantly improved survival versus those that did not, MS: 17 months versus 11 months, $p=0.041$. Jeremic B et al. Role of radiation therapy in the combined-modality treatment of patients with extensive disease small-cell lung cancer: a randomized study. J Clin Oncol. 1999;17:2092–9.

24. The correct answer is B. In contrast to the Auperin meta-analysis for PCI with limited-stage small-cell lung cancer, a complete response was not required for those with extensive-stage small-cell lung cancer – ANY response was acceptable. Brain imaging was not required as a standard staging or follow-up procedure, unless symptoms indicative of brain metastases were present. Acceptable dose/fractionation schemes were 20 Gy in 5 or 8 fractions, 24 Gy in 12 fractions, 25 Gy in 10 fractions, or 30 Gy in 10 or 12 fractions. There was a 5.4 % survival benefit at 3 years seen with PCI in limited-stage small-cell lung cancer. At 1 year, survival after PCI for extensive-stage small-cell lung cancer was 27.1 % versus 13.3 %. Slotman BJ et al. Prophylactic cranial irradiation in extensive small-cell lung cancer. N Engl J Med. 2007;357:664–72.

25. The correct answer is B. The National Lung Screening Trial randomized 53, 454 participants at high risk for the development of lung cancer (history of 30 pack years smoking or former smoker quit within 15 years) to undergo three screenings at yearly intervals by either low-dose CT or chest radiograph. The incidence of lung cancer was 645 cases per 100,000 by low-dose CT, with 247 deaths from lung cancer versus 572 cases per 100,000 in the chest x-ray group, with 309 deaths. The death rate from any cause was reduced by 6.7 % compared to the radiograph group. The National Lung Screening Trial Research Team. N Engl J Med. 2011;365:395–409.

26. The correct answer is B. Mediastinal prevascular lymph nodes are level 3. Edge SB, Byrd DR, Compton CC, et al. editors. Lung. AJCC cancer staging handbook. 7th ed.. New York: Springer; 2010.

27. The correct answer is C. Lymph nodes in mediastinal level 5 (aortopulmonary window) are best evaluated through a Chamberlain procedure, also known as an anterior mediastinotomy. Lymph nodes adjacent to the trachea, levels 2L, 2R, 4R, 4L, and 7, are best evaluated by cervical mediastinoscopy. EUS-FNA can be performed for mediastinal nodes that can be accessed from the esophagus, particularly levels 7, 8, and 9. CT-guided biopsies are used most frequently to evaluate peripheral parenchymal lung nodules. Wagner H. Non-small cell lung cancer. In: Gunderson LL, Tepper JE, editors. Clinical radiation oncology. 3rd ed. Philadelphia: Elsevier Saunders; 2012. p. 805–38.

28. The correct answer is C. Tumors in the left upper lobe frequently drain to the contralateral paratracheal and anterior mediastinal lymph nodes. Baird A et al. The pathways of lymphatic spread of carcinoma of the lung. Br J Surg. 1965; 52:868–72.

29. The correct answer is B. Nodules in different lobes of the ipsilateral lung are now classified as T4 in the AJCC 7th edition. There were classified at M1 in the prior edition. T2 tumors are subclassified by size: T2a (>3 cm to ≤5 cm) or T2b (>5 cm to ≤7 cm). Edge SB, Byrd DR, Compton CC, et al. editors. Lung. AJCC cancer staging handbook. 7th ed. New York: Springer; 2010.

30. The correct answer is A. In the AJCC 7th edition, supraclavicular lymph node metastases, whether they are ipsilateral or contralateral, are classified as N3. T2 tumors are subclassified by size: T2a (>3 cm to ≤5 cm) or T2b (>5 cm to ≤7 cm). Edge SB, Byrd DR, Compton CC, et al. editors. Lung. AJCC cancer staging handbook. 7th ed. New York: Springer; 2010.

31. The correct answer is C. In the AJCC 7th edition, T3 tumors are classified as those >7 cm; directly invading pleura, chest wall, diaphragm, or phrenic nerve; with associated atelectasis of the entire lobe; invasion of the distal 2 cm of the mainstem bronchus without involvement of the carina; or separate tumor nodules in the same lobe. Ipsilateral hilar lymph node involvement is classified as N1. Pleural effusions are classified as M1a in the AJCC 7th edition; they were previously T4. M1b refers to distant metastases. Edge SB, Byrd DR, Compton CC, et al. editors. Lung. AJCC cancer staging handbook. 7th ed. New York: Springer; 2010.

32. The correct answer is B. Adenocarcinoma most commonly (75 %) presents in a peripheral location and can arise out of old tuberculosis scars. It has the slowest doubling time of non-small-cell lung cancer subtypes, and stage-for-stage has worse outcomes than squamous cell carcinoma. Wagner H. Non-small cell lung cancer. In: Gunderson LL, Tepper JE, editors. Clinical radiation oncology. 3rd ed. Philadelphia: Elsevier Saunders; 2012. p. 805–38. Arai T et al. Tumor doubling time and prognosis in lung cancer patients: evaluation from chest films and clinical follow-up study. Jpn. J Clin Oncol. 1994;24(4):199–204.

33. The correct answer is A. Of the listed subtypes of lung cancer, bronchioalveolar carcinoma is least related to smoking. Ebbert JO et al. Clinical features of bronchioalveolar carcinoma with new histologic and staging definitions. J Thoracic Oncol. 2010;5(8):1213–20. Wagner H. Non-small cell lung cancer. In: Gunderson LL, Tepper JE, editors. Clinical radiation oncology. 3rd ed. Philadelphia: Elsevier Saunders; 2012. p. 805–38.

34. The correct answer is D. More than 5,000 patients with inoperable bronchogenic carcinoma of the lung were entered in Veterans Administration Lung Group Protocols 9-15. Through these, the three most important prognostic factors affecting survival were found to be Karnofsky performance status, extent of disease, and weight loss in the previous 6 months. Stanley KE et al. Prognostic factors for survival in patients with inoperable lung cancer. J Natl Cancer Inst. 1980;65(1):25–32.

35. The correct answer is B. Participants in the Lung Cancer Study Group trial were randomized to undergo lobectomy versus limited resection for T1N0M0 lung cancer. There was significantly improved local control in those that underwent lobectomy; cancer mortality was increased in those that underwent limited resection, 62 % versus 55 %. Those that underwent wedge resection had a three-fold increase in local recurrence; those that underwent segmental resec-

tion had a 2.4-fold increase in local recurrence. Of those that underwent limited resection, none required postoperative ventilation >24 h. While the intent of the study was to show the equivalence of limited resection and lobectomy, given the increased local recurrence and cancer mortality associated with limited resection, the conclusion of the study was that lobectomy should remain the standard surgical treatment. Ginsberg R, Rubenstein L. Randomized trial of lobectomy versus limited resection for T1N0 non-small cell lung cancer. Lung Cancer Study Group. Ann Thorac Surg. 1995;60:615–23.

36. The correct answer is A. There is data showing that SBRT is an excellent therapy for medically inoperable early-stage lung tumors. While RTOG 0618, a phase II trial of SBRT in the treatment of medically operable stage I/II NSCLC, has completed accrual, for now, surgical resection remains the gold standard for operable NSCLC. Regarding the optimal surgery for resection of early-stage NSCLC, CALGB 140503 is an open phase III study looking at lobectomy versus sublobar resection for peripheral NSCLC tumors <2 cm. RTOG 1021/ACOSOG Z4099 is currently enrolling on a phase III trial comparing sublobar resection +/− brachytherapy versus SBRT in high-risk surgical patients with stage I NSCLC.

37. The correct answer is D. The Mountain data include clinical, surgical, pathologic, and follow-up data from 5319 combined consecutive patients with lung cancer (4351 treated at M.D. Anderson Cancer Center and 968 from the Reference Classification for Anatomic and Pathologic Classification of Lung Cancer database). The 5-year overall survival of a cT1N0 lung cancer is 61 %. Mountain CF. Revisions in the international lung cancer system for staging lung cancer. Chest. 1997;111(6):1710–7.

38. The correct answer is C. The Mountain data include clinical, surgical, pathologic, and follow-up data from 5319 combined consecutive patients with lung cancer (4351 treated at M.D. Anderson Cancer Center and 968 from the Reference Classification for Anatomic and Pathologic Classification of Lung Cancer database). The 5-year overall survival of a pT1N0 lung cancer is 67 %. Mountain CF. Revisions in the international lung cancer system for staging lung cancer. Chest. 1997;111(6):1710–7.

39. The correct answer is C. RTOG 0236 was a phase II study in which early-stage, medically inoperable NSCLC was treated with SBRT (prescription dose 20 Gy × 3 fractions without heterogeneity corrections). Both T1 and T2 tumors were included. Three-year primary tumor control rate was excellent (97.6 %), though there was a 22 % 3-year distant failure rate. Three-year overall survival was 55.8 %. Timmerman R et al. Stereotactic body radiation therapy for inoperable early stage lung cancer. JAMA. 2010;303(11):1070–6.

40. The correct answer is C. Describing their experience in which 257 patients with operable stage I NSCLC were treated with hypofractionated radiation (doses ranging 18–75 Gy at the isocenter in 1–22 fractions), Onishi et al. reported that

those treated with a dose of BED ≥ 100 Gy has statistically decreased 5-year local recurrence (8.4 % vs. 42.9 %, $p < 0.001$) and statistically increased 5-year overall survival (70.8 % vs. 30.2 %, $p < 0.05$). With these higher reported overall survivals, it is important to remember that these are operable patients. Onishi H et al. Hypofractionated stereotactic radiotherapy (HypoFXSRT) for stage I non-small cell lung cancer: updated results of 257 patients in a Japanese multi-institutional study. J Thora Oncol. 2007;2(7):S94–100.

41. The correct answer is B. The original PORT Meta-analysis published in 1998 included both published and unpublished trials ($n = 9$). Postoperative radiotherapy doses ranged from 30 to 60 Gy, and postoperative radiotherapy was associated with a 7 % absolute detriment in overall survival. This effect was seen mostly in N0/N1 patients. The role in N2 disease is less clear, while there is no benefit, there is no detriment seen. PORT Meta-analysis Trialists' Group. The Lancet. 1998;352(9124):257–63.

42. The correct answer is C. In the LCSG 773 trial, 210 patients with either T1-2/N1 or T3 or T, any N2 squamous cell carcinoma of the lung were randomized after surgery to observation or postoperative radiotherapy (50 Gy). The addition of postoperative radiotherapy improved local control for all patients, even those with only N1 disease, but there was no overall survival benefit. In N2 patients, there was a trend towards improved survival. Weisenburger TH et al. The lung cancer study group: effects of postoperative mediastinal radiation on completely resected stage II and stage II epidermoid cancer of the lung. N Engl J Med. 1986;315:1377–81.

43. The correct answer is D. The Medical Research Council (MRC) Trial of postoperative radiotherapy randomized 308 patients with R0 resected (negative margins) pT1-2/N1-2 lung cancer to either observation or postoperative radiotherapy (40 Gy/15 fractions). The addition of postoperative radiotherapy did not show any benefit in patients with N1 disease. However, subset analysis of those with N2 disease showed improved local control and a 1-month gain in median survival (17.6 months vs. 16.2 months). Stephens RJ et al. The role of postoperative radiotherapy in non-small-cell lung cancer: a multicentre randomised trial in patients with pathologically stage T1-2, N1-2, M0 disease. Medical Research Council Lung Cancer Working Party. Br J Cancer. 1996;74(4):632–9.

44. The correct answer is A. The International Adjuvant Lung Cancer Trial (IALT) randomized 1867 patients after surgery to observation versus chemotherapy with a cisplatin doublet. The second agent (etoposide, vindesine, vinblastine, vinorelbine) was given as per institutional preference. Radiation therapy was permitted after the completion of chemotherapy. Adjuvant chemotherapy was associated with a 4 % absolute benefit in 5-year OS (44 % vs. 40 %, $p < 0.03$), and this benefit was present for all stage groups. Arriagada R et al. for the International Adjuvant Lung Cancer Trial (IALT) Group. Cisplatin-based adjuvant chemotherapy in patients with completely resected non-small-cell lung cancer. N Engl J Med. 2004;350:351–60.

45. The correct answer is D. CALGB 9633 randomized postoperative T2N0M0 tumors to observation versus 4 cycles of adjuvant carboplatin/paclitaxel. Eighty-six percent of patients were able to receive all 4 cycles, and of these patients, 66 % were able to receive the full doses. Neutropenia was the predominant grade 3/4 toxicity. Looking at all the T2 tumors, there was no survival benefit to adjuvant chemotherapy. On subset analysis, those with tumors ≥4 cm who received chemotherapy did demonstrate a significant improvement in overall survival. Strauss GM et al. Adjuvant paclitaxel plus carboplatin compared with observation in stage IB non-small-cell lung cancer: CALGB 9633 with the cancer and leukemia group B, radiation therapy oncology group, and North central cancer treatment group study groups. J Clin Oncol. 2008;(26):5043–51.

46. The correct answer is B. The preoperative trial reported by Rosell et al. randomized 60 patients with stage IIIA NSCLC to either undergo preoperative chemotherapy with 3 cycles of mitomycin, ifosfamide, and cisplatin followed by surgery or surgery alone. All patients received postoperative mediastinal radiation to 50 Gy. Median survival was improved in those that received combined therapy, 26 versus 8 months ($p < 0.001$). Median disease-free survival was also improved: 20 versus 5 months ($p < 0.001$), as was the rate of local recurrence, 56 % versus 74 %. Rosell R et al. A randomized trial comparing preoperative chemotherapy plus surgery with surgery alone in patients with non-small cell lung cancer. N Engl J Med. 1994;330(3):153–8.

47. The correct answer is D. The CALBG 8433 trial as reported by Dillman et al. randomized patients with stage III NSCLC—either by clinical or surgical staging – to receive either induction cisplatin on d 1 and 29 or vinblastine on d 1,8, 15, 22, and 29 + radiotherapy to 60 Gy versus definitive radiotherapy alone to 60 Gy. As reported in the JNCI with more than 7 years of follow-up, the addition of induction chemotherapy improved median survival to 13.7 m compared to 9.6 m ($p = 0.012$). Dillman RO et al. J Natl Cancer Institute. 1996;88:1210–5.

48. The correct answer is C. Intergroup 0139 randomized patients with stage IIIA NSCLC with ipsilateral N2 nodes to undergo either definitive chemoradiation (cisplatin/etoposide × 2 cycles concurrent to 61 Gy) followed by two additional cycles of cisplatin/etoposide versus preoperative chemoradiation with 2 cycles of concurrent cisplatin/etoposide to 45 Gy, then resection if there was no progression, followed by two additional cycles of cisplatin/etoposide. There was no difference in survival between the two arms, though progression-free survival and local control were both improved with the addition of surgery. No differences were noted in the first site of progression. On exploratory analysis, those that underwent lobectomy rather than pneumonectomy were found to have significantly improved survival (MS, 33.6 months vs. 21.7 months). Neutropenia was the most common grade 3 or 4 toxicity; esophagitis was the second most common grade 3 or 4 toxicity. Albain KS et al. Radiotherapy plus chemotherapy with or without surgical resection for stage III non-small-cell lung cancer: a phase III randomised controlled trial. Lancet. 2009;374(9687):379–86.

49. The correct answer is A. Intergroup 0139 randomized patients with stage IIIA NSCLC with ipsilateral N2 nodes to undergo either definitive chemoradiation (cisplatin/etoposide × 2 cycles concurrent to 61 Gy) followed by two additional cycles of cisplatin/etoposide versus preoperative chemoradiation with 2 cycles of concurrent cisplatin/etoposide to 45 Gy, then resection if there was no progression, followed by two additional cycles of cisplatin/etoposide. There was no difference in survival between the two arms, though progression-free survival and local control were both improved with the addition of surgery. No differences were noted in the first site of progression. On exploratory analysis, those that underwent lobectomy rather than pneumonectomy were found to have significantly improved survival (MS, 33.6 months vs. 21.7 months). Neutropenia was the most common grade 3 or 4 toxicity; esophagitis was the second most common grade 3 or 4 toxicity. Albain KS et al. Radiotherapy plus chemotherapy with or without surgical resection for stage III non-small-cell lung cancer: a phase III randomised controlled trial. Lancet. 2009;374(9687):379–86.

50. The correct answer is A. RTOG 73-01 established 60 Gy as the standard dose for locally advanced NSCLC. In this randomized study, 365 patients with unresectable NSCLC were randomized to one of four arms: 40 Gy split course, 40 Gy continuous, 50 Gy continuous, and 60 Gy continuous. Survival was worst in the split-course arm, 10 % at 2 years. There was a dose response noted in terms of increased tumor regression and decreased intrathoracic recurrence, with increasing dose. The most frequent complications were pneumonitis, pulmonary fibrosis, and dysphagia from transient esophagitis. RTOG 94-10 reported by Curran et al. established the survival benefit of concurrent chemoradiation with standard fractionation over sequential chemotherapy then radiation. Perez CA et al. A Prospective randomized study of various irradiation doses and fractionation schedules in the treatment of inoperable non-oat-cell carcinoma of the lung. Cancer. 1980;45:2744–53. Curran WJ et al. Sequential vs. concurrent chemoradiation for stage iii non-small cell lung cancer: randomized phase III trial RTOG 9410. J Natl Cancer Inst. 2011;103:1–9.

51. The correct answer is D. Treatment of an upper lobe tumor is least likely to increase the risk of pneumonitis, likely due to the decreased volume of lung treated. All the others increase the risk of pneumonitis. Lind P et al. Receiver operating characteristic curves to assess predictors of radiation-induced symptomatic lung injury. Int J Radiat Oncol Biol Phys. 2002;54:340–7. Yamada M et al. Risk factors for pneumonitis following chemoradiotherapy for lung cancer. Eur J Cancer. 1998;34:71–5.

52. The correct answer is C. Amifostine, trade name Ethyol®, is a thioester that scavenges free radicals. It is usually delivered IV or SC shortly prior to radiotherapy. Hypotension is the most common side effect observed. While it has been shown to decrease xerostomia when treating H&N tumors, there was no statistically significant improvement in measured grade 3 esophagitis in a phase III study with concurrent irradiation, carboplatin, and paclitaxel. Movsas

B et al. Randomized trial of amifostine in locally advanced non-small cell lung cancer patients receiving chemotherapy and hyperfractionated radiation: radiation therapy oncology group trial 98-01. J Clin Oncol. 2005;23(10):2145–54.

53. The correct answer is D. In RTOG 98-01, 243 patients with stage II–IIIA/B non-small-cell lung cancer first received induction carboplatin/paclitaxel on days 1 and 22, followed by concurrent chemoradiation to 69.6 Gy/1.2 Gy BID with weekly carboplatin and paclitaxel with or without amifostine (500 mg/m^2, four times per week). The majority of patients randomized to amifostine (72 %) received amifostine either per protocol or with only a minor deviation. There was no difference in the rate of grade 3 esophagitis (30 % vs. 34 %, $p=0.9$) with the addition of amifostine. Movsas B et al. Randomized trial of amifostine in locally advanced non-small cell lung cancer patients receiving chemotherapy and hyperfractionated radiation: radiation therapy oncology group trial 98-01. J Clin Oncol. 2005;23(10):2145–54.

54. The correct answer is D. RTOG 0617 is a 4-arm study with two purposes: (1) ascertain benefit of dose escalation and (2) ascertain benefit of addition of anti-EGFR therapy with cetuximab to standard chemotherapy. Patients with stage IIIA or B NSCLC were stratified according to RT technique (3D-CRT vs. IMRT), Zubrod performance status (0 vs. 1), use of PET staging (yes vs. no), and histology (squamous vs. non-squamous) to one of four arms: (1) chemoRT to 60 Gy, (2) chemoRT to 74 Gy, (3) chemoRT + cetuximab to 60 Gy, and (4) chemoRT + cetuximab to 74 Gy. Standard chemotherapy in all arms consisted of carboplatin (AUC=2/week) and paclitaxel (45 mg/m^2/week). Cetuximab was given as a loading dose of 400 mg/m^2 on day 1, then weekly at 250 mg/m^2 each subsequent week. All arms were to subsequently receive 2 cycles of consolidation chemotherapy with or without cetuximab depending on their randomization. Critical structure constraints included keeping the total lung V20 ≤ 37 %. A planned early analysis showed that the high-dose arm had crossed the futility boundary and the dose escalation phase of the study was closed. When comparing survival between the high- and low-dose arms, survival was found to be greater in the low-dose arms, 1-year OS: 70.4 % versus 81 %, though toxicity was not different between the two dose groups. It is suggested that effects on the normal lung and heart are responsible for the findings. Despite closure of the dose escalation phase of the study, the cetuximab portion of the study is still open. RTOG 0617 Protocol- PI Jeffrey Bradley. A Randomized Phase III Comparison of Standard-Dose (60 Gy) versus High dose (74 Gy) Conformal Radiotherapy with Concurrent and Consolidation Carboplatin/Paclitaxel +/− Cetuximab (IND#103444) in Patients with Stage IIIA/IIIB Non-Small Cell Lung Cancer. Version 6/30/2011. Cox JD. Are the results of RTOG 0617 mysterious? Int J Radiat Oncol Biol Phys. 2012;82(3):1042–4.

55. The correct answer is B. RTOG 0617 is a 4-arm study with two purposes: (1) ascertain benefit of dose escalation and (2) ascertain benefit of addition of anti-EGFR therapy with cetuximab to standard chemotherapy. Patients with stage IIIA or B NSCLC were stratified according to RT technique (3D-CRT vs. IMRT), Zubrod performance status (0 vs. 1), use of PET staging (yes vs. no), and histology (squamous vs. non-squamous) to one of four arms: (1) chemoRT to 60 Gy, (2) chemoRT to 74 Gy, (3) chemoRT+cetuximab to 60 Gy, and (4) chemoRT + cetuximab to 74 Gy. Chemotherapy in all arms consisted of carboplatin (AUC = 2/week) and paclitaxel (45 mg/m^2/week). Cetuximab was given as a loading dose of 400 mg/m^2 on day 1, then weekly at 250 mg/m^2 each subsequent week. All arms were to subsequently receive 2 cycles of consolidation chemotherapy with or without cetuximab depending on their randomization. Critical structure constraints included keeping the total lung V20 ≤ 37 %. A planned early analysis showed that the high-dose arm had crossed the futility boundary and the dose escalation phase of the study was closed. When comparing survival between the high- and low-dose arms, survival was found to be greater in the low-dose arms, 1-year OS: 70.4 % versus 81 %, though toxicity was not different between the two dose groups. It is suggested that effects on the normal lung and heart are responsible for the findings. Despite closure of the dose escalation phase of the study, the cetuximab portion of the study is still open. RTOG 0617 Protocol- PI Jeffrey Bradley. A Randomized Phase III Comparison of Standard-Dose (60 Gy) versus High dose (74 Gy) Conformal Radiotherapy with Concurrent and Consolidation Carboplatin/Paclitaxel +/− Cetuximab (IND#103444) in Patients with Stage IIIA/IIIB Non-Small Cell Lung Cancer. Version 6/30/2011. Cox JD. Are the results of RTOG 0617 mysterious? Int J Radiat Oncol Biol Phys. 2012;82(3):1042–4.

56. The correct answer is C. The LAMP trial randomized 257 patients to one of three arms: (1) induction carbo/taxol × 2 cycles, with radiation alone to post-chemotherapy volume (63 Gy) starting on day 42; (2) induction carbo/taxol × 2 cycles, followed by concurrent chemoradiation to 63 Gy, concurrent chemo = weekly taxol with q3week carbo × 2 cycles; and (3) concurrent chemoradiation followed by 2 cycles of consolidative chemotherapy, concurrent chemo = weekly taxol with q3week carbo × 2 cycles. Arm two was closed after an early interim analysis. Those patients in the consolidative chemotherapy arm had the highest percentage of completion of the scheduled radiotherapy dose (81 % vs. 76 % and 70 % in the other two arms). Neutropenia was the most common grade 3 or 4 toxicity. There was increased esophagitis in the concurrent chemoradiation arms. With a median follow-up of 39.6 months, there was no difference in MS between the arms, 13 versus 12.7 versus 16.3 months. There was a trend for improved survival in the concurrent chemoradiation followed by consolidative chemotherapy arm. Belani CP et al. J Clin Oncol. 2005;23(25):5883–91.

57. The correct answer is D. The LAMP trial randomized 257 patients to one of three arms: (1) induction carbo/taxol × 2 cycles, with radiation alone to post-chemotherapy volume (63 Gy) starting on day 42; (2) induction carbo/taxol × 2 cycles, followed by concurrent chemoradiation to 63 Gy, concurrent chemo = weekly taxol with q3week carbo × 2 cycles; and (3) concurrent chemoradiation followed by 2 cycles of consolidative chemotherapy, concurrent chemo = weekly taxol with q3week carbo × 2 cycles. Arm two was closed after an early interim analysis. Those patients in the consolidative chemotherapy arm had the highest percentage of completion of the scheduled radiotherapy dose (81 % vs. 76 % and 70 % in the other two arms). Neutropenia was the most common grade 3 or 4 toxicity. There was increased esophagitis in the concurrent chemoradiation arms. With a median follow-up of 39.6 months, there was no difference in MS between the arms, 13 versus 12.7 versus 16.3 months. There was a trend for improved survival in the concurrent chemoradiation followed by consolidative chemotherapy arm. Belani CP, et al. J Clin Oncol. 2005;23(25): 5883–91.

58. The correct answer is B. Rosenzweig et al. reported their experience of treating NSCLC with involved nodal rather than elective nodal irradiation in an effort to decrease toxicity while treating the GTV to a higher dose. Involved nodes were defined as lymph nodes pathologically proven to be involved and radiographically ≥15 mm in the short axis on CT. With a median follow-up of 21 months, they reported 11 of 171 patients (6.4 %) failing in the elective nodal region, with a median time of 4 months to failure. Two-year actuarial rates of elective nodal and primary control were 91 % and 38 %, respectively. Rosenzweig KE et al. Elective nodal irradiation in the treatment of non-small-cell lung cancer with three-dimensional conformal radiation therapy. Int J Radiat Oncol Biol Phys. 2001;50(3):681–5.

59. The correct answer is C. The Hoosier Oncology Group Phase III study of concurrent chemoradiation with cisplatin/etoposide to 59.4 Gy with or without consolidation docetaxel × 3 cycles in eligible stage IIIA/IIIB NSCLC patients showed no survival benefit compared to observation after definitive chemoradiation. Of those randomized to consolidation docetaxel, 80.8 % completed all three planned cycles. There was increased toxicity in the docetaxel arm, with 10.9 % experiencing febrile neutropenia and 9.6 % experiencing grade 3–5 pneumonitis, compared to 1.4 % in the observation arm. More patients required hospitalization in the docetaxel arm (28.8 %) compared to the observation arm (8.1 %). Median survival was not improved with docetaxel 21.2 months versus 23.2 months in the observation arm ($p = 0.883$). Hanna N et al. Phase III study of cisplatin, etoposide, and concurrent chest radiation with or without consolidation docetaxel in patients with inoperable stage III non-small cell lung cancer: the Hoosier oncology group and U.S. oncology. J Clin Oncol. 2008;26(35): 5755–60.

60. The correct answer is D. RTOG 94-10 was the phase III trial that established concurrent chemoradiation as the standard of care for advanced non-small-cell lung cancer. In this study, 610 patients with medically or surgically inoperable stage II–IIIB NSCLC were randomized to one of three arms: (1) induction cisplatin 100 mg/m² on days 1 and 29/vinblastine 5 mg/m² weekly then 63 Gy starting Day 50 (Dillman 8433 arm); (2) cisplatin 100 mg/m² on days 1 and 29/vinblastine 5 mg/m² weekly with radiation to 63 Gy starting on day 1 (concurrent chemoRT arm); and (3) cisplatin 50 mg/m² on days 1, 8, 29, and 36/etoposide 50 mg BID x 10 days on RT days 1-5, 8-12, with radiation to 69.6 Gy in 1.2 Gy BID fractions starting on day 1 (concurrent hyperfractionated arm). With a median follow-up of 11 years, Curran et al. reported improved median survival in the concurrent chemoRT arms. Median survivals were 14.6, 17.0, and 15.6 months in the respective arms. Acute grade 3–5 non-hematologic toxicities were greater in the concurrent chemoradiation arms, with grade 3 or worse esophagitis worst in the hyperfractionated arm. Late esophagitis rates were similar between the arms at 1–4 %. Curran WJ et al. Sequential vs. concurrent chemoradiation for stage III non-small cell lung cancer: randomized phase III trial of RTOG 9410. J Natl Cancer Inst. 2011;103:1–9.

61. The correct answer is B. RTOG 94-10 was the phase III trial that established concurrent chemoradiation as the standard of care for advanced non-small-cell lung cancer. In this study, 610 patients with medically or surgically inoperable stage II–IIIB NSCLC were randomized to one of three arms: (1) induction cisplatin 100 mg/m² on days 1 and 29/vinblastine 5 mg/m² weekly then 63 Gy starting Day 50 (Dillman 8433 arm); (2) cisplatin 100 mg/m² on days 1 and 29/vinblastine 5 mg/m² weekly with radiation to 63 Gy starting on day 1 (concurrent chemoRT arm); and (3) cisplatin 50 mg/m² on days 1, 8, 29, and 36/etoposide 50 mg BID × 10 days on RT days 1–5, 8–12, with radiation to 69.6 Gy in 1.2 Gy BID fractions starting on day 1 (concurrent hyperfractionated arm). With a median follow-up of 11 years, Curran et al. reported improved median survival in the concurrent chemoRT arms. Median survivals were 14.6, 17.0, and 15.6 months in the respective arms. Acute grade 3–5 non-hematologic toxicities were greater in the concurrent chemoradiation arms, with grade 3 or worse esophagitis worst in the hyperfractionated arm. Late esophagitis rates were similar between the arms at 1–4 %. Curran WJ et al. Sequential vs. concurrent chemoradiation for stage III non-small cell lung cancer: randomized phase III trial of RTOG 9410. J Natl Cancer Inst. 2011; 103:1–9.

62. The correct answer is B. RTOG 88-08 enrolled 452 patients and randomized them to one of three regimens for locally advanced, surgically unresectable stage II–IIIB NSCLC: (1) standard radiotherapy 60 Gy/30 fx, (2) induction cisplatin/vinblastine followed by standard radiotherapy (60 Gy/30 fx) starting on day 50, and (3) twice daily radiotherapy (69.2 Gy/BID 1.2 Gy fractions). More than 95 % of patients were stage IIIA or IIIB, and over two thirds had a KPS ≥80.

Median survival was highest in the concurrent chemoradiation arm 13.8 months and statistically improved to the other two arms, 11.4 months RT alone and 12.3 months hyperFX ($p=0.03$). Sause WT et al. Radiation Therapy Oncology Group (RTOG) 88-08 and Eastern Cooperative Oncology Group (ECOG) 4588: preliminary results of a phase III trial in regionally advanced, unresectable non-small-cell lung cancer. J Natl Cancer Inst. 1995;87(3):198–205.

63. The correct answer is D. Schaake-Koning et al. randomized 331 patients with unresectable non-small-cell lung cancer to one of three treatment arms: (1) split-course RT alone, 30 Gy, then 25 Gy; (2) split-course RT with weekly cisplatin; and (3) split-course RT with daily cisplatin. The addition of chemotherapy improved both local control and overall survival, but significantly increased acute toxicity. There was no benefit to daily cisplatin compared to weekly cisplatin. Schaake-Koning C et al. Effects of concomitant cisplatin and radiotherapy on inoperable non-small cell lung cancer. N Engl J Med. 1992;326:524–30.

64. The correct answer is A. Continuous hyperfractionated accelerated radiation treatment was studied in the United Kingdom by the Medical Research Council. In this trial, an aggressive TID hyperfractionation regimen to 54 Gy in 12 days was compared to standard 60 Gy/30 fractions. The CHART regimen was found to confer a survival advantage compared to conventional fractionation with 1-year survival improved from 55 % to 63 % and 2-year survival improving from 20 % to 29 %. While there was increased acute toxicity, there was no increase in late toxicity. Saunders M et al. Continuous hyperfractionated accelerated radiotherapy (CHART) versus conventional radiotherapy in non-small-cell lung cancer: a randomised multicentre trial. Lancet 1997;350(9072):161–5.

65. The correct answer is D. Radiation pneumonitis is treated with a slow taper of prednisone, prescribed at either 1 mg/kg/day or 60 mg/day. Along with prednisone, trimethoprim-sulfamethoxazole should be given for PCP prophylaxis.

66. The correct answer is B. The symptom of sudden electric shocks extending down the spine with head flexion, infrequently associated with treatment of non-small-cell lung cancer, is known as Lhermitte's syndrome. Nelson's syndrome is enlargement of a pituitary adenoma in a patient with Cushing's disease after removal of the adrenals – results from loss of feedback inhibition of cortisol. Lemierre's syndrome is when an oropharyngeal infection is complicated by internal jugular vein thrombosis and metastatic lung abscesses. Ring enhancement is seen in the internal jugular vein on CT. Garcin syndrome is extensive unilateral cranial palsies associated with malignancy in the nasopharynx or base of skull.

67. The correct answer is C. RTOG 0214 randomized 356 patients (target accrual 1058) with stage III NSCLC without disease progression after surgery and/or radiation with or without chemotherapy to either receive prophylactic cranial

irradiation (30 Gy in 15 fractions) versus observation. Patients were stratified according to stage (IIIA vs. IIIB), histology (squamous vs. non-squamous), and therapy (surgery vs. none). The study was closed early due to poor accrual. While PCI in patients with treated NSCLC did improve the rate of brain metastasis, it did not improve overall survival nor disease-free survival. One-year OS between the two arms was not statistically different, 75.6 % PCI versus 76.9 % obs ($p=0.86$), nor was disease-free survival. The 1-year rates of brain metastases were significantly different, 7.7 % PCI versus 18 % obs ($p=0.004$). Gore EM et al. Phase III comparison of prophylactic cranial irradiation versus observation in patients with locally advanced non-small- cell lung cancer: primary analysis of radiation therapy oncology group study RTOG 0214. J Clin Oncol. 2011;29(3):272–8.

68. The correct answer is C. The SWOG 0023 trial randomized patients with stage IIIA/B NSCLC after definitive chemoRT and 3 cycles of adjuvant docetaxel to observation versus gefitinib. Concurrent chemotherapy consisted of 2 cycles of cisplatin/etoposide. Total radiotherapy dose delivered was 61 Gy. The addition of gefitinib did not improve progression-free nor median survival. MS was 23 months in the gefitinib group versus 35 months in the observation group. Kelly K et al. J Clin Oncol. 2007, ASCO Annual Meeting Proceedings Part I. Vol 25, No. 18S (June 20 Supplement), 2007:7513.

69. The correct answer is A. Ramella et al. published their experience of treating 97 patients with NSCLC treated with 3D-CRT and chemotherapy, incorporating ipsilateral lung dosimetric planning constraints in an effort to predict and minimize radiation pneumonitis. After 3D-CRT treatment planning, patients were only treated if total lung V20 ≤31 %, V30 ≤18 %, and mean lung dose ≤20 Gy. After treatment, total lung and ipsilateral lung dose-volume histogram parameters and total dose delivered were correlated with pneumonitis incidence in an effort to develop additional dosimetric constraints to minimize pneumonitis. They found that the most statistically significant factors predicting pneumonitis were V20ipsilateral (V20 ipsi), V30 ipsilateral (V30ipsi), and planning target volume. Those patients exceeding these ipsilateral constraints were classified as the high-risk group, whereas those meeting ipsilateral criteria were classified as low risk. Risk of pneumonitis for each of the constraints by risk group is listed in Table 4.1.

Table 4.1 Risk of pneumonitis by ipsilateral lung DVH parameters

	Low-risk	High-risk	Low-risk	High-risk
	V20ipsi ≤52 %	V20ipsi >52 %	V30ipsi≤ 39 %	V30ipsi >39 %
Risk of pneumonitis	9 %	46 %	8 %	38 %

Adapted from Ramella et al. Risk of grade 2 pneumonitis by ipsilateral lung DVH parameters. Int J Radiat Oncol Biol Phys. 2010;76(1):110–5.

70. The correct answer is B. Of the listed histologic subtypes, large cell is a subtype of adenocarcinoma, not malignant mesothelioma. Rengan R, Bonner Millar LP, Thomas CR Jr. Uncommon thoracic tumors. In: Gunderson LL, Tepper JE, editors. Clinical radiation oncology. 3rd ed. Philadelphia: Elsevier Saunders; 2012. p. 859–902.

71. The correct answer is A. Of the listed histologic subtypes of malignant pleural mesothelioma, epithelioid type has the best prognosis. Rengan R, Bonner Millar LP, Thomas CR Jr. Uncommon thoracic tumors. In: Gunderson LL, Tepper JE, editors. Clinical radiation oncology. 3rd ed. Philadelphia: Elsevier Saunders; 2012. p. 859–902.

72. The correct answer is C. Pass et al. described their results from a cohort study comparing 69 patients with asbestos-related nonmalignant pulmonary disease, 45 patients without asbestos exposure, and 76 patients with surgically staged pleural mesothelioma. In this study, they found that osteopontin, a suggested biomarker for pleural mesothelioma, could be identified by enzyme-linked immunoabsorbent assay (ELISA). As such, serum osteopontin levels in persons with exposure to asbestos could be used to identify early-stage (stage I) pleural mesothelioma, as serum osteopontin levels were significantly higher in those with pleural mesothelioma than in the group without exposure to asbestos. Calcitonin is a biomarker for medullary thyroid cancer. Chromogranin A is a biomarker of neuroendocrine tumors. Nuclear matrix protein 22 is a biomarker used to monitor response to treatment in bladder cancer. Pass H et al. Asbestos exposure, pleural mesothelioma, and serum osteopontin levels. N Engl J Med. 2005;353(15):1564–73.

73. The correct answer is D. Of the listed chemotherapy doublets, only cisplatin/ pemetrexed is approved by the FDA and was shown in a phase III trial of unresectable malignant pleural mesothelioma to improve survival compared to cisplatin alone (12.1 months vs. 9.3 months, $p = 0.02$). Cisplatin/gemcitabine is an option for chemotherapy as recommended by the NCCN after it was shown in phase II studies to improve median survival. Carboplatin/pemetrexed is also an acceptable NCCN recommended therapy as it was found in two phase II studies to improve median survival. Cisplatin/etoposide has a role in treating non-small-cell lung cancer, not malignant pleural mesothelioma. Vogelzang NJ et al. Phase III study of pemetrexed in combination with cisplatin versus cisplatin alone in patients with malignant pleural mesothelioma. J Clin Oncol. 2003;21:2636–44. Van Haarst et al. Multicentre phase II study of gemcitabine and cisplatin in malignant pleural mesothelioma. Br J Cancer. 2002;86:342–5. Nowak AK et al. A multicentre phase II study of cisplatin and gemcitabine for malignant mesothelioma. Br J Cancer. 2002;87:491–96. Ceresoli GL et al. Phase II study of pemetrexed plus carboplatin in malignant pleural mesothelioma. J Clin Oncol. 2006;24:1443–8. Castagneto B et al. Phase II study of pemetrexed in combination with carboplatin in patients with malignant pleural mesothelioma (MPM). Ann Oncol. 2008;19:370–3.

74. The correct answer is C. The role of radiotherapy in the treatment of malignant pleural mesothelioma (MPM) is limited. While there may be a role as part of multimodality therapy in resectable MPM, there is little role in unresectable disease, as high-dose radiation to the entire hemithorax has NOT shown to improve survival and carries with it significant toxicity. In resected MPM, total adjuvant radiotherapy dose should fall between 50 and 60 Gy, depending on margin status. A retrospective review showed that survival may be dose dependent, with those receiving >40 Gy living longer than those receiving <40 Gy. In those that have undergone pleural intervention, adjuvant radiotherapy to the tract site is recommended – 700 cGy × 3. Baldini EH et al. Radiation therapy options for malignant pleural mesothelioma. Semin Thorac Cardiovasc Surg. 2009;21:159–63. Gupta V et al. Patterns of local and nodal failure in malignant pleural mesothelioma after extrapleural pneumonectomy and photon- electron radiotherapy. J Thorac Oncol. 2009;4:746–50. Rusch VW et al. A phase II trial of surgical resection and adjuvant high-dose hemithoracic radiation for malignant pleural mesothelioma. J Thorac Cardiovasc Surg. 2001;122:788–95. Manegold C et al. Second-line (post-study) chemotherapy received by patients treated in the phase III trial of pemetrexed plus cisplatin versus cisplatin alone in malignant pleural mesothelioma. Ann Oncol. 2005;16:923–7. Di Salvo et al. Prevention of malignant seeding at drain sites after invasive procedures (surgery and/or thoracoscopy) by hypofractionated radiotherapy in patients with pleural mesothelioma. Acta Oncol. 2008;47:1094–8.

75. The correct answer is C. Di Salvo et al. reported their experience of treating the tract sites of 32 patients that had undergone surgery and/or thoracoscopy for diagnosis, staging, or talc pleurodesis. In this retrospective review, at a mean follow-up of 13.6 months, there were no local recurrences after treating the sites with 700 cGy × 3 fractions. RTOG grade 1 toxicity erythema was reported in 11 of the patients. Di Salvo M et al. Prevention of malignant seeding at drain sites after invasive procedures (surgery and/or thoracoscopy) by hypofractionated radiotherapy in patients with pleural mesothelioma. Acta Oncol. 2008;47: 1094–8.

76. The correct answer is B. While contralateral mediastinal involvement, diaphragmatic invasion, and distant metastatic disease preclude surgery, the presence of multiple pleural plaques in the ipsilateral lung does not constitute unresectability. Rengan R, Bonner Millar LP, Thomas CR Jr. Uncommon thoracic tumors. In: Gunderson LL, Tepper JE, editors. Clinical radiation oncology. 3rd ed. Philadelphia: Elsevier Saunders; 2012. p. 859–902.

Chapter 5
Tumors of the Mediastinum

Celine Bicquart Ord and Charles R. Thomas, Jr.

Questions

1. What is the most common tumor of the anterior mediastinum?
   A. Thymic carcinoma
   B. Thymoma
   C. Non-seminomatous germ cell tumor
   D. Thymic carcinoid tumor

2. Which of the following subtypes of thymic carcinoma has the best prognosis?
   A. Clear cell
   B. Sarcomatoid
   C. Basaloid
   D. Anaplastic

3. All of the following are risk factors for the development of thymic tumors, except:
   A. Childhood thymic irradiation
   B. EBV infection
   C. Familial cytogenetic abnormalities
   D. HPV infection

C.B. Ord, MD (✉)
Department of Radiation Oncology, Scott & White Memorial Hospital,
2401 S. 31st Street, Temple, TX 76508, USA
e-mail: cord@sw.org

C.R. Thomas Jr., MD (✉)
Department of Radiation Medicine, Oregon Health & Science University, Knight Cancer Institute,
181 SW Sam Jackson Park Road, KPV4, Portland, OR 97239-3098, USA
e-mail: thomasch@ohsu.edu; thomas@gmail.com

C.B. Ord et al. (eds.), *Radiation Oncology Study Guide*,
DOI 10.1007/978-1-4614-6400-6_5, © Springer Science+Business Media New York 2013

4. What percentage of patients with thymoma is associated with myasthenia gravis?
   A. 20 %
   B. 40 %
   C. 60 %
   D. 80 %

5. What percentage of patients with myasthenia gravis have an associated thymic neoplasm?
   A. <5 %
   B. 10 %
   C. 20 %
   D. 30 %

6. Patients with which of the following thymoma-associated autoimmune diseases will have a more favorable prognosis?
   A. Myasthenia gravis
   B. Red cell aplasia
   C. Hypogammaglobulinemia
   D. Lupus erythematosus

7. Which of the following histologic subtypes of thymoma has the best prognosis?
   A. Cortical
   B. Organoid
   C. Mixed
   D. Medullary

8. Which one of the following anatomical structures is not found in the anterior compartment of the mediastinum?
   A. Pulmonary vessels
   B. Superior vena cava
   C. Thymus
   D. Aortic arch

9. What percentage of thymoma is incidentally found on chest radiograph?
   A. 10 %
   B. 30 %
   C. 50 %
   D. 70 %

10. The Masaoka staging system for thymoma is based on:
    A. Clinical staging
    B. Both clinical and pathological findings at the time of surgery
    C. Pathological findings at the time of surgery
    D. Pathological findings at the time of surgery and histologic subtype

11. What Masaoka stage would be most appropriate for a thymoma that has been completely resected and found to have macroscopic invasion into the pericardium?
    A. Masaoka stage I
    B. Masaoka stage II
    C. Masaoka stage III
    D. Masaoka stage IV

12. Which of the following would be the preferred treatment option for a stage III/IVa unresectable thymoma?
    A. Preoperative chemotherapy, then surgery
    B. Preoperative chemoradiation, then surgery
    C. Definitive chemoradiation
    D. Hospice

Answers and Rationales

1. The correct answer is B. Thymoma is the most common tumor of the anterior mediastinum. Davis RD et al. Primary cysts and neoplasms of the mediastinum: recent changes in clinical presentation, methods of diagnosis, management, and results. Ann Thorac Surg. 1987;44:229–37. Mullen B et al. Primary anterior mediastinal tumors in children and adults. Ann Thorac Surg. 1986;42:338–45.

2. The correct answer is C. Of the listed subtypes of thymic carcinoma, the basaloid subtype has the best prognosis, with a lower incidence of local recurrence and metastasis. The clear cell, sarcomatoid, and anaplastic subtypes have a higher propensity for local invasion and subsequent metastasis. Ritter JH et al. Primary carcinomas of the thymus gland. Semin Diagn Pathol. 1999;16:18–31. Ogawa K et al. Treatment and prognosis of thymic carcinoma: a retrospective analysis of 40 cases. Cancer. 2002;94:3115–9.

3. The correct answer is D. Childhood thymic radiation, EBV infection, and familial cytogenetic abnormalities are all risk factors for the development of thymic tumors. One series reported 30 % of thymic carcinomas were associated with MEN types 1 and 2. Other studies showed translocation of chromosomes 15 and 19 [t(15;19)(q15:p13)] in young adult and pediatric patients with high-grade thymic carcinoma. Benign thymomas can also be associated with deletion of the short arm of chromosome 6. Rosai J et al. Mediastinal endocrine neoplasm in patients with multiple endocrine adenomatosis: a previously unrecognized association. Cancer. 1972;29:1075–83. Kubonishi I et al. Novel t(15;19) (q15; p13)chromosome abnormality in a thymic carcinoma. Cancer Res. 1991;51:3327–8. Herens C et al. Deletion of (6)(p22p25) is a recurrent anomaly of thymoma: report of a second case and review of the literature. Cancer Genet Cytogenet. 2003;146:66–9.

4. The correct answer is B. While myasthenia gravis frequently accompanies thymoma, a diagnosis of thymoma or thymic carcinoma subsequent to myasthenia gravis is less common. Thymomas are frequently associated with autoimmune disorders, particularly myasthenia gravis, occurring in 30–45 % of cases. Myasthenia gravis is less commonly associated with thymic neoplasms, occurring in 10–15 % of cases of thymoma or thymic carcinoma. Lara PN Jr. Malignant thymoma: current status and future directions. Cancer Treat Rev. 2000;26:127–31. Detterbeck PC et al. Thymic tumors. Ann Thorac Surg. 2004;1860–969. Morganthaler TI et al. Thymoma. Mayo Clin Proc. 1993;68:1110–23. Souadijan JV et al. The spectrum of diseases associated with thymoma. Coincidence or syndrome? Arch Intern Med. 1974;134:374–9.

5. The correct answer is B. While myasthenia gravis frequently accompanies thymoma, a diagnosis of thymoma or thymic carcinoma subsequent to myasthenia gravis is less common. Thymomas are frequently associated with autoimmune disorders, particularly myasthenia gravis, occurring in 30–45 % of cases. Myasthenia gravis is less commonly associated with thymic neoplasms, occurring in 10–15 % of cases of thymoma or thymic carcinoma. Lara PN Jr. Malignant thymoma: current status and future directions. Cancer Treat Rev. 2000;26:127–31. Detterbeck PC et al. Thymic tumors. Ann Thorac Surg. 2004;1860–9. Morganthaler TI et al. Thymoma. Mayo Clin Proc. 1993;68:1110–23. Souadijan JV et al. The spectrum of diseases associated with thymoma. Coincidence or syndrome? Arch Intern Med. 1974;134:374–9.

6. The correct answer is A. Of the listed autoimmune disorders associated with thymoma, myasthenia gravis has the best prognosis, perhaps because it leads to earlier discovery of a small thymoma. Following thymectomy, myasthenic symptoms will show interval improvement. The other listed autoimmune disorders that can be associated with thymoma portend a poorer prognosis. Maggi G et al. Thymoma: results of 241 operated cases. Ann Thorac Surg. 1991;51:152–6. Blumberg D et al. Thymoma: a multivariate analysis of factors predicting survival. Ann Thorac Surg. 1995;60:908–14. Murakawa T et al. Thymoma associated with pure red-cell aplasia: clinical features and prognosis. Asian Cardiovasc Thorac Ann. 2002;10:150–4.

7. The correct answer is D. Of the listed histologic subtypes, medullary type has the best prognosis, with a relatively benign clinical course. One series showed no recurrences in medullary or mixed thymomas (types A and AB, respectively), despite capsular invasion. In this same series, organoid and cortical thymomas (types B1 and B2) showed a low but significant risk of relapse, despite minimal invasion. Thymic carcinomas are type C and have the most malignant clinical course. Rosai J et al. Tumors of the thymus. In atlas of tumor pathology, series 2, fascicle 34. Washington, DC: Armed Forces Institute of Pathology; 1976. p. 55–99.

8. The correct answer is A. Of the listed structures, the pulmonary vessels are not found in the anterior but middle compartment of the mediastinum.

9. The correct answer is C. Approximately half of thymoma tumors are incidentally found on chest radiograph performed for another reason. Bonner L, Rengan R, Thomas CR Jr. Uncommon thoracic malignancies. In: Gunderson LL, Tepper JE, editors. Clinical radiation oncology. 3rd ed. Philadelphia: Elsevier Saunders; 2011. p. 859–89.

10. The correct answer is C. The Masaoka staging system for thymoma takes into account the pathological findings at the time of surgery. Masaoka A et al. Follow-up study of thymomas with special reference to their clinical stages. Cancer. 1981; 45: 2485–92.

11. The correct answer is C. Macroscopic invasion into adjacent organs is stage III. Masaoka A. Staging system of thymoma. J Thorac Oncol. 2010;5:S304–12.

12. The correct answer is B. Unresectable thymoma can be treated with preoperative chemoradiotherapy. Bonner L, Rengan R, Thomas CR, Jr. Uncommon thoracic malignancies. In Gunderson LL, Tepper JE, editors. Clinical radiation oncology. 3rd ed. Philadelphia: Elsevier Saunders; 2011. p 859–89.

Chapter 6
Breast Cancer

Celine Bicquart Ord and Charlotte Dai Kubicky

Questions

1. Breast cancer is the most common cancer in incidence in women and is the
   _____ in terms of cause of cancer deaths.
   A. First
   B. Second
   C. Third
   D. Fourth

2. All of the following are risk factors for the development of breast cancer,
   except:
   A. Age
   B. Nulliparity
   C. Family history
   D. Age at last pregnancy

3. What percentage of breast cancers are associated with a germline mutation?
   A. 5 %
   B. 10 %
   C. 15 %
   D. 20 %

C.B. Ord, MD (✉)
Department of Radiation Oncology, Scott & White Memorial Hospital,
2401 S. 31st Street, 76508 Temple, TX, USA
e-mail: celineord@gmail.com

C.D. Kubicky, MD, PhD
Department of Radiation Medicine, Oregon Health Science University,
3181 SW Sam Jackson Park Road, KPV4, 97239 Portland, OR, USA
e-mail: charlottedai@gmail.com

C.B. Ord et al. (eds.), *Radiation Oncology Study Guide*,
DOI 10.1007/978-1-4614-6400-6_6, © Springer Science+Business Media New York 2013

4. Which of the following is NOT a feature of Cowden's syndrome, which exhibits an increased risk of breast cancer?
   A. Germline PTEN mutation
   B. Increased risk of endometrial cancer
   C. Increased risk of non-small cell lung cancer
   D. Increased risk of non-medullary thyroid cancer

5. According to the retrospective study by Rebbeck et al. (NEJM 2002), looking at the efficacy of prophylactic oophorectomy in women who are BRCA mutation carriers, all of the following are true, except:
   A. A cohort of BRCA carriers who underwent prophylactic oophorectomy was compared to age-matched BRCA controls.
   B. Those that underwent surgery were less likely to use post-oophorectomy hormone replacement.
   C. There was a reduction in the risk of ovarian cancer with the use of prophylactic oophorectomy.
   D. There was a reduction in the risk of breast cancer with the use of prophylactic oophorectomy.

6. "Removal of the breast tissue alone with no lymph node dissection" describes which type of mastectomy?
   A. Total mastectomy
   B. Modified radical mastectomy
   C. Radical mastectomy
   D. Skin-sparing mastectomy

7. Regarding mastectomies, which of the following is NOT true?
   A. A skin-sparing mastectomy preserves both the skin of the breast and the nipple/areolar complex.
   B. A radical mastectomy includes dissection of the level III lymph nodes.
   C. A modified radical mastectomy does not remove the pectoralis major or level III lymph nodes.
   D. The radical mastectomy is also known as the Halsted mastectomy.

8. Regarding axillary lymph node levels, which of the following is not true?
   A. Level I nodes are located medial to the pectoralis major.
   B. Level I nodes are located lateral to the pectoralis minor.
   C. Rotter's nodes are located in level II.
   D. Rotter's nodes are located beneath pectoralis major and minor.

9. Regarding chemoprevention, which of the following is NOT true according to the NSABP P-1 trial published by Fisher et al.?
   A. Tamoxifen reduced the relative risk of invasive breast cancer by ~50 %.
   B. Tamoxifen reduced the relative risk of noninvasive breast cancer by ~50 %.
   C. There was no increased risk of uterine cancer.
   D. Individuals with atypical ductal hyperplasia (ADH) had the greatest benefit.

10. Which of the following is true regarding the NSABP-P2 STAR trial by Vogel et al.?
   A. Raloxifene was as effective as tamoxifen in reducing invasive cancers in premenopausal women.
   B. Raloxifene was inferior to tamoxifen in reducing invasive cancers in premenopausal women.
   C. Raloxifene was inferior to tamoxifen in reducing invasive cancers in postmenopausal women.
   D. Raloxifene was as effective as tamoxifen in reducing invasive cancers in postmenopausal women.

11. All of the following are FALSE regarding the NSABP-P2 STAR trial by Vogel et al., except:
   A. There were no differences in the incidence of uterine cancer between the arms.
   B. There were no differences in the incidence of embolic events between the arms.
   C. There were fewer osteoporotic fractures in the raloxifene arm.
   D. There were similar numbers of stroke and heart disease between the arms.

12. Regarding the Early Breast Cancer Trialists' Collaborative Group study of tamoxifen, all of the following are true, except:
   A. At 5 years, there was a nearly 50 % reduction in local recurrence.
   B. At 5 years, there was a 26 % reduction in mortality.
   C. At 5 years, there was no reduction in contralateral breast cancer.
   D. ER-negative tumors yielded small overall benefits.

13. Regarding the Early Breast Cancer Trialists' Collaborative Group study of tamoxifen, what was the absolute increase in overall survival at 10 years in lymph node-negative patients?
   A. 6 %
   B. 8 %
   C. 11 %
   D. 13 %

14. Regarding the Early Breast Cancer Trialists' Collaborative Group study of tamoxifen, what was the absolute increase in overall survival at 10 years in lymph node-positive patients?
   A. 6 %
   B. 8 %
   C. 11 %
   D. 13 %

15. A BI-RADS category 0 assignment on a mammogram indicates:
    A. A negative mammogram, with a recommendation for review of prior studies or completion of additional studies
    B. A negative mammogram, with a recommendation for routine screening
    C. Incomplete assessment, with a recommendation for review of prior studies or completion of additional studies
    D. Incomplete assessment, with a recommendation for short-term follow-up mammogram in 6 months

16. Ductal carcinoma in situ (DCIS) comprises what percentage of breast cancer?
    A. 20 %
    B. 30 %
    C. 40 %
    D. 50 %

17. What percentage of mammographically detected breast cancers are DCIS?
    A. 25 %
    B. 35 %
    C. 45 %
    D. 55 %

18. Which of the following is incorrect regarding DCIS?
    A. Malignant cells are confined within the basement membrane.
    B. It is E-cadherin negative.
    C. One-third of patients with DCIS develop invasive disease within 10 years.
    D. The lower the grade of DCIS, the higher the likelihood of ER positivity.

19. Which of the following is true regarding HER2?
    A. DCIS is more likely to overexpress HER2 compared to invasive ductal carcinoma.
    B. Use of trastuzumab, an HER2-targeted monoclonal antibody, cannot be given concurrently with radiotherapy.
    C. Fluorescence in situ hybridization is used most commonly to detect HER2 expression.
    D. HER2 overexpression is least commonly associated with large cell, comedo-type DCIS.

20. Which of the molecular subtype descriptions is incorrect?
    A. Luminal A: ER/PR positive, Her2neu negative
    B. Luminal B: ER/PR positive, Her2neu positive
    C. Basal-like: ER/PR negative, Her2neu positive
    D. Basal-like: ER/PR negative, Her2neu negative

21. All of the following statements regarding BRCA-associated breast cancers are true, except:
    A. There is an association with ovarian cancer in BRCA-1 tumors.
    B. BRCA-1 tumors have more ER + tumors than BRCA-2 tumors.
    C. The lifetime risk for development of breast cancer is 60–80 % with either mutation.
    D. BRCA-2 tumors are more commonly associated with male breast cancer.

22. What percentage of male breast cancers are ER positive?
    A. 20–30 %
    B. 40–50 %
    C. 60–70 %
    D. 80–90 %

23. Which statement is false regarding medullary carcinoma of the breast?
    A. Histologically, a plasma cell infiltrate can be seen.
    B. They are typically ill-defined lesions.
    C. Lymph node metastases are not infrequent.
    D. The majority of tumors are ER negative.

24. What is not true regarding Oncotype DX®?
    A. It is a 21-gene expression profiling assay.
    B. It predicts a prognostic category (low vs. intermediate vs. high) in terms of distant metastasis-free survival (DMFS) and overall survival (OS).
    C. It requires fresh-frozen tissue and on-site processing.
    D. Those patients with a high (≥31) Oncotype DX recurrence score derive the greatest benefit from chemotherapy.

25. What percentage of Paget's disease of the breast is associated with an underlying malignancy?
    A. <5 %
    B. 25 %
    C. 50 %
    D. >95 %

26. What percentage of Paget's disease of the breast is associated with a mass at diagnosis?
    A. <5 %
    B. 25 %
    C. 50 %
    D. <95 %

27. All of the following regarding the Oncotype DX® for DCIS assay are true, except:
    A. The recurrence score predicts 10-year local recurrence.
    B. The recurrence score predicts 10-year overall survival.
    C. It uses the same five reference genes as the assay for invasive disease.
    D. It can be performed on core samples.

28. What clinical TNM stage is a 2.0 cm invasive ductal carcinoma with a palpable ipsilateral internal mammary LN without detectable axillary lymph nodes?
    A. T1N2b
    B. T1N3b
    C. T2N2b
    D. T2N3b

29. The maximum dimensions of isolated nodal tumor cell clusters and micrometastases are _____ and _____, respectively.
    A. 0.02 mm and 0.2 mm
    B. 0.2 mm and 2.0 mm
    C. 0.02 mm and 2.0 mm
    D. 0.2 mm and 2.0 cm

30. What is the correct 7th edition AJCC T stage for a breast cancer that is accompanied by skin edema and chest wall invasion?
    A. T4a
    B. T4b
    C. T4c
    D. T4d

31. What is the 7th edition AJCC clinical nodal stage for positive axillary nodes and internal mammary nodes?
    A. N2b
    B. N3a
    C. N3b
    D. N3c

32. What is the 7th edition AJCC clinical nodal stage for positive infraclavicular lymph nodes?
    A. N2b
    B. N3a
    C. N3b
    D. N3c

33. Which axillary level contains the greatest number of lymph nodes?
    A. Level I.
    B. Level II.
    C. Level III.
    D. They contain an equal number of lymph nodes.

34. What percentage of clinically negative lymph nodes are pathologically positive after axillary lymph node dissection?
    A. 15 %
    B. 30 %
    C. 45 %
    D. 60 %

35. In which quadrant of the breast is primary breast cancer most common?
    A. Upper outer
    B. Upper inner
    C. Lower outer
    D. Lower inner

36. Historically, what is the incidence of internal mammary lymph node positivity in an upper outer quadrant tumor without positive axillary lymph nodes?
    A. 5 %
    B. 10 %
    C. 20 %
    D. 50 %

37. Historically, what is the incidence of internal mammary lymph node positivity in an upper outer quadrant tumor with positive axillary lymph nodes?
    A. 5 %
    B. 10 %
    C. 20 %
    D. 50 %

38. All of the following statements regarding NSABP-04 are correct, except:
    A. Women with clinically LN-positive breast cancer were randomized to radical mastectomy versus total mastectomy + RT.
    B. There was no difference in terms of disease-free survival, distant metastasis-free survival, or overall survival among women with clinically LN-negative breast cancer.
    C. There was no difference in terms of disease-free survival, distant metastasis-free survival, or overall survival among women with clinically LN-positive breast cancer.
    D. Internal mammary lymph nodes were not included in the radiation field.

39. Which patients were included in NSABP B-17?
    A. Patients with DCIS after undergoing lumpectomy with margin requirement unspecified.
    B. Patients with invasive ductal carcinoma after undergoing lumpectomy with margin requirement unspecified.
    C. Patients with DCIS after undergoing lumpectomy with negative margins.
    D. Patients with invasive ductal carcinoma after undergoing lumpectomy with negative margins.

40. Regarding NSABP B-17, all of the following are true, except:
   A. At 12 years follow-up, RT reduced invasive local failure, but not noninvasive failure.
   B. At 12 years follow-up, RT reduced noninvasive and invasive failures.
   C. There was no difference in DM or OS.
   D. At 15 years follow-up, the benefit of RT in reducing invasive local failures persists.

41. What was the total radiotherapy dose to the whole breast in NSABP B-17?
   A. 45 Gy
   B. 50 Gy
   C. 60 Gy
   D. 66 Gy

42. According to EORTC 10853, features associated with increased local recurrence include all of the following, except:
   A. Age ≤ 45
   B. Intermediate to high grade
   C. Cribriform growth pattern
   D. Omission of radiation

43. Regarding NSABP B-24, all of the following are true, except:
   A. Approximately one-quarter of patients had positive margins.
   B. ER status was unknown.
   C. Tamoxifen was given at 20 mg daily × 5 years.
   D. Overall mortality decreased with the addition of tamoxifen.

44. Regarding NSABP B-24, which randomized patients with DCIS after lumpectomy and RT to +/− tamoxifen, which of the following is true?
   A. The addition of tamoxifen improved mortality by probable cause.
   B. Invasive in-breast tumor recurrence was associated with a greater risk of all-cause death.
   C. Noninvasive recurrence was associated with a greater risk of breast cancer mortality.
   D. Invasive contralateral recurrence was not associated with an increase in mortality risk.

45. In the UKCCR-randomized trial of DCIS s/p lumpectomy randomized to RT, tamoxifen, both, or neither, which of the following is false?
   A. RT reduced local failures (noninvasive and invasive) 14% to 6%.
   B. Tamoxifen yielded an ipsilateral breast local control benefit in addition to RT.
   C. Tamoxifen reduced the overall incidence of DCIS.
   D. Negative margins were required for enrollment.

46. Which of the findings from the ECOG 5194 observational DCIS study is false?
    A. Omission of RT can be considered in low-grade DCIS excised with clear margins ≥3 mm.
    B. The 5 years IBTR in Group 1 (G1-2, <2.5 cm) was 6.1 %
    C. The 5 years IBTR in Group 2 (G3, <1 cm) was 15.3 %.
    D. Excision alone is adequate for high-risk DCIS with clear margins ≥3 mm.

47. All of the following are differences between the ECOG 5194 and Wong et al. Harvard DCIS observational studies, except:
    A. Tamoxifen was allowed only in the ECOG study.
    B. Margins were required to be ≥3 mm in both studies.
    C. The Harvard study included mostly small, low-intermediate-grade DCIS.
    D. Only the ECOG study required "sequential tissue processing."

48. All of the following are parameters of the Van Nuys Prognostic Index (VNPI) of DCIS by Silverstein et al., except:
    A. Age
    B. Margin status
    C. Grade
    D. ER status

49. Each of the following VNPI parameters would be scored "3 points," except:
    A. <0.1 cm margins
    B. 4.1 cm tumor size
    C. 40 years old
    D. Grade 3 with comedonecrosis

50. Which of the following is a definite contraindication to breast-conservation therapy?
    A. Multicentricity
    B. Lymph node involvement
    C. Multifocality
    D. Extensive intraductal component

51. Which of the following is a relative contraindication to breast-conservation therapy?
    A. Previous breast/chest RT
    B. Pregnancy
    C. Systemic lupus erythematosus
    D. Persistently positive margins on excision

52. Which of the following is not an appropriate therapy for LCIS?
    A. Observation
    B. Tamoxifen
    C. Mastectomy
    D. Lumpectomy + radiation

53. Regarding NSABP B-06, all of the following are true, except:
    A. All arms underwent axillary dissection.
    B. Node-positive patients received melphalan and 5-fluorouracil chemotherapy.
    C. The occurrence of tumor in the ipsilateral breast after lumpectomy was considered to be a cosmetic failure.
    D. No ER receptor status data is known.

54. What is correct regarding outcomes from the Milan I trial comparing radical mastectomy (RM) versus quadrantectomy + 60 Gy RT?
    A. Local control was better in the RM arm, as was overall survival.
    B. Local control was better in the quadrantectomy + RT arm, as was overall survival.
    C. Local control was better in the RM arm, with no difference in overall survival.
    D. Local control was better in the quadrantectomy + RT arm, with no difference in overall survival.

55. Regarding the CALGB C9343 trial comparing tamoxifen versus tamoxifen + RT in patients ≥70 years with small tumors, all of the following are true, except:
    A. All patients were ER + .
    B. The addition of RT decreased local failure rates.
    C. The 5-year mastectomy-free survival did not differ between the two arms.
    D. Overall survival did not differ between the two arms.

56. Regarding the 14-year follow-up data of the three-arm NSABP B-21 trial comparing tamoxifen versus placebo + RT versus tamoxifen + RT in small ≤1 cm tumors, all of the following are true, except:
    A. There was no difference in OS between the three arms.
    B. Tamoxifen decreased ipsilateral breast tumor recurrence (IBTR).
    C. Tamoxifen decreased contralateral breast primaries.
    D. RT improved local control only in conjunction with tamoxifen.

57. Regarding NSABP B-18, all of the following are true, except:
    A. Neoadjuvant chemotherapy increased the ability of patients to undergo breast-conservation therapy.
    B. Neoadjuvant chemotherapy improved disease-free survival.
    C. Neoadjuvant chemotherapy did not improve overall survival.
    D. Pathological complete response was a significant predictor for disease-free survival.

58. What were the pathological complete response rates in the preop AC and AC + T chemotherapy arms in the latest update of NSABP B-18 and B-27, respectively?
    A. 13 % and 26 %
    B. 26 % and 13 %
    C. 15 % and 32 %
    D. 32 % and 15 %

59. Which one of the following is not one of Haagensen's grave signs?
    A. Skin edema
    B. Palpable lymph nodes
    C. Chest fixation
    D. Ulceration

60. What is the most common site of locoregional failure after a mastectomy?
    A. Chest wall
    B. Axilla
    C. Supraclavicular fossa
    D. Internal mammary lymph nodes

61. All of the following characteristics of inflammatory breast carcinoma are correct, except:
    A. It usually presents with rapid onset erythema, warmth, and edema of breast.
    B. Pathological confirmation of tumor in the dermal lymphatic is not required.
    C. Patients can still be candidates for BCT if a complete response is obtained after neoadjuvant chemotherapy.
    D. An underlying mass is frequently not appreciated on clinical examination.

62. What percentage of inflammatory breast cancer has a palpable mass at diagnosis?
    A. 20 %
    B. 30 %
    C. 40 %
    D. 50 %

63. What percentage of inflammatory breast cancer has a normal mammogram?
    A. 5 %
    B. 10 %
    C. 15 %
    D. 20 %

64. Regarding the Danish 82b postmastectomy trial, which of the following is true?
    A. Patients were postmenopausal.
    B. The median number of lymph nodes dissected was 9.
    C. The internal mammary lymph nodes were treated with radiation.
    D. There was a 20 % benefit in overall survival with the addition of postmastectomy radiation.

65. Regarding the Danish 82b postmastectomy trial, all of the following are true, except:
    A. Disease-free survival improved with the addition of postmastectomy RT.
    B. Overall survival improved with the addition of postmastectomy RT.
    C. More than 50 % of recurrences were on the chest wall.
    D. Tamoxifen was not allowed.

66. Regarding the Danish 82c postmastectomy trial, all of the following are true, except:
    A. Patients were postmenopausal.
    B. Tamoxifen was given for 5 years.
    C. Locoregional recurrences were decreased in the RT + tamoxifen arm.
    D. There was ~10 % benefit in overall survival with the addition of postmastectomy radiation.

67. In the British Columbia postmastectomy trial, all of the following are true, except:
    A. Patients were premenopausal.
    B. Radiation consisted of 48–50 Gy to the chest wall, supraclavicular fossa, axilla, and internal mammary LNs.
    C. The median number of lymph nodes dissected was 11.
    D. There was an improvement in breast cancer-specific survival with radiation.

68. Regarding the Canadian Hypofractionation study by Whelan et al., all of the following are true, except:
    A. Ductal carcinoma in situ was excluded.
    B. Boosts ranged from 10 to 16 Gy.
    C. Tumors >5 cm were excluded.
    D. Use of tamoxifen was allowed.

69. Regarding outcomes of the Canadian Hypofractionation study by Whelan et al., all of the following are true, except:
    A. There was no difference in local recurrence between the arms.
    B. There was no difference in overall survival between the arms.
    C. There was better "good/excellent" cosmesis in the standard fractionation arm.
    D. There was no difference in disease-free survival between the arms.

70. All are true comparing the schemas of the UK START A and B trials, except:
    A. START A compared different fraction sizes delivered over the same amount of weeks.
    B. START A compared different fraction sizes delivered over different amounts of weeks.
    C. START B compared different fraction sizes delivered over different amounts of weeks.
    D. Boosts were allowed in both trials.

71. Regarding the UK START B trial, which of the following is correct?
    A. Patients were randomized to receive 50 Gy/25 versus 39 Gy/13.
    B. There was a higher rate of late toxicity in the hypofractionated arm.
    C. There was a statistically significant improvement in overall survival in the hypofractionated arm.
    D. There was a higher 5-year rate of distant relapse in the hypofractionated arm.

72. Regarding the UK START A trial, which of the following is correct?
    A. Patients in the hypofractionation arms had improved cosmesis compared to the standard fractionation arm.
    B. Local control did not differ between the arms.
    C. There was a greater number of confirmed symptomatic lung fibrosis in the 50 Gy arm.
    D. No supraclavicular fossa radiation was allowed.

73. Which one of the following is not an Accelerated Partial Breast Irradiation (APBI) technique?
    A. Intraoperative x-rays
    B. Permanent Ir-192 seed placement
    C. 3DCRT
    D. Balloon brachytherapy

74. Which of the following is the correct dose fractionation pairing for balloon APBI?
    A. Balloon brachytherapy 2.67 BID × 5 days
    B. Balloon brachytherapy 3.4 Gy BID × 5 days
    C. Balloon brachytherapy 3.5 Gy BID × 5 days
    D. Balloon brachytherapy 3.85 Gy BID × 5 days

75. All of the following are "cautionary" criteria for APBI according to the ASTRO consensus statement, except:
    A. Age 59
    B. Extensive intraductal component ≤3 cm
    C. A 2.0 cm tumor
    D. <2 mm margins

76. Regarding the NCIC-CTG MA.20 trial comparing whole breast versus whole breast + regional node irradiation after breast-conserving surgery, at 5 years of follow-up, which of the following is not true?
    A. Internal mammary nodes were included in the regional nodes irradiated.
    B. There was a statistically significant improvement in both distant DFS and overall DFS.
    C. There was a statistically significant improvement in both locoregional DFS and distant DFS.
    D. There was a statistically significant improvement in both overall DFS and overall survival.

77. Regarding the NSABP B-32 trial comparing sentinel lymph node biopsy (SLNB) + axillary lymph node dissection (ALND) versus SLNB alone, all of the following are correct, except:
    A. Clinically positive axillary LNs were excluded.
    B. 99 % of LNs were in levels I/II.
    C. The technical success was 97 %.
    D. The mean number of lymph nodes removed was 3.

78. Regarding outcomes of the NSABP B-32 trial comparing sentinel lymph node biopsy (SLNB) + axillary lymph node dissection (ALND) versus SLNB alone, all of the following are correct, except:
    A. Deficit of 10 % or more in shoulder range of motion was less in the SLNB alone group.
    B. DFS was longer in the SLNB + ALND group.
    C. There was no difference in OS between the groups.
    D. There was less arm volume increase in the SLNB alone group.

79. Regarding the ACOSOG Z0011 trial in which patients with positive sentinel lymph nodes were randomized to receive subsequent axillary dissection versus no further axillary surgery, all of the following are true, except:
    A. Following breast-conserving surgery, all patients received whole breast irradiation.
    B. Those with three or fewer positive sentinel nodes were eligible.
    C. Negative margins (at ink) were required for randomization.
    D. Axillary dissection required removal of at least ten lymph nodes.

80. Regarding the ACOSOG Z0011 trial in which patients with positive sentinel lymph nodes were randomized to receive subsequent axillary dissection versus no further axillary surgery, all of the following are true, except:
    A. Approximately one-quarter of patients who underwent axillary dissection had additional positive axillary lymph nodes.
    B. The majority of patients had estrogen-receptor-positive disease.
    C. The majority of patients had two positive SLNs.
    D. The superior border of the tangential fields treated was not clearly defined.

81. Regarding the NSABP B-20 trial in which women were randomized to tamoxifen +/− chemotherapy, which of the following is correct?
    A. Patients were required to have pathologically negative nodes.
    B. One of the three arms was a tamoxifen + CF chemotherapy arm.
    C. The addition of chemotherapy improved disease-free survival, but not overall survival.
    D. Patients were not required to have ER + breast cancer.

82. Regarding the NSABP B-28 trial in which patients with lymph node-positive breast cancer were randomized to receive taxane-based chemotherapy, all of the following are true, except:
    A. Both arms received Adriamycin and cyclophosphamide chemotherapy.
    B. The addition of paclitaxel improved locoregional recurrence and disease-free survival.
    C. The addition of paclitaxel improved locoregional recurrence and overall survival.
    D. Patients with estrogen-receptor-positive tumors also received tamoxifen for 5 years.

83. All are conclusions from the Early Breast Cancer Trialists' Collaborative Group study regarding chemotherapy, except:
    A. There is a larger benefit for chemotherapy in node-positive versus node-negative women.
    B. The addition of chemotherapy benefits all women in terms of death.
    C. Women >50 years gain the most benefit.
    D. Anthracycline-based chemotherapy is better than CMF chemotherapy.

84. All of the following regarding exemestane are true, except:
    A. It is associated with a statistically significant decrease in invasive breast cancers.
    B. Compared with placebo, there is no increased risk of bisphosphonate therapy use.
    C. Compared with placebo, there are no increased self-reported menopause-related vasomotor and sexual symptoms.
    D. Compared with placebo, there is no increased risk of cardiovascular events.

85. All of the following are observations from the Early Breast Cancer Trialists' Collaborative Group study regarding radiotherapy, except:
    A. Radiation after breast-conserving surgery produces a significant absolute improvement in 15-year local control.
    B. Radiation after mastectomy with axillary clearance in lymph node-positive disease produces a significant absolute improvement in 15-year local control.
    C. The addition of radiotherapy, at 15 years, conferred an additional 20 % absolute benefit in local control and 5 % absolute benefit in breast cancer mortality.
    D. There is no excess mortality from heart disease in those treated with radiotherapy.

86. Regarding the EORTC boost trial, all of the following are true, except:
    A. Negative margins were required only for invasive disease; DCIS was allowed at the margin.
    B. Patients were randomized to +/− 16 Gy boost after whole breast radiotherapy.
    C. Addition of a 16 Gy boost benefited all groups except those >60 years old.
    D. There was a slight increased rate of severe fibrosis in those that received the boost.

87. Regarding the Lyon boost trial, all of the following are true, except:
    A. Patients were randomized after radiotherapy to receive a 16 Gy boost.
    B. Patients were randomized after radiotherapy to receive a 10 Gy boost.
    C. Addition of a boost reduced local recurrence.
    D. There was no worsened cosmesis in the boost arm.

Answers and Rationales

1. The correct answer is B. Although number one in cancer incidence, breast cancer is the second leading cause of cancer deaths. Lung cancer is the second most common but leading cause of cancer deaths among US women. Jemal A, Siegel R, Xu J, Ward E. Cancer statistics, 2010. CA Cancer J Clin. 2010;60:277–300.

2. The correct answer is D. Age is the most important risk factor for the development of breast cancer. Nulliparity, family history, and age at first pregnancy are also risk factors. Buchholz TA. Breast cancer overview. In: Gunderson LL, Tepper JE, editors. Clinical radiation oncology. 3rd ed. Philadelphia: Elsevier Saunders; 2012. p. 1299–309.

3. The correct answer is B. Ten percent of breast cancer cases are associated with a germline mutation, including p53 (Li Fraumeni), BRCA 1, BRCA2. Buchholz TA. Breast cancer overview. In: Gunderson LL, Tepper JE, editors. Clinical radiation oncology. 3rd ed. Philadelphia: Elsevier Saunders, 2012. p. 1299–309.

4. The correct answer is C. Cowden's Syndrome is a rare hereditary cancer syndrome due to a mutation in the PTEN tumor suppressor gene on chromosome 10. It is associated with multiple hamartomatous and/or cancerous lesions. The lifetime risks for various cancers are breast cancer, 25–50 %; non-medullary thyroid cancer, 3–10 %; and endometrial cancer, 5–10 %. There is no increased risk of NSCLC. Skin cancers, renal cell carcinomas, colorectal cancer, brain tumors, and vascular malformations are also occasionally seen. Pilarski R. Cowden syndrome: a critical review of the clinical literature. J Genet Couns. 2009;18:13–27. Starink TM et al. The Cowden syndrome: a clinical and genetic study in 21 patients. Clin Genet. 1986;29:222–33.

5. The correct answer is B. In Rebbeck's retrospective study, 259 women with BRCA mutations, no personal history of breast or ovarian cancer, and had undergone prophylactic oophorectomy were age-matched to a cohort of 292 women with BRCA mutations. Those that underwent prophylactic oophorectomy were more likely to use post-oophorectomy hormone-replacement therapy (47.9 % vs. 19.9 %, $p < 0.001$). There was a 96 % reduction in the risk of ovarian cancer with prophylactic oophorectomy, as well as a 53 % reduction in the risk of breast cancer (HR 0.47, 95 % CI .29–.77). Rebbeck et al. Prophylactic oophorectomy in carriers of BRCA1 or BRCA2 mutations. N Engl J Med. 2002;346(21):1616–22.

6. The correct answer is A. In a total mastectomy, there is removal of only the breast with NO axillary dissection. Whereas a radical mastectomy removes pectoralis major, a modified radical mastectomy preserves it; and both remove levels I–II. The Halstead mastectomy (radical) also removes level III. Buchholz

TA. Breast cancer overview. In: Gunderson LL, Tepper, JE, editors. Clinical radiation oncology. 3rd ed. Philadelphia: Elsevier Saunders, 2012. p. 1299–309.

7. The correct answer is A. A skin-sparing mastectomy preserves only the skin of the breast, a total skin-sparing mastectomy preserves both the skin of the breast and the nipple/areolar complex. A radical mastectomy includes dissection of the level III lymph nodes. A modified radical mastectomy does not remove the pectoralis major or level III lymph nodes. The radical mastectomy is named for William Stewart Halsted, the first surgeon to perform a radical mastectomy. Buchholz TA. Breast cancer overview. In: Gunderson LL, Tepper, JE, editors. Clinical radiation oncology. 3rd ed. Philadelphia: Elsevier Saunders, 2012. p. 1299–309.

8. The correct answer is A. Level I axillary lymph nodes are located inferior/lateral to the pectoralis minor. Level II nodes are located directly beneath the pectoralis minor muscle. Rotter's nodes are considered level II and are located between the pectoralis major and minor muscles. Level III nodes are located superior/medial to pectoralis minor. Buchholz TA. Breast cancer overview. In: Gunderson LL, Tepper, JE, editors. Clinical radiation oncology. 3rd ed. Philadelphia: Elsevier Saunders, 2012. p. 1299–309.

9. The correct answer is C. In the NSABP P-1 chemoprevention trial, 13,388 patients at elevated risk for breast cancer were randomized to receive either placebo or tamoxifen × 5 years. At 69 months follow-up, tamoxifen reduced the relative risk of both invasive and noninvasive breast cancer by ~50 %, though the ARRs were only 2 % and 0.9 %, respectively. The greatest benefit (4–5×) was seen in patients with ADH. There was an increased risk of stage I uterine cancers (HR = 2.53). With 7 years follow-up, the relative risk reduction in invasive cancer was 43 % and in noninvasive cancer was 37 %. Tamoxifen also led to a 32 % reduction in osteoporotic fractures. Fisher B, Constantino JP, et al. J Natl Cancer Inst. 2005;22:1652–62.

10. The correct answer is D. In the NSABP-P2 STAR trial, 19,747 postmenopausal women at increased risk of breast cancer were randomized to tamoxifen 20 mg qd versus raloxifene 60 mg qd × 5 years. There was no difference in the incidence of invasive cancer in each arm, 0.4 %, though there were fewer noninvasive cases with tamoxifen. Vogel VG et al. Effects of tamoxifen vs. raloxifene on the risk of developing invasive breast cancer and other disease outcomes: the NSABP study of tamoxifen and raloxifene (STAR) P-2 Trial. JAMA. 2006;295(23):2727–41.

11. The correct answer is D. In the NSABP-P2 STAR trial, 19,747 postmenopausal women at increased risk of breast cancer were randomized to tamoxifen 20 mg qd versus raloxifene 60 mg qd × 5 years. Raloxifene reduced the risk of uterine

cancer, cataracts, and thromboembolic events, though there were similar numbers of osteoporotic fractures, stroke, and heart disease. Vogel VG et al. Effects of tamoxifen vs. raloxifene on the risk of developing invasive breast cancer and other disease outcomes: the NSABP study of tamoxifen and raloxifene (STAR) P-2 Trial. JAMA. 2006;295(23):2727–41.

12. The correct answer is C. In the initial results of the EBCTCG study of tamoxifen published in 1998, those with ER + tumors yielded a significant benefit from tamoxifen. At 5 years, there was a 47 % reduction in local recurrence, a 47 % reduction in contralateral breast cancer, and a 26 % reduction in mortality. ER-negative tumors yielded a very small benefit from tamoxifen. Early Breast Cancer Trialists' Collaborative Group. Tamoxifen for early breast cancer: An overview of the randomised trials. Lancet. 1998;351(9114):1451–67.

13. The correct answer is A. In the initial results of the EBCTCG study of tamoxifen published in 1998, those with ER + tumors and positive lymph nodes yielded a significant benefit from tamoxifen. In lymph node-positive tumors, there was an 11 % absolute increase in survival at 10 years. Lymph node-negative tumors yielded less of a benefit with a 6 % absolute increase in survival at 10 years. Early Breast Cancer Trialists' Collaborative Group. Tamoxifen for early breast cancer: an overview of the randomised trials. Lancet. 1998;351(9114):1451–67.

14. The correct answer is C. In the initial results of the EBCTCG study of tamoxifen published in 1998, those with ER + tumors and positive lymph nodes yielded a significant benefit from tamoxifen. In lymph node-positive tumors, there was an 11 % absolute increase in survival at 10 years. Lymph node-negative tumors yielded less of a benefit with a 6 % absolute increase in survival at 10 years. Early Breast Cancer Trialists' Collaborative Group. Tamoxifen for early breast cancer: an overview of the randomised trials. Lancet. 1998; 351(9114):1451–67.

15. The correct answer is C. The Breast Imaging Reporting and Data System (BI-RADS) provides standardized classification for mammographic studies. BI-RADS category 0 indicates incomplete assessment, with a recommendation for review of prior studies or completion of additional studies. BI-RADS category 1 indicates a negative mammogram, with a recommendation for continuation of routine screening. BI-RADS category 2 indicates a benign finding, with a recommendation for continuation of routine screening. BI-RADS category 3 indicates a probably benign finding, with a recommendation for short-term follow-up mammogram at 6 months, then every 6–12 months for 1–2 years. BI-RADS category 4 indicates a suspicious abnormality, with a recommendation for further characterization with biopsy (preferably needle biopsy). BI-RADS category 5 indicates a highly suspicious malignancy, with a recommendation for biopsy and treatment as necessary. BI-RADS category 6 indicates known malignancy, with a recommendation to ensure treatment is

completed. American College of Radiology (ACR) Breast Imaging Reporting and Data System Atlas (BI-RADS Atlas). Reston, VA. © American College of Radiology; 2003.

16. The correct answer is A. DCIS comprises approximately 15–20 % of all breast cancer. Arthur DW, Vicini FA. Noninvasive breast cancer. In Gunderson LL, Tepper JE, editors. Clinical radiation oncology. 3rd ed. Philadelphia: Elsevier Saunders; 2012. p. 1311–20.

17. The correct answer is A. Approximately 20–25 % of mammographically detected breast cancers are DCIS. The percentage does statistically differ by age. In those women age 40–49, the percentage is 28.2 % versus 20.5 % in women age 60–84. Ernster VL et al. Detection of ductal carcinoma in situ in women undergoing screening mammography. J Natl Canc Inst. 2002;94(20):1546–54.

18. The correct answer is B. The hallmark of DCIS is the confinement of malignant cells within the basement membrane. DCIS and invasive ductal carcinoma are E-cadherin positive as opposed to lobular carcinoma in situ and invasive lobular carcinoma, which are E-cadherin negative. Approximately 90 % of low-grade DCIS is ER+, compared to ~25 % of high-grade DCIS. One-third of patients with DCIS will develop invasive disease within 10 years. Arthur DW, Vicini FA. Noninvasive breast cancer. In: Gunderson LL, Tepper JE, editors. Clinical radiation oncology. 3rd ed. Philadelphia: Elsevier Saunders; 2012. p. 1311–20.

19. The correct answer is A. Compared to invasive ductal carcinoma, DCIS is more likely to overexpress HER2. HER2 expression is most commonly evaluated by immunohistochemistry, with subsequent reflex testing performed with FISH. The Intergroup Study 0011 reported HER2 overexpression in 56 % of pure DCIS (77 % of comedo subtype) and only 11 % in IDC alone. A study from the Netherlands also showed that of 45 patients with DCIS, 45 % overexpressed HER2, and all of these DCIS cases were large cell, comedo growth type. NSABP B-43 is a study currently enrolling patients with HER2-positive DCIS s/p lumpectomy and randomized to receive radiation +/– concurrent trastuzumab × 2 doses. Allred DC et al. HER2 in node-negative breast cancer: prognostic significance of overexpression influenced by the presence of in situ carcinoma. J Clin Oncol. 1992;10:566–605. Van de Vijver MJ et al. Association with comedo-type ductal carcinoma in situ and limited prognostic value in stage II breast cancer. N Eng J Med. 1988;319:1239–45.

20. The correct answer is C. The basal-like subtype is triple negative—ER/PR negative, Her2neu negative. The luminal B subtype can be either ER/PR positive, Her2neu positive, or ER/PR positive, Her2neu negative with a high Ki67 index. Buchholz TA. Breast cancer overview. In: Gunderson LL, Tepper JE, editors. Clinical radiation oncology. 3rd ed. Philadelphia: Elsevier Saunders, 2012. p. 1299–309.

21. The correct answer is B. With both BRCA-1 tumors and BRCA-2 tumors, there is a 60–80 % chance of developing breast cancer. BRCA-1-associated tumors have a 30–40 % risk of developing ovarian cancer. BRCA-2 tumors tend to be more commonly ER + and associated with male breast cancer. Petrucelli N, Daly MB. *BRCA1* and *BRCA2* hereditary breast and ovarian cancer. In: Pagon RA, Bird TD, editors. Gene reviews. Seattle, WA: University of Washington; 2011. p. 1453–61.

22. The correct answer is D. Male breast cancers are overwhelmingly (80–90 %) ER positive. Buchholz TA. Breast cancer overview. In: Gunderson LL, Tepper JE, editors. Clinical radiation oncology. 3rd ed. Philadelphia: Elsevier Saunders, 2012. p. 1299–309.

23. The correct answer is B. Medullary carcinoma of the breast involves large cells with pleomorphic nuclei with a frequent lymphoid/plasma cell infiltrate. The tumors are frequently well circumscribed, and lymph node metastases are not infrequent. Most are ER/PR negative; only 10 % are ER positive. The current thinking is that these cancers should be treated just as other invasive ductal carcinomas. Young JS et al. Asynchronous bilateral medullary carcinoma of the breast. South Med J. 1997;90(4):423–5. Reinfuss M et al. Typical medullary carcinoma of the breast: a clinical and pathological analysis of 52 cases. J Surg Oncol. 1995;60(2):89–94.

24. The correct answer is C. Oncotype DX® is a 21-gene expression profiling assay that differs from MammaPrint® in that it can assay a fixed specimen, precluding the need for on-site testing. The assay assigns a recurrence score, which falls into one of three prognostic categories: low risk (<18), intermediate risk (18–30), and high risk (≥31). The recurrence score (RS) predicts the magnitude of chemotherapy benefit. In their analysis of the 21-gene assay (Oncotype DX®) recurrence score for 651 ER+, pLN- patients treated with tamoxifen ± chemotherapy on NSABP B-21, Paik et al. found that the greatest chemotherapy benefit was seen in high-RS patients. Paik S, Tang G, Shak S, et al. Gene expression and benefit of chemotherapy in women with node-negative, estrogen receptor- positive breast cancer. J Clin Oncol. 2006;24(23):3723–34.

25. The correct answer is D. Over 95 % of Paget's disease is associated with an underlying malignancy. Arthur DW, Vicini FA. Noninvasive breast cancer. In: Gunderson LL, Tepper JE, editors, Clinical radiation oncology. 3rd ed. Philadelphia: Elsevier Saunders, 2012. p. 1311–20.

26. The correct answer is C. Paget's disease of the breast is associated with a mass at diagnosis approximately 50 % of the time. Arthur DW, Vicini FA. Noninvasive breast cancer. In: Gunderson LL, Tepper JE, editors, Clinical radiation oncology. 3rd ed. Philadelphia: Elsevier Saunders, 2012. p. 1311–20.

27. The correct answer is B. The Oncotype DX® for DCIS is a 12-gene profiling assay that seeks to identify a proportion of patients with DCIS, for whom radiation after lumpectomy will have a small absolute risk reduction, thus precluding the need for radiotherapy. The assay uses the same 5 reference genes and can be performed on a core sample. The assay was validated in the low-risk ECOG 5194 DCIS observational study population. The recurrence score predicts 10-year local recurrence and was found on multivariate analysis to be an independent predictor of ipsilateral breast event, in addition to menopausal status, and tumor size. Solin L et al. Quantitative multigene RT-PCR assay for predicting recurrence risk after surgical excision alone without irradiation for Ductal Carcinoma In Situ (DCIS): a prospective validation study of the DCIS score from ECOG E5194. 34th Annual San Antonio Breast Cancer Symposium Abstract S4-6.

28. The correct answer is A. A 2.0 cm invasive ductal carcinoma with a palpable ipsilateral internal mammary LN without detectable axillary lymph nodes is cT1N2b. A tumor ≤20 mm is T1; >20 mm is T2. A palpable ipsilateral IM lymph node in the absence of axillary LNs is N2b; in the setting of present axillary LNs, it would be N3b. Edge SB, Byrd DR, Compton CC, et al., editors. Breast. AJCC cancer staging handbook. 7th ed. New York, NY: Springer, 2010.

29. The correct answer is B. The maximum dimensions of isolated tumor cell clusters and micrometastases are 0.2 and 2.0 mm, respectively. Edge SB, Byrd DR, Compton CC, et al., editors. Breast. AJCC cancer staging handbook. 7th ed. New York, NY: Springer, 2010.

30. The correct answer is C. Invasion of the chest wall with presence of skin edema is clinical stage T4c. Inflammatory breast cancer is cT4d. Edge SB, Byrd DR, Compton CC, et al., editors. Breast. AJCC cancer staging handbook. 7th ed. New York, NY: Springer, 2010.

31. The correct answer is C. The AJCC stage of positive axillary nodes in conjunction with positive internal mammary lymph nodes is cN3b. Edge SB, Byrd DR, Compton CC, et al., editors. Breast. AJCC cancer staging handbook. 7th ed. New York, NY: Springer, 2010.

32. The correct answer is B. Infraclavicular lymph nodes are AJCC clinical stage N3a. Edge SB, Byrd DR, Compton CC, et al. editors. Breast. AJCC cancer staging handbook. 7th ed. New York, NY: Springer, 2010.

33. The correct answer is B. Axillary level II contains the greatest number of lymph nodes. Danforth DN Jr. et al. Complete axillary lymph node dissection for stage I–II carcinoma of the breast. J Clin Oncol. 1986;4(5):655–62.

34. The correct answer is B. Approximately 1/3 of clinically negative lymph nodes are pathologically positive. Voogd AC et al. The risk of nodal metastases in breast cancer patients with clinically negative lymph nodes: a population-based analysis. Breast Cancer Res Treat. 2000;62(1):63–9.

35. The correct answer is A. In one series, almost half (48 %) of primary breast tumors were found in the upper outer quadrant, with the fewest primary tumors occurring in the lower inner quadrant. Spratt J, Donegan W. Cancer of the breast. Philadelphia: WB Saunders, 1971.

36. The correct answer is A. The incidence of positive internal mammary nodes in an upper outer quadrant tumor with a negative axilla is 5 %. Recht A. Breast cancer: stages I and II. In: Gunderson LL, Tepper JE, editors. Clinical radiation oncology. 3rd ed. Philadelphia: Elsevier Saunders, 2012. p. 1321–38.

37. The correct answer is C. The incidence of positive internal mammary nodes in an upper outer quadrant tumor with a positive axilla is 20 %. Historically, the incidence of positive internal mammary nodes in an inner quadrant tumor with a positive and negative axilla is 50 % and 10 %, respectively. Recht A. Breast cancer: stages I and II. In: Gunderson LL, Tepper JE, editors. Clinical radiation oncology. 3rd ed. Philadelphia: Elsevier Saunders, 2012. p. 1321–38.

38. The correct answer is D. NSABP-04 was a large randomized trial initiated to answer the question of whether less extensive surgery ± radiation would be as effective as the radical mastectomy. Women with breast cancer and clinically negative axillary LNs were randomized to one of three arms: radical mastectomy versus total mastectomy + RT versus total mastectomy alone. Women with breast cancer and clinically positive axillary LNs were randomized to one of two arms: radical mastectomy versus total mastectomy + RT. Women with clinically negative ALNs who subsequently developed pathologically positive axillary LNs subsequently underwent axillary dissection. No women received adjuvant systemic therapy. Radiation consisted of 50 Gy delivered in 25 fractions to the chest wall; 45 Gy in 25 fractions was delivered to the internal mammary and supraclavicular LNs. Those women with positive nodes received an additional boost dose of 10–20 Gy. The 25-year data published by Fisher et al. in the NEJM in 2002 showed no significant differences in disease-free survival or overall survival regardless of LN status, showing no benefit to radical mastectomy. Fisher B et al. Twenty-five-year follow-up of a randomized trial comparing radical mastectomy, total mastectomy, and total mastectomy followed by irradiation. N Engl J Med. 2002;347(8):567–75.

39. The correct answer is C. NSABP B-17 was a randomized trial initiated to define the role of radiation after lumpectomy for DCIS. 818 patients s/p lumpectomy for DCIS with negative margins were randomized to observation versus

postoperative RT (50 Gy). With 12 years follow-up, RT reduced noninvasive local failure 15 % to 8 %, as well as invasive failures 17 % to 8 %. There were no DM or OS differences. The 15-year update in the JNCI in 2011 showed that RT reduced ipsilateral invasive in-breast tumor recurrences, 19.4 % to 8.9 %, and ipsilateral noninvasive in-breast tumor recurrences, 15.7 % to 8.8 %. Wapnir IL et al. Long-term outcomes of invasive ipsilateral breast tumor recurrences after lumpectomy in NSABP B-17 and B-24 randomized clinical trials for DCIS. J Natl Cancer Inst. 2011;103(6):478–88.

40. The correct answer is A. NSABP B-17 was a randomized trial initiated to define the role of radiation after lumpectomy for DCIS. 818 patients s/p lumpectomy for DCIS with negative margins were randomized to observation versus postoperative RT (50Gy). With 12 years follow-up, RT reduced noninvasive local failure 15 % to 8 %, as well as invasive failures 17 % to 8 %. There were no DM or OS differences. The 15-year update in the JNCI in 2011 showed that RT reduced ipsilateral invasive in-breast tumor recurrences, 19.4 % to 8.9 %, and ipsilateral noninvasive in-breast tumor recurrences, 15.7 % to 8.8 %. Wapnir IL et al. Long-term outcomes of invasive ipsilateral breast tumor recurrences after lumpectomy in NSABP B-17 and B-24 randomized clinical trials for DCIS. J Natl Cancer Inst. 2011;103(6):478–88.

41. The correct answer is B. NSABP B-17 was a randomized trial initiated to define the role of radiation after lumpectomy for DCIS. 818 patients s/p lumpectomy for DCIS with negative margins were randomized to observation versus postoperative RT. Whole breast radiation dose was 50 Gy; the study was later modified so that an additional 10 Gy boost was permitted to the lumpectomy cavity. Wapnir IL et al. Long-term outcomes of invasive ipsilateral breast tumor recurrences after lumpectomy in NSABP B-17 and B-24 randomized clinical trials for DCIS. J Natl Cancer Inst. 2011;103(6):478–88.

42. The correct answer is A. EORTC 10853 was a randomized trial initiated to define the role of radiation after lumpectomy for DCIS. 1010 patients s/p lumpectomy for DCIS with negative margins (tumor cells not at margin) were randomized to observation versus postoperative RT (50 Gy). With a median follow-up of 10.5 years, RT reduced noninvasive local failure 14 % to 7 %, as well as invasive failures 13 % to 8 %. There were no DM or OS differences. On multivariate analysis, features significantly associated with increased local recurrence were age ≤40 years, G2-3 DCIS, cribriform or solid pattern, doubtful margins, and omission of RT. Bijker N, Meijnen P, Peterse JL et al. Breast-conserving treatment with or without radiotherapy in ductal carcinoma in situ: 10-year results of European Organisation for Research and Treatment of Cancer randomized phase III trial 10853—a study by the EORTC Breast Cancer Cooperative Group and EORTC Radiotherapy Group. J Clin Oncol. 2006; 24(21):3381–7.

43. The correct answer is D. NSABP B-24 randomized 1,804 patients with DCIS s/p lumpectomy and 50 Gy RT to placebo versus 20 mg daily tamoxifen × 5 years. Approximately 25 % of patients had positive margins; ER status was unknown. In the latest update in 2011, there was a 32 % reduction in the risk of invasive in-breast tumor recurrence (I-IBTR) with the addition of tamoxifen to radiotherapy. The addition of tamoxifen to lumpectomy and radiation also reduced contralateral events by 32 %. Two-thirds (67 %) of these events were invasive. The addition of tamoxifen did not result in improved overall mortality. Wapnir IL et al. Long-term outcomes of invasive ipsilateral breast tumor recurrences after lumpectomy in NSABP B-17 and B-24 randomized clinical trials for DCIS. J Natl Cancer Inst. 2011;103(6):478–88.

44. The correct answer is B. NSABP B-24 randomized 1,804 patients with DCIS s/p lumpectomy and 50 Gy RT to placebo versus 20 mg daily tamoxifen × 5 years. Approximately 25 % of patients had positive margins; ER status was unknown. In the latest update in 2011, there was a 32 % reduction in the risk of invasive in-breast tumor recurrence (I-IBTR) with the addition of tamoxifen to radiotherapy. The addition of tamoxifen to lumpectomy and radiation also reduced contralateral events by 32 %. Two-thirds (67 %) of these events were invasive. The addition of tamoxifen did not result in improved overall mortality. Regarding mortality, I-IBTR was found to increase the risk of all-cause death, as well as breast cancer death. Noninvasive IBTR did not increase overall or breast cancer mortality risk. Contralateral invasive recurrence was also associated with an increase in mortality risk. Wapnir IL et al. Long-term outcomes of invasive ipsilateral breast tumor recurrences after lumpectomy in NSABP B-17 and B-24 randomized clinical trials for DCIS. J Natl Cancer Inst. 2011;103(6):478–88.

45. The correct answer is B. The UKCCR randomized 1,701 patients with DCIS s/p lumpectomy with negative margins to one of four arms: RT (50 Gy), tamoxifen (20 mg qd × 5 years), RT + tamoxifen, or neither. At a median follow-up of 53 months, rates of all breast events were 8 %, 18 %, 6 %, and 22 %, respectively. Looking at those randomized to RT versus no RT, RT reduced either noninvasive or invasive local failures from 14 % to 6 %. In contrast to NSABP-24, however, there was no additional benefit of tamoxifen in terms of ipsilateral invasive events, though it did decrease the overall incidence of DCIS. Notably, whereas 33.5 % of the women in NSABP-24 were <50 years old, only 9.5 % of the women in UKCCR were <50 years old. Houghton J et al. Radiotherapy and tamoxifen in women with completely excited ductal carcinoma in situ of the breast in the UK, Australia, and New Zealand: randomised control trial. Lancet. 2003;363(9378):95–102.

46. The correct answer is D. ECOG 5194 was a prospective study to determine the risk of IBTR after local excision without radiation. Women s/p lumpectomy with a clear margin of ≥3 mm were stratified into two cohorts and observed: Group 1 (G1-2, <2.5 cm) or Group 2 (G3, <1.0 cm). Tamoxifen was allowed. Pathologic

assessment was rigorous, with required complete sequential tissue processing. 5 years IBTR was 6.1 % in Group 1 and 15.3 % in Group 2, suggesting that excision alone is inadequate in the higher risk DCIS, but may be adequate in those with low-risk DCIS with clear ≥3 mm margins. Hughes LL et al. Local excision alone without irradiation for ductal carcinoma in situ of the breast: a trial of the Eastern Cooperative Oncology Group. J Clin Oncol. 2009;27(32):5319–24.

47. The correct answer is B. The Harvard DCIS observational study by Wong et al. prospectively sought to determine the risk of IBTR after local excision without radiation. Women were observed s/p lumpectomy with a clear margin of ≥1 cm. Tumors were <2.5 cm and mostly G1-2. Tamoxifen was NOT allowed. There were ten patients (6 %) with grade 3 tumors. Between 7 and 63 months after study entry, there were 13 local recurrences, corresponding to a 5 years IBTR was 12 % and meeting the predetermined stopping rules. The study was closed to accrual with the conclusion that despite wide margins in early stage tumors, there is a substantial risk for LR without radiation. Wong JS et al. Prospective study of wide excision alone for ductal carcinoma in situ of the breast. J Clin Oncol. 2006;24(7):1031–6.

48. The correct answer is D. Based on the retrospective review of 706 patients s/p BCT with or without RT, Silverstein created a prognostic index to predict the benefit of RT depending on pathological characteristics. Pathologic assessment was very rigorous and comprehensive in this study. Four parameters were scored 1–3: age (>60, 40–60, <40), margins (≥1 cm, 0.1–0.9 cm, <0.1 cm), grade (non-high grade without necrosis, non-high grade with necrosis, high grade), and tumor size (≤1.5 cm, 1.5–4.0 cm, ≥4. cm). Total scores were then grouped into three categories: low risk (≤6), intermediate (7–9), high (10–12). Ten-year local recurrence by group was low, 3 % with or without RT; intermediate, 21 % with RT; and high, 41 % with RT, prompting recommendations for no adjuvant RT in the low-risk group, RT in the intermediate risk group, and mastectomy in the high-risk group. An update was published in 2010, with the goal of achieving a 12-year LR of <20 %. Silverstein MJ. An argument against routine use of radiotherapy for ductal carcinoma in situ. Oncology 2003;(11):1511–23. Silverstein MJ, Lagios MD. Choosing treatment for patients with ductal carcinoma in situ: fine tuning the University of Southern California/Van Nuys Prognostic Index. J Natl Cancer Inst Monogr. 2010;(41):193–6.

49. The correct answer is C. Based on the retrospective review of 706 patients s/p BCT with or without RT, Silverstein created a prognostic index to predict the benefit of RT depending on pathological characteristics. Pathologic assessment was very rigorous and comprehensive in this study. Four parameters were scored 1–3: age (>60, 40–60, <40), margins (≥1 cm, 0.1–0.9 cm, <0.1 cm), grade (non-high grade without necrosis, non-high grade with necrosis, high grade), and tumor size (≤1.5 cm, 1.5–4.0 cm, ≥4.1 cm). Age of 40 years is scored "2 points." Silverstein MJ. An argument against routine use of radiotherapy for ductal

carcinoma in situ. Oncology. 2003;(11):1511–23. Silverstein MJ, Lagios MD. Choosing treatment for patients with ductal carcinoma in situ: fine tuning the University of Southern California/Van Nuys Prognostic Index. J Natl Cancer Inst Monogr. 2010;(41):193–6.

50. The correct answer is A. While multifocality (multiple foci of tumor in the same quadrant) is not a contraindication to BCT, multicentricity is (multiple foci in different breast quadrants). Lymph node involvement itself is not a contraindication to BCT nor is EIC independently (though it may be more difficult to obtain negative margins on resection). Recht A. Breast cancer: stages I and II. In: Gunderson LL, Tepper JE, editors. Clinical radiation oncology. 3rd ed. Philadelphia: Elsevier Saunders; 2012. p. 1321–38.

51. The correct answer is C. All of the listed choices are absolute contraindications except systemic lupus erythematosus. An additional absolute contraindication is diffuse suspicious or malignant-appearing microcalcifications. Relative contraindications include active connective tissue diseases involving the skin (SLE and scleroderma), tumors >5 cm, focally positive margin, women <35 years, or premenopausal women with a known BRCA1/2 mutation. NCCN Guidelines. Version 2.2011.

52. The correct answer is D. LCIS increases the risk of developing invasive carcinoma by 9–12 times. The risk of developing invasive cancer is 25 % at 20 years; this risk is reduced with tamoxifen. Lifelong close observation and prophylactic bilateral simple mastectomy are also viable treatment options. There is no role for radiation in the treatment of LCIS. Arthur DW, Vicini FA. Noninvasive breast cancer. In: Gunderson LL, Tepper JE, editors. Clinical radiation oncology. 3rd ed. Philadelphia: Elsevier Saunders; 2012. p. 1311–20.

53. The correct answer is D. NSABP B-06 randomized 1,851 patients with stage I/II (<4 cm) breast cancer to one of three arms: total mastectomy + ALN, lumpectomy + ALND, and lumpectomy + ALND + 50 Gy RT. All patients had negative margins. ER status data was available for ~3/4 of the women, with ~2/3 being ER+. Sixty-two percent of women were node negative; those with positive nodes underwent adjuvant melphalan + 5-FU. Twenty-year follow-up data was published in the NEJM in 2002. There were no differences observed between the arms in terms of DFS, OS, or DM-free survival. LR was scored differently between the mastectomy and lumpectomy arms. Recurrence in the chest wall or mastectomy scar was classified as a local recurrence. Recurrence in the ipsilateral breast after lumpectomy was not classified as a local failure, as the mastectomy arm was not at risk for this event; it was instead classified as a cosmetic failure. The addition of RT decreased LR in the lumpectomy arm from 39 % to 14 %. Fisher B et al. Twenty-year follow-up of a randomized trial comparing total mastectomy, lumpectomy, and lumpectomy plus irradiation for the treatment of invasive breast cancer. N Engl J Med. 2002;347(16):1233–41.

54. The correct answer is C. The Milan I trial randomized 701 patients with T1N0 invasive breast cancer to radical mastectomy versus quadrantectomy + 50 Gy RT + 10 Gy boost. Approximately 25 % of patients were LN + and subsequently received CMF chemotherapy. Twenty-year local recurrence was 2 % (RM) versus 9 % BCT. True in-quadrant recurrences were comparable (10 BCT, 8RM) as was OS (41 % in both groups), and DFS (~75 % in both groups), suggesting that BCT is an excellent treatment option for women with small breast cancers. Veronesi U et al. Twenty-year follow-up of a randomized study comparing breast-conserving surgery with radical mastectomy for early breast cancer. N Engl J Med. 2002;347(16):1227–32.

55. The correct answer is A. CALGB C9343 randomized 636 women $\geq$70 years with pT1N0 tumors to tamoxifen (20 mg daily × 5 years) versus tamoxifen + RT (45 Gy + boost). 97 % of patients were ER+. There were 3 % that were either ER negative or had unknown ER status. The addition of RT did improve LR at 10 years from 9 % to 2 %, but there was no difference in time to mastectomy or OS (63 % vs. 61 %). Hughes KS et al. Lumpectomy plus tamoxifen with or without irradiation in women 70 years of age or older with early breast cancer. N Engl J Med. 2004;351(10):971–7. Hughes KS. ASCO. 2010 Abstract #507.

56. The correct answer is D. NSABP B-21 randomized 1009 women with small $\leq$1 cm tumors to one of three arms: tamoxifen versus RT + placebo versus RT + tamoxifen. At 8 years, local recurrence was 16 % with tamoxifen alone, 9 % with RT alone, and 3 % with RT + tamoxifen. Though RT + tamoxifen did result in a greater reduction in the hazard rate of IBTR (81 %), RT alone still resulted in a 49 % lower hazard rate of IBTR. Moreover, RT reduced IBTR below the level achieved with tamoxifen alone. Tamoxifen reduced the incidence of contralateral breast cancers from 5.4 % to 2.2 %. There was no difference in survival between the three groups (93–94 %). Fisher B et al. Tamoxifen, radiation therapy, or both for prevention of ipsilateral breast tumor recurrence after lumpectomy in women with invasive breast cancers of one centimeter or less. J Clin Oncol. 2002:20(20):4149–59.

57. The correct answer is B. In NSABP B-18, 1,493 patients were randomized to undergo either preoperative or postoperative chemotherapy with Adriamycin and cyclophosphamide (AC). Those that underwent lumpectomy also received postoperative radiotherapy; postmastectomy RT was not allowed. While neoadjuvant chemotherapy did increase the percentage of patients undergoing breast-conservation therapy (68 % vs. 60 %), this did not result in disease-free or overall survival improvement. The pathological complete response rate (pCR) after neoadjuvant AC was 13 %. Those with a pCR did have significantly improved disease-free and overall survival, compared to those that did not. Rastogi P et al. Pre-operative chemotherapy: updates of National Surgical Adjuvant Breast and Bowel Project Protocols B-18 and B-27. J Clin Oncol. 2008;26(16):2793.

58. The correct answer is A. In NSABP B-27, 2,344 patients were randomized to one of three arms: preop AC; preop AC, then T (docetaxel), then surgery; and preop AC, then surgery, then T. While the addition of T to preop AC did not improve disease-free or overall survival, it did increase the pCR rate to 26 %. Those with a pCR did have significantly improved disease-free and overall survival, compared to those that did not. Rastogi P et al. Pre-operative chemotherapy: updates of National Surgical Adjuvant Breast and Bowel Project Protocols B-18 and B-27. J Clin Oncol. 2008;26(16):2793.

59. The correct answer is B. Haagensen's grave signs are a group of clinical signs described by Haagensen and Stout, in a review of patients treated for breast cancer at their hospital. There are five grave signs: (1) skin ulceration, (2) fixation of tumor to chest wall, (3) axillary nodes >2.5 cm in diameter, (4) edema of <1/3 of the skin of the breast, and (5) fixed/matted axillary nodes. The presence of two or more signs signifies inoperability. Palpable lymph nodes alone are not a grave sign. Buchholz TA. Breast cancer: postmastectomy radiation therapy, locally advanced disease, and inflammatory breast cancer. In: Gunderson LL, Tepper JE, editors. Clinical radiation oncology. 3rd ed. Philadelphia: Elsevier Saunders; 2012. p. 1339–53.

60. The correct answer is A. The chest wall is the most common site of locoregional failure. Buchholz TA. Breast cancer: postmastectomy radiation therapy, locally advanced disease, and inflammatory breast cancer. In: Gunderson LL, Tepper JE, editors. Clinical radiation oncology. 3rd ed. Philadelphia: Elsevier Saunders; 2012. p. 1339–53.

61. The correct answer is C. Inflammatory carcinoma is a clinical diagnosis, and pathological confirmation of tumor in the dermal lymphatics is NOT required. It presents with a rapid onset of erythema, warmth, and breast edema, and a mass is frequently not detected on clinical examination. Despite achieving a complete response with neoadjuvant chemotherapy, BCT is still contraindicated in inflammatory breast carcinoma. Buchholz TA. Breast cancer: postmastectomy radiation therapy, locally advanced disease, and inflammatory breast cancer. In: Gunderson LL, Tepper JE, editors. Clinical radiation oncology. 3rd ed. Philadelphia: Elsevier Saunders; 2012. p. 1339–53.

62. The correct answer is D. Fifty percent of inflammatory breast cancers have an associated mass at diagnosis. Perez CA et al. Management of locally advanced carcinoma of the breast. II. Inflammatory Carcinoma. Cancer 1994;74: 466–76.

63. The correct answer is A. Five percent of inflammatory cancer has a normal mammogram at diagnosis. Perez CA et al. Inflamm Breast Cancer 1994;74:466–76.

64. The correct answer is C. The Danish 82b trial randomized 1,708 premenopausal women s/p modified radical mastectomy with a median of seven dissected LNs, to receive either (1) adjuvant CMF chemotherapy alone, (2) CMF + RT, or (3) CMF + tamoxifen (enrollment in this group was later stopped due to higher mortality). Radiation (48–50 Gy) was given to the chest wall, SCF, and axillary and internal mammary nodes. The addition of radiotherapy decreased LRF from 32 % to 9 %, translating into ~10 % OS benefit (10-year OS, 54 % vs. 45 %). Disease-free survival was also improved. Over 50 % of recurrences were on the chest wall. Overgaard M et al. Postoperative radiotherapy in high-risk premenopausal with breast-cancer who receive adjuvant chemotherapy. Danish Breast Cancer Cooperative Group 82b Trial. N Engl J Med. 1997;337(14):949–55.

65. The correct answer is D. The Danish 82b trial randomized 1,708 premenopausal women s/p modified radical mastectomy with a median of seven dissected LNs, to receive either (1) adjuvant CMF chemotherapy alone, (2) CMF + RT, or (3) CMF + tamoxifen (enrollment in this group was later stopped due to higher mortality). Radiation (48–50 Gy) was given to the chest wall, SCF, and axillary and internal mammary nodes. The addition of radiotherapy decreased LRF from 32 % to 9 %, translating into ~10 % OS benefit (10-year OS, 54 % vs. 45 %). Disease-free survival was also improved. Over 50 % of recurrences were on the chest wall. Overgaard M et al. Postoperative radiotherapy in high-risk premenopausal with breast-cancer who receive adjuvant chemotherapy. Danish Breast Cancer Cooperative Group 82b Trial. N Engl J Med. 1997;337(14):949–55.

66. The correct answer is B. The Danish 82c trial randomized 1,375 postmenopausal women s/p modified radical mastectomy to receive either tamoxifen 30 mg daily × 1 year or tamoxifen + RT. Radiation (48–50 Gy) was given to the chest wall, SCF, and axillary and internal mammary nodes. The addition of radiotherapy decreased LRF from 35 % to 8 %, translating into ~10 % OS benefit (10-year OS, 45 % vs. 36 %). Overgaard M et al. Postoperative radiotherapy in high-risk postmenopausal with breast-cancer patients given adjuvant tamoxifen: Danish Breast Cancer Cooperative Group DBCG 82c Randomised Trial. Lancet. 1999;353(9165):1641–8.

67. The correct answer is B. The British Columbia trial randomized 318 premenopausal women s/p modified radical mastectomy with a median of 11 dissected LNs, and pathologically positive LNs, to receive either adjuvant CMF chemotherapy alone or CMF + RT. Radiation (37.5 Gy) was given to the chest wall, SCF, and axillary and internal mammary nodes. The addition of radiotherapy decreased LRF from 26 % to 10 %, translating into ~10 % OS benefit (20-year OS, 47 % vs. 37 %). Breast cancer-specific survival was also improved with radiotherapy (53 % vs. 38 %). Ragaz J et al. Locoregional radiation therapy in patients high-risk breast cancer receiving adjuvant chemotherapy: 20-year results of the British Columbia Randomized Trial. J Natl Cancer Inst. 2005;97(2):116–26.

68. The correct answer is B. The Canadian Hypofractionation trial by Whelan et al. randomized 1,234 women s/p lumpectomy for invasive breast cancer and negative ALND to receive whole breast radiotherapy by either standard fractionation RT (50 Gy in 25 fractions) or hypofractionation (42.5 Gy in 16 fractions). No boost was given. Tumors >5 cm were excluded, as were patients with a breast width >25 cm at the posterior border of the medial and lateral tangents. Patients were stratified according to age, tumor size, adjuvant systemic therapy, and center. Ten-year local recurrence was 6.7 % (standard) versus 6.2 % (hypofractionated), and good-excellent cosmesis was 71.3 % (standard) versus 69.8 % (hypofractionated). There was no difference in either overall or disease-free survival. Whelan TJ et al. Long-term results of hypofractionated radiotherapy for breast cancer. N Engl J Med. 2010;362:513–20.

69. The correct answer is C. The Canadian Hypofractionation trial by Whelan et al. randomized 1,234 women s/p lumpectomy for invasive breast cancer and negative ALND to receive whole breast radiotherapy by either standard fractionation RT (50 Gy in 25 fractions) or hypofractionation (42.5 Gy in 16 fractions). No boost was given. Tumors >5 cm were excluded, as were patients with a breast width >25 cm at the posterior border of the medial and lateral tangents. Patients were stratified according to age, tumor size, adjuvant systemic therapy, and center. There were no differences in either local control or cosmesis. Ten-year local recurrence was 6.7 % (standard) versus 6.2 % (hypofractionated), and good-excellent cosmesis was 71.3 % (standard) versus 69.8 % (hypofractionated). There was no difference in either overall or disease-free survival. Whelan TJ et al. Long-term results of hypofractionated radiotherapy for breast cancer. N Engl J Med. 2010;362:513–20.

70. The correct answer is B. The UK START A randomized 2,236 women with pT1-3, N0-1 invasive breast cancer to receive whole breast radiotherapy via one of three arms: (1) standard fractionation (SF—50 Gy/25) versus (2) 41.6 Gy/13 versus (3) 39 Gy/13. All were treated over 5 weeks—different fraction sizes were treated over the same treatment period. The UK START B randomized 2,215 women to receive whole breast radiotherapy via either standard fractionation (SF—50 Gy/25) or accelerated hypofractionation (AH—40 Gy/15). This trial looked at true accelerated hypofractionation-different treatment periods. Both trials allowed boosts. START Trialists' Group. The UK Standardisation of Breast Radiotherapy (START) Trial A of radiotherapy hypofractionation for treatment of early breast cancer: a randomised trial. Lancet. 2008;9(4):331–41. START Trialists' Group. The UK Standardisation of Breast Radiotherapy (START) Trial B of radiotherapy hypofractionation for treatment of early breast cancer: a randomised trial. Lancet. 2008;371(9618):1098–107.

71. The correct answer is C. The UK START B randomized 2,215 women with pT1-3, N0-1 invasive breast cancer to receive whole breast radiotherapy via either standard fractionation (SF—50 Gy/25) or accelerated hypofractionation (AHF—40 Gy/15). Boosts were allowed (51 %). After a median follow-up of 6 years,

local control was similar between the two groups, 2.2 % (AHF) versus 3.3 % (SF). There was a lower rate of distant relapse in the AHF arm, leading to higher rates of DFS and OS in the AHF arm. The survival difference was unexpected, and unexplained by known factors, and may disappear with longer follow-up. To assess breast appearance, photographs were taken at baseline and then at 2 and 5 years. At 5 years, there was little change in breast appearance (photographically) in the AHF group, as indicated by a hazard ratio of 0.83 (95 % CI 0.66–1.004, $p=0.06$). START Trialists' Group. The UK Standardisation of Breast Radiotherapy (START) Trial B of radiotherapy hypofractionation for treatment of early breast cancer: a randomised trial. Lancet. 2008;371(9618):1098–107.

72. The correct answer is B. The UK START A randomized 2,236 women with pT1-3, N0-1 invasive breast cancer to receive whole breast radiotherapy via one of three arms: standard fractionation (SF—50 Gy/25) versus 41.6 Gy/13 versus 39 Gy/13. Supraclavicular fossa radiotherapy was permitted. All were treated over 5 weeks—different fraction sizes were treated over the same treatment period. 5-year LRR did not differ between the arms (3.6 % vs. 3.5 % vs. 5.2 %). There were fewer late effects in the 39 Gy/13 fractions arm, but no differences between the 41.6 and 50 Gy arms. START Trialists' Group. The UK Standardisation of Breast Radiotherapy (START) Trial A of radiotherapy hypofractionation for treatment of early breast cancer: a randomised trial. Lancet. 2008;9(4):331–41.

73. The correct answer is B. Of the choices listed, permanent Ir-192 seed placement is not an APBI technique. Intraoperative x-rays were the studied technique of the TARGIT trial in which 2,232 women were randomized after lumpectomy to receive either whole breast radiotherapy or a single fraction of 20 Gy to the lumpectomy cavity via 50 kV x-rays. At 4 years, there was no difference in local recurrence between the arms (1.2 % APBI vs. 0.95 % WB). Radiotherapy toxicity was less in the APBI group (0.5 % vs. 2.1 %, $p=0.002$). 3DCRT and balloon brachytherapy are both allowed techniques on the NSABP-39 trial; interstitial brachytherapy is the third allowed APBI technique. Vaidya JS et al. Targeted intraoperative radiotherapy versus whole breast radiotherapy for breast cancer: TARGIT A Trial: an international prospective, randomised, non-inferiority phase 3 trial. Lancet. 2010;375(9735):91–102.

74. The correct answer is B. All fractionation for APBI is 3.4 Gy BID × 5 days, with the exception of 3.85 Gy BID × 5 days using the 3DCRT technique. Recht A. Breast cancer: stages I and II. In: Gunderson LL, Tepper JE, editors. Clinical radiation oncology. 3rd ed. Philadelphia: Elsevier Saunders; 2012. p. 1321–38.

75. The correct answer C. The ASTRO Consensus Statement for APBI was released in 2009. A 2.0 cm tumor is pT1 and would thus be in the suitable category. The other listed criteria are "cautionary" for APBI. Smith BD et al. Accelerated partial breast irradiation consensus statement from the American Society for Radiation Oncology (ASTRO). Int J Radiat Oncol Biol Phys. 2009;74(4): 987–1001.

76. The correct answer is D. MA.20 randomized 1,832 women with either high-risk node-negative or node-positive breast cancer treated with breast-conserving surgery and adjuvant chemotherapy and/or endocrine therapy to receive either whole breast irradiation (50 Gy +/− boost) or WBI + regional node irradiation (RNI) (45 Gy to supraclavicular, high axillary, and internal mammary). Ten percent of subjects were node negative, 85 % had 1–3 positive LNs, 5 % had >4 positive nodes. Ninety-one percent received adjuvant chemotherapy; 71 % received adjuvant endocrine therapy. With a median follow-up of 62 months, the addition of RNI was found to statistically significantly improve locoregional DFS, distant DFS, and overall DFS. There was a trend towards improved OS ($p=0.07$), notable with only 5 years follow-up. Whelan, et al. NCIC-CTG MA.20: an intergroup trial of regional nodal irradiation in early breast cancer. ASCO 2011 Meeting—Abstract LBA1003.

77. The correct answer is D. NSABP B-32 randomized 5,611 women with operable invasive breast cancer and clinically negative axillae to either SLNB + immediate completion ALND (group 1) versus SLNB alone with ALND only if no sentinel LN identified or SLN + (group 2). Technical success of SLNB was 97 %, and 99 % of LNs were in axillary levels I/II. The mean number of LNs removed was 2.1. There was no difference in the incidence of SLNs between groups (26 %). The SLN false-negative rate was 10 %. Overall accuracy was 97 %, with a negative predictive value of 96.1 %. Morbidity and deficit in shoulder range of motion, arm edema volume, and sensory deficits were all decreased in the SLNB group (group 2). Survival data was published in 2010. There was no difference in OS, DFS, or regional control between the two arms. Eight-year Kaplan-Meier estimates for OS were 91.8 % (group 1) versus 90.3 % (group 2). Krag DN et al. Technical outcomes of sentinel-lymph node resection and conventional axillary-lymph node dissection in patients with clinically node-negative breast cancer: results from the NSABP B-32 randomised phase III trial. Lancet Oncol. 2007;8(10):881–8. Ashikaga T et al. Morbidity results from the NSABP B-32 trial comparing sentinel lymph node dissection versus axillary dissection. J Surg Oncol. 2010;102(2):111–8. Krag DN et al. Sentinel-lymph node resection compared with conventional axillary-lymph node dissection in patients with clinically node-negative breast cancer: overall survival findings from the NSABP B-32 randomised phase 3 trial. Lancet Oncol. 2010;11(10):927–33.

78. The correct answer is B. NSABP B-32 randomized 5,611 women with operable invasive breast cancer and clinically negative axillae to either SLNB + immediate completion ALND (group 1) versus SLNB alone with ALND only if no sentinel LN identified or SLN + (group 2). Technical success of SLNB was 97 %, and 99 % of LNs were in axillary levels I/II. The mean number of LNs removed was 2.1. There was no difference in the incidence of SLNs between groups (26 %). The SLN false-negative rate was 10 %. Overall accuracy was 97 %, with a negative predictive value of 96.1 %. Morbidity and deficit in shoulder range of motion, arm edema volume, and sensory deficits were all decreased in the SLNB group (group 2). Survival data was published in 2010.

There was no difference in OS, DFS, or regional control between the two arms. Eight-year Kaplan-Meier estimates for OS were 91.8 % (group 1) versus 90.3 % (group 2). Krag DN et al. Technical outcomes of sentinel-lymph node resection and conventional axillary-lymph node dissection in patients with clinically node-negative breast cancer: results from the NSABP B-32 randomised phase III trial. Lancet Oncol. 2007;8(10):881–8. Ashikaga T et al. Morbidity results from the NSABP B-32 trial comparing sentinel lymph node dissection versus axillary dissection. J Surg Oncol. 2010;102(2):111–8. Krag DN et al. Sentinel-lymph node resection compared with conventional axillary-lymph node dissection in patients with clinically node-negative breast cancer: overall survival findings from the NSABP B-32 randomised phase 3 trial. Lancet Oncol. 2010;11(10):927–33.

79. The correct answer is B. ACOSOG Z0011 randomized 891 women with pT1-2 invasive breast cancer without palpable adenopathy, and either 1–2 positive sentinel LNs to undergo or not, and without completion axillary dissection of at least ten axillary LNs. The median age was 55 years, and the majority (82 %) had estrogen-receptor-positive tumors. The majority (71 %) had only one positive SLN. Of those randomized to undergo completion axillary dissection, 27 % were found to have additional positive axillary lymph nodes. Following surgery, patients on both arms underwent tangential whole breast irradiation, though the superior border of the tangential fields is unknown. With tangents, a significant portion of axillary levels I and II can be treated, and this can be further increased with the use of high tangents. This was a non-inferiority study with a primary endpoint of OS. With a median follow-up of 6.3 years, those that did not undergo axillary dissection despite having positive SLNs did not experience inferior disease-free or overall survival. Giuliano et al. Axillary dissection vs. no axillary dissection in women with invasive breast cancer and sentinel node metastasis. JAMA. 2011;305(6):569–75.

80. The correct answer is C. ACOSOG Z0011 randomized 891 women with pT1-2 invasive breast cancer without palpable adenopathy, and either 1–2 positive sentinel LNs to undergo or not, and without completion axillary dissection of at least ten axillary LNs. The median age was 55 years, and the majority (82 %) had estrogen-receptor-positive tumors. The majority (71 %) had only one positive SLN. Of those randomized to undergo completion axillary dissection, 27 % were found to have additional positive axillary lymph nodes. Following surgery, patients on both arms underwent tangential whole breast irradiation, though the superior border of the tangential fields is unknown. With tangents, a significant portion of axillary levels I and II can be treated, and this can be further increased with the use of high tangents. This was a non-inferiority study with a primary endpoint of OS. With a median follow-up of 6.3 years, those that did not undergo axillary dissection despite having positive SLNs did not experience inferior disease-free or overall survival. Giuliano et al. Axillary dissection vs. no axillary dissection in women with invasive breast cancer and sentinel node metastasis. JAMA. 2011;305(6):569–75.

81. The correct answer is A. NSABP B-20 randomized 2,306 patients s/p surgery with pathologically negative, ER + breast cancers to one of three arms: tamoxifen alone versus tamoxifen + MF versus tamoxifen + CMF. There was no tamoxifen + CF arm. NSABP B-20 randomized 2,306 patients s/p surgery with pathologically node-negative, ER + breast cancers to one of three arms: tamoxifen alone versus tamoxifen + MF versus tamoxifen + CMF. There was no tamoxifen + CF arm. The addition of chemotherapy to tamoxifen improved not only DFS (90 % vs. 85 %, $p = 0.0001$) but also OS (97 % vs. 87 %, $p = 0.03$) with 5 years follow-up. The benefit of chemotherapy persisted regardless of tumor size, ER/PR level, and patient age, though the group that benefited most was that ≤49 years. There was no subgroup that did not benefit. Fisher B et al. Tamoxifen and chemotherapy for lymph node-negative, estrogen receptor-positive breast cancer. J Natl Cancer Inst. 1997;89(22):1673–82.

82. The correct answer is C. NSABP B-28 randomized 3,060 patients s/p surgery with pathologically node-positive breast cancer to one of two arms: AC × 4 cycles versus AC × 4 cycles + paclitaxel × 4 cycles. The addition of paclitaxel chemotherapy to AC improved not only locoregional recurrence but also DFS (76 % vs. 72 %, $p = 0.006$) with 5 years follow-up. There was no OS benefit. Those patients with ER + tumors (approximately 2/3 of the patients) also received TAM × 5 years. No interaction was seen between treatment effect and receptor status of use of TAM. Mamounas et al. Paclitaxel after doxorubicin plus cyclophosphamide as adjuvant chemotherapy for node-positive breast cancer: results from NSABP B-28. J Clin Oncol. 2005;23(16):3686–96.

83. The correct answer is C. The Early Breast Cancer Trialists' Collaborative Group meta-analysis regarding chemotherapy included data from over 18,000 women. It showed that all women derive benefit in terms of death from 6 months of chemotherapy, with women <50 years gaining more benefit. The risk of reduction of death is 38% for those <50 years, compared to 20 % in those >50 years, irrespective of ER status, nodal status, or other tumor characteristics. Node-positive patients derive more benefit than node-negative patients (11 % vs. 7 % absolute gain in survival). Anthracycline chemotherapy is superior to CMF chemotherapy with an improvement in 5-year survival from 69 % to 72 %. Early Breast Cancer Trialists' Collaborative Group. Polychemotherapy for early breast cancer: an overview of the randomised trials. Early Breast Cancer Trialists' Collaborative Group. Lancet. 1998;352(9132):930–42. Early Breast Cancer Trialists' Collaborative Group. Effects of chemotherapy and hormonal therapy for early breast cancer on recurrence and 15-year survival: an overview of the randomised trials. Lancet. 2005;365(9472):1687–717.

84. The correct answer is C. A randomized, placebo-controlled, double-blind trial from Goss et al. showed that at a median follow-up of 35 months, there was a 65 % relative reduction in the annual incidence of invasive breast cancer (0.19 % vs. 0.55 %) with the use of exemestane. There were no differences in terms of

increased skeletal fractures, bisphosphonate therapy use, or cardiovascular events. Quality of life was assessed 1 week before randomization, and then 6 and 12 months, and then yearly after randomization. Menopausal symptoms were more common in those women taking exemestane. Goss, et al. Exemestane for breast-cancer prevention in postmenopausal women. N Engl J Med. 2011;364(25):2381–91.

85. The correct answer is D. The Early Breast Cancer Trialists' Collaborative Group study was a meta-analysis of 78 randomized trials published in 2005, including 42,000 women. Radiation after both breast-conserving surgery and mastectomy was found to confer a significant absolute local control improvement of 20 %, which translated into a 5 % absolute benefit in breast cancer mortality, at 15 years. This benefit was observed in addition to and independent of systemic therapy. In terms of non-breast cancer mortality, radiation did increase the risk of heart disease mortality (RR 1.27), as well as lung cancer mortality (RR 1.78). However, this excess non-breast cancer mortality is still less than the improvement in breast cancer-specific mortality. Early Breast Cancer Trialists' Collaborative Group. Effects of radiotherapy and of differences in the extent of surgery for early breast cancer on local recurrence and 15 year survival: an overview of the randomized trials. Lancet. 2005;366: 2087–106.

86. The correct answer is C. The EORTC boost trial randomized 5,318 patients with stage I/II breast cancer after lumpectomy with negative margins and whole breast radiotherapy (50 Gy) to +/− 16 Gy boost. DCIS at the margin was ignored. Two-hundred fifty-one patients with microscopically positive margins were randomized to 10Gy vs. 26Gy. Median age was 55 years. With 10 years of follow-up, the addition of a 16 Gy boost decreased LF from 10.2 % to 6.2 %. The benefit was seen in all age groups, though it was the greatest in those ≤40 years old (23.9 % vs. 13.5 %) and smallest in those >60 years. The boost was associated with higher rates of severe fibrosis (4.4 % vs. 1.6 %, $p < 0.0001$). Survival at 10 years was 82 % in both arms. Bartelink H et al. Impact of a higher radiation dose on local control and survival in breast-conserving therapy of early breast cancer: 10-year results of the randomized boost versus no boost EORTC 22881–10882 trial. J Clin Oncol. 2007;25(22):3259–65.

87. The correct answer A. The Lyon boost trial randomized 1,024 patients with early stage breast cancer after lumpectomy, ALND, and whole breast radiotherapy (50 Gy) to +/− 10 Gy boost. With 5 years follow-up, the addition of a 10 Gy boost decreased LF from 4.5 % to 3.6 %. There was no difference in self-assessed cosmesis between the two arms, though the boost group did have a higher rate of grade 1 and 2 telangiectasias (12.4 % vs. 5.9 %). Romestaing P et al. Role of a 10 Gy boost in the conservative treatment of early breast cancer: results of a randomized clinical trial in Lyon, France. J Clin Oncol. 1997;15(3):963–8.

Chapter 7
Upper Gastrointestinal Cancers

Faisal Siddiqui, Celine Bicquart Ord, and Charles R. Thomas, Jr.

Questions

1. What is the approximate number of new annual cases of esophageal cancer in the United States?
   A. 7,000
   B. 12,000
   C. 17,000
   D. 25,000

2. Which of the following is not a risk factor for the development of esophageal cancer?
   A. Plummer–Vinson syndrome
   B. Tobacco and alcohol
   C. Tylosis
   D. *H. pylori* infection

F. Siddiqui, MD, PhD (✉)
Department of Radiation Medicine, Oregon Health & Science University,
3181 Sam Jackson Park Road, KPV4, Portland, OR 97229, USA
e-mail: siddiqui@ohsu.edu

C.B. Ord, MD
Department of Radiation Oncology, Scott & White Memorial Hospital, Temple, TX 76508, USA
e-mail: cord@sw.org

C.R. Thomas Jr., MD
Department of Radiation Medicine, Knight Cancer Institute, Oregon Health &
Science University, 3181 SW Sam Jackson Park Road, KPV4, 97239-3098 Portland, OR, USA
e-mail: thomasch@ohsu.edu; thomas@gmail.com

C.B. Ord et al. (eds.), *Radiation Oncology Study Guide*,
DOI 10.1007/978-1-4614-6400-6_7, © Springer Science+Business Media New York 2013

3. The mid-thoracic esophagus begins at which distance from the upper incisors?
   A. 15–20 cm
   B. 20–25 cm
   C. 25–30 cm
   D. 30–40 cm

4. What is the correct 7th edition AJCC TNM stage for a 3 cm distal esophagus adenocarcinoma that invades the muscularis mucosa, and is found to have two involved regional lymph nodes, with no evidence of distant metastatic disease?
   A. T1N0M0
   B. T2N2M0
   C. T2N1M0
   D. T3N2M0

5. All of the following are components of a transhiatal esophagectomy, except:
   A. Cervical anastomosis
   B. Gastric conduit in esophageal bed
   C. Celiotomy
   D. Thoracotomy

6. In the CALGB 9781 trial (Tepper et al.) in which patients were randomized to surgery alone versus neoadjuvant chemoRT followed by surgery, what was the reported 5-year overall survival benefit seen with the addition of neoadjuvant therapy?
   A. 12 %
   B. 18 %
   C. 23 %
   D. 30 %

7. What were the chemotherapy agents and total radiotherapy doses employed in the CALGB 9781 trial?
   A. Cisplatin, 5-FU, and 50.4 Gy
   B. Cisplatin, etoposide, and 45 Gy
   C. Cisplatin, paclitaxel, and 54 Gy
   D. Cisplatin, 5-FU, and 45 Gy

8. What was the pathologic complete response rate seen in those that underwent neoadjuvant chemoRT in CALGB 9781?
   A. 5 %
   B. 15 %
   C. 40 %
   D. 45 %

9. The phase III study, RTOG 85-01 (Herskovic et al.), randomized patients with esophageal cancer to:
   A. Surgery alone versus neoadjuvant chemoRT
   B. Surgery alone versus neoadjuvant chemotherapy
   C. Surgery alone versus radiation alone
   D. Radiation alone versus chemoRT

10. What was the radiation dose employed in the control arm of RTOG 85-01?
   A. 45 Gy
   B. 50.4 Gy
   C. 60 Gy
   D. 64 Gy

11. What was the 5-year overall survival in the control arm of RTOG 85-01?
   A. 32 %
   B. 26 %
   C. 8 %
   D. 0 %

12. Which of the following is the esophageal dose escalation study that did not show a benefit for increasing radiation dose?
   A. INT 0123 (Minsky et al.)
   B. RTOG 92-07 (Gaspar et al.)
   C. RTOG 02-46 (Swisher et al.)
   D. EORTC (Bosset et al.)

13. What was the radiation dose employed in the high-dose arm of the esophageal dose escalation study (Minsky et al.)?
   A. 60 Gy
   B. 63 Gy
   C. 64.8 Gy
   D. 66 Gy

14. Which was an arm of the neoadjuvant therapy for esophageal cancer as reported by Walsh et al.?
   A. Weekly cisplatin + radiation, then surgery
   B. Continuous 5-FU + radiation, then surgery
   C. Cisplatin/5-FU + radiation, then surgery
   D. Carboplatin/paclitaxel + radiation, then surgery

15. What was the total radiation dose/fractionation of the Walsh neoadjuvant trial?
   A. 45 Gy in 25 fractions
   B. 40 Gy in 15 fractions
   C. 42.7 Gy in 16 fractions
   D. 50.4 Gy in 28 fractions

16. What was the pathological complete response rate in those that underwent neoadjuvant therapy prior to surgery in the Walsh neoadjuvant trial?
    A. 8 %
    B. 14 %
    C. 22 %
    D. 30 %

17. The CROSS group/Dutch study (van Hagen et al.) randomized patients to surgery versus neoadjuvant chemoRT followed by surgery. The neoadjuvant chemotherapy and RT was:
    A. Cisplatin/5-FU and 50.4 Gy
    B. Carboplatin/paclitaxel and 50.4 Gy
    C. Cisplatin/5-FU and 41.4 Gy
    D. Carboplatin/paclitaxel and 41.4 Gy

18. The CROSS group/Dutch study showed a benefit for neoadjuvant chemoradiation compared to surgery alone. The median overall survival advantage for neoadjuvant chemoRT followed by surgery was:
    A. 49 months versus 24 months.
    B. 18 months versus 12 months.
    C. There was no overall survival advantage with neoadjuvant chemoRT.
    D. There was actually a survival detriment to neoadjuvant chemoRT.

19. What was the pathological complete response rate in those that underwent neoadjuvant chemoradiation in the CROSS trial?
    A. 5 %
    B. 20 %
    C. 30 %
    D. 35 %

20. What was the most common grade 3 toxicity seen in those undergoing neoadjuvant chemoradiation in the CROSS trial?
    A. Anemia
    B. Anorexia
    C. Leukopenia
    D. Duodenal perforation

21. In which subsite of the stomach is gastric cancer least commonly found?
    A. Antrum
    B. Lesser curvature of the body
    C. Greater curvature of the body
    D. Cardia

22. What percentage of those with gastric cancer undergo potentially curative surgery?
    A. 90 %
    B. 75 %
    C. 50 %
    D. 25 %

23. All are true statements regarding the GITSG trial for locally advanced gastric cancer, except:
    A. Patients were randomized to chemoradiation versus chemotherapy alone.
    B. Maintenance MeCCNU + 5-FU was given in the experimental arm.
    C. Resection of the primary tumor was not allowed.
    D. Overall survival improved with the addition of radiation.

24. The MAGIC trial (Cunningham et al.) randomized patients to surgery alone versus surgery with perioperative chemotherapy. What were the chemotherapy agents?
    A. Cisplatin, 5-FU
    B. Epirubicin, carboplatin, paclitaxel
    C. Epirubicin, cisplatin, 5-FU
    D. Epirubicin, cyclophosphamide, 5-FU

25. The MAGIC trial (Cunningham et al.) randomized patients to surgery alone versus surgery with perioperative chemotherapy and demonstrated that:
    A. Perioperative chemotherapy with surgery improved 5-year overall survival from 23 % to 36 %.
    B. Perioperative chemotherapy did not impact progression-free survival.
    C. Perioperative chemotherapy with surgery was more toxic than surgery alone.
    D. There was not a significant T-stage downstaging benefit with perioperative chemotherapy.

26. Histologies of gastric cancer in order of decreasing prevalence are:
    A. Adenocarcinoma, squamous cell carcinoma, lymphoma, carcinoid, malignant stromal cell
    B. Squamous cell carcinoma, adenocarcinoma, lymphoma, carcinoid, malignant stromal cell
    C. Lymphoma, adenocarcinoma, squamous cell carcinoma, carcinoid, malignant stromal cell
    D. Adenocarcinoma, lymphoma, carcinoid, malignant stromal cell, squamous cell carcinoma

27. The SWOG 9008/INT 0116 trial (MacDonald et al.) randomized patients to:
    A. Surgery alone versus surgery with perioperative chemotherapy
    B. Surgery alone versus surgery followed by adjuvant chemoradiation
    C. Surgery alone versus neoadjuvant chemotherapy followed by surgery
    D. Surgery alone versus definitive chemoradiation.

28. In the SWOG 9008/INT 0116 trial (MacDonald et al.), the percent of patients undergoing D0 and D2 resection, respectively, was:
    A. 50 %, 10 %
    B. 50 %, 30 %
    C. 30 %, 50 %
    D. 10 %, 50 %

29. All of the following are true regarding the SWOG 9008/INT 0116 trial (MacDonald et al.), regarding the addition of adjuvant therapy to resected gastric cancer, except:
    A. Those with gastroesophageal junction tumors were not excluded.
    B. The addition of adjuvant therapy improved 3-year overall survival.
    C. Chemotherapy consisted of cisplatin and 5-FU.
    D. Diffuse-type gastric carcinoma does not yield a benefit from adjuvant therapy.

30. Gastric adenocarcinoma has been subdivided into the intestinal-type and diffuse-type (Lauren's classification). Which of the following statements is false?
    A. Intestinal-type is associated with an older population and is more common in men.
    B. Intestinal-type is associated with *H. pylori* infection.
    C. Diffuse-type is associated with a precancerous lesion.
    D. Diffuse-type has a poorer prognosis than intestinal-type.

31. Which of the following is not a risk factor for the development of gastric cancer?
    A. Cigarette smoking
    B. *H. pylori* infection
    C. Chronic gastritis
    D. Gastroesophageal reflux disease

32. Imatinib, used in the treatment of gastrointestinal stromal tumors (GISTs), targets:
    A. *RET*
    B. *ras*
    C. *raf*
    D. *kit*

33. Gastrointestinal tumors with which mutation respond best to imatinib?
    A. Exon 9
    B. Exon 11
    C. Exon 13
    D. Exon 17

34. Which of the following is not known to be a risk factor for the development of pancreatic cancer?
    A. Cigarette smoking
    B. High-fat diet
    C. Exposure to radiation
    D. Coffee drinking

35. In adults, the pancreas lies at approximately which vertebral level?
    A. T10–T11
    B. T12–L1
    C. L1–L2
    D. L2–L3

36. The most common histology of pancreatic cancer is:
    A. Adenocarcinoma
    B. Intraductal carcinoma
    C. Squamous cell carcinoma
    D. Cystadenocarcinoma

37. Which of the following is not a common presenting symptom of pancreatic cancer?
    A. Abdominal pain
    B. Nausea and vomiting
    C. Migratory thrombophlebitis (Trousseau sign)
    D. Weight loss

38. What is the most common genetic mutation seen in pancreatic cancer?
    A. *kras*
    B. *RET*
    C. *p53*
    D. *braf*

39. Which of the following has important prognostic value in pancreatic cancer?
    A. CA-125
    B. CEA
    C. CA 19–9
    D. AFP

40. What percentage of pancreatic cancers are resectable at diagnosis?
    A. >90 %
    B. 75 %
    C. 50 %
    D. <25 %

41. What percentage of patients with pancreatic cancer present with distant metastases at diagnosis?
    A. 75 %
    B. 50 %
    C. 25 %
    D. 10 %

42. The GITSG 9173 trial (Kalser et al.) of postoperative therapy for resected pancreatic cancer demonstrated an overall survival benefit with adjuvant therapy. The 2-year overall survivals with and without adjuvant therapy were, respectively:
    A. 55 % versus 26 %
    B. 42 % versus 15 %
    C. 19 % versus 5 %
    D. 32 % versus 19 %

43. The GITSG 9173 trial (Kalser et al.) of postoperative chemoradiation in resected pancreatic cancer employed which dose of radiation?
    A. 45 Gy in 25 fractions at 1.8 Gy/fraction
    B. 50 Gy in 25 fractions at 2 Gy/fraction
    C. Split course with 20 Gy in 10 fractions, a 2-week break, then another 20 Gy in 10 fractions
    D. Split course with 18 Gy in 10 fractions, a 2-week break, then another 18 Gy in 10 fractions

44. Which of the following was an arm of the RTOG 97-04 trial for resected pancreatic cancer?
    A. Surgery followed by adjuvant gemcitabine + concurrent radiation
    B. Surgery followed by adjuvant 5-FU + concurrent radiation
    C. Surgery followed by induction gemcitabine, then concurrent radiation with gemcitabine, then adjuvant gemcitabine
    D. Surgery followed by induction gemcitabine, then concurrent radiation with 5-FU, then adjuvant gemcitabine

45. What was the 3-year overall survival of the experimental arm in RTOG 97-04?
    A. 20 %
    B. 30 %
    C. 40 %
    D. 50 %

46. The CONKO-001 trial (Neuhaus et al.) randomized patients after resection of pancreatic cancer to:
    A. Gemcitabine alone versus observation
    B. Fluorouracil alone versus observation
    C. Concurrent chemoradiation versus radiation alone
    D. Concurrent chemoradiation versus chemotherapy alone

47. The CONKO-001 trial showed:
    A. Improved disease-free, but not overall survival in the experimental arm
    B. No disease-free or overall survival benefit in the experimental arm
    C. Improved disease-free and overall survival in the experimental arm
    D. Worse disease-free and overall survival in the experimental arm

48. GITSG 9273 randomized patients with locally unresectable pancreatic cancer to one of three arms. Which one of the following was not one of these arms?
    A. 60 Gy alone
    B. 40 Gy + concurrent 5-FU
    C. 50 Gy + concurrent 5-FU
    D. 60 Gy + concurrent 5-FU

49. The ESPAC trial of adjuvant therapy for resected cancer randomized patients in a 2×2 design to observation, chemoradiotherapy, chemotherapy alone, or both. The total radiation dose employed in this trial was:
    A. 20 Gy
    B. 45 Gy
    C. 50.4 Gy
    D. 54 Gy

50. The ESPAC trial of adjuvant therapy for resected cancer randomized patients in a 2×2 design to observation, chemoradiotherapy, chemotherapy alone, or both. What was the published conclusion from this trial?
    A. There is no benefit for adjuvant therapy.
    B. There is a survival benefit only for chemotherapy + chemoradiotherapy.
    C. There is a survival benefit only for chemoradiotherapy alone.
    D. There is a survival benefit only for chemotherapy.

51. In treating a resected head of pancreas tumor with postoperative radiation, which of the following does not need to be included in the radiation field?
    A. Splenic hilum
    B. Duodenal bed
    C. Porta hepatis
    D. Pancreaticoduodenal lymph nodes

52. In treating a resected tail of pancreas tumor with postoperative radiation, which of the following does not need to be included in the radiation field?
    A. Splenic hilum
    B. Duodenal bed
    C. Pancreaticoduodenal lymph nodes
    D. Lateral suprapancreatic lymph nodes

53. Screening for patients at high risk of hepatocellular carcinoma should include:
    A. Triple phase liver CT scan, abdominal ultrasound, and serum alpha-fetoprotein
    B. Triple phase liver CT scan and serum alpha-fetoprotein
    C. Liver ultrasound and serum alpha-fetoprotein
    D. CT scan without contrast and complete metabolic panel

54. According to the AJCC 7th edition, what is the correct stage for a patient with a solitary hepatocellular carcinoma measuring 4.2 cm in largest dimension with a single positive lymph node?
    A. Stage IIIA
    B. Stage IIIB
    C. Stage IVA
    D. Stage IVB

55. Which of the following is not a component of Child–Pugh scoring?
    A. Encephalopathy
    B. Serum alkaline phosphatase
    C. Albumin
    D. Prothrombin time

56. What percentage of those undergoing cholecystectomy for cholelithiasis are incidentally found to have gallbladder cancer?
    A. 50 %
    B. 40 %
    C. 25 %
    D. 10 %

57. Which of the following does not predict a favorable outcome in resectable gallbladder cancer?
    A. Papillary histology
    B. Younger age
    C. Adjuvant radiation
    D. Neoadjuvant chemotherapy

58. All of the following are risk factors for cholangiocarcinoma, except:
    A. Ulcerative colitis
    B. Primary sclerosing cholangitis
    C. Hepatitis B or C infection
    D. Cholecystectomy

59. The most common location for extrahepatic cholangiocarcinoma is:
    A. Cystic duct
    B. Pancreatic duct
    C. Bifurcation of the common hepatic duct
    D. Ampulla of Vater

60. Which of the following is not a subtype of bile duct adenocarcinoma?
    A. Sclerosing
    B. Nodular
    C. Clear-cell
    D. Papillary

61. Carcinoid tumors stain for all of the following, except:
    A. Myoglobin
    B. Neuron-specific enolase
    C. Synaptophysin
    D. Chromogranin

62. What is the most common site of carcinoid tumor?
    A. Liver
    B. Appendix
    C. Ileum
    D. Duodenum

63. What is the most common tumor of the small bowel?
    A. Squamous cell carcinoma
    B. Carcinoid
    C. Lymphoma
    D. Adenocarcinoma

Answers and Rationales

1. The correct answer is C. In the United States, the approximate number of new annual cases of esophageal cancer is 17,500, with 15,000 annual deaths. http://www.cancer.gov/cancertopics/types/esophageal

2. The correct answer is D. In fact, *H. pylori* is considered protective for esophageal cancer, especially adenocarcinoma. Plummer–Vinson syndrome is the thin growth of excess tissue in the esophagus that leads to obstructive symptoms and dysphagia with resultant increase in esophageal squamous cell carcinoma. It is associated with glossitis and iron-deficiency anemia. Tylosis esophageal cancer is associated with a locus on chromosome 17q25 and is associated with sporadic causes of squamous cell esophageal carcinoma and Barrett's adenocarcinoma. Other risk factors are obesity, gastroesophageal reflux disease, lack of dietary fiber, and lack of fruits and vegetables in the diet. Risk JM, Mills HS, Garde J, et al. The tylosis esophageal cancer (TOC) locus: more than just a familial cancer gene. Dis Esophagus. 1999;12(3):173–6. Blackstock AW, Russo S. Cancer of the esophagus. In: Gunderson LL, Tepper JE editors., Clinical radiation oncology. 3rd ed. .Philadelphia: Elsevier Saunders; 2012. p. 839–58.

3. The correct answer is C. The esophagus is divided by endoscopic measurements from the upper incisors. The cervical esophagus extends from 15 to 20 cm, the upper thoracic esophagus extends from 20 to 25 cm, the middle thoracic extends from 25 to 30 cm, and the lower thoracic esophagus extends from 30 to 40 cm. These distances correspond to anatomical landmarks: cervical esophagus starts at the distal hypopharynx to the sternal notch, the upper thoracic esophagus extends from sternal notch to the azygos vein, the midthoracic esophagus extends from the azygos vein to the inferior pulmonary vein, and the lower thoracic esophagus extends to the gastroesophageal junction. Blackstock AW,, Russo S. Cancer of the esophagus. In: Gunderson LL, Tepper JE, editors. Clinical radiation oncology. 3rd ed. Philadelphia: Elsevier Saunders; 2012. p. 839–58.

4. The correct answer is C. Invasion of the muscularis propria is denoted as T2. N1 describes involvement of 1–2 regional LNs. This would be stage IIB. T-staging for esophageal cancer is defined by depth of invasion, while N staging denotes number of involved regional lymph nodes. The most recent edition of AJCC staging now subdivides the staging of esophageal cancer by histology-squamous cell carcinoma versus adenocarcinoma. For squamous cell carcinoma, tumor location is a component of the staging whereas it is independent of location for adenocarcinoma. Both now take grade of tumor into account in stage groupings. Edge SB, Byrd DR, Compton CC, et al., editors. Esophagus and esophagogastric junction. AJCC cancer staging handbook. 7th ed. New York, NY: Springer; 2010.

5. The correct answer is D. All of the listed choices are components of transhiatal esophagectomy, except for thoracotomy. The major advantage of this approach is the avoidance of combined thoracoabdominal incision and mediastinitis associated with an intrathoracic esophageal anastomotic leak. Orringer MB, Sloan H. Esophagectomy with thoracotomy. J Thorac Cardiovasc Surg. 1978;76(5):643–54.

6. The correct answer is C. CALGB 9781 randomized 56 patients with resectable esophageal cancer to surgery alone versus neoadjuvant chemoradiation (cisplatin and 5-FU with 50.4 Gy in 28 fractions) followed by surgery. The addition of neoadjuvant chemoRT to surgery improved 5-year overall survival from 16 % to 39 % (23 % benefit). Median survival improved from 1.8 y to 4.5 y. Patients who underwent neoadjuvant therapy had a pathologic complete response rate of 40 %. Tepper J. et al. Phase III trial of trimodality therapy with cisplatin, fluorouracil, radiotherapy, and surgery compared with surgery alone for esophageal cancer: CALGB 9781. J Clin Oncol. 2008;26:1086–92.

7. The correct answer is A. Cisplatin 100 mg/m² bolus IV infusion was given during 30 min on days 1 and 29. 5-FU 1,000 mg/m²/day was administered as a continuous IV infusion for 96 h after completion of cisplatin on day 1–day 4 and then again on day 29–day 32. Radiotherapy (50.4 Gy in 28 fractions) was begun within 24 h of administration of chemotherapy, with the final 5.4 Gy delivered as a boost. Radiation fields extended 5 cm beyond the proximal and distal extent of the tumor and radially 2 cm beyond the apparent mass. Supraclavicular lymph nodes were included if the tumor extended 2 cm above the carina. If the primary tumor was in the distal third of the esophagus or the celiac nodes were involved, the radiation fields were enlarged to include this target. Surgery was performed 3–8 weeks after completion of chemoradiation. Tepper J et al. Phase III trial of trimodality therapy with cisplatin, fluorouracil, radiotherapy, and surgery compared with surgery alone for esophageal cancer: CALGB 9781. J Clin Oncol. 2008;26:1086–92.

8. The correct answer is C. CALGB 9781 randomized 56 patients with resectable esophageal cancer to surgery alone versus neoadjuvant chemoradiation (cisplatin and 5-FU with 50.4 Gy in 28 fractions) followed by surgery. The addition of neoadjuvant chemoRT to surgery improved 5-year overall survival from 16 % to 39 % (23 % benefit). Median survival improved from 1.8 y to 4.5 y. Patients who underwent neoadjuvant therapy had a pathologic complete response rate of 40 %. Tepper J. et al. Phase III trial of trimodality therapy with cisplatin, fluorouracil, radiotherapy, and surgery compared with surgery alone for esophageal cancer: CALGB 9781. J Clin Oncol. 2008;26:1086–92.

9. The correct answer is D. RTOG 8501 randomized 121 patients with unresectable esophageal cancer to chemoradiation versus radiation alone. In the radiation alone arm, radiation was delivered to a total of 64 Gy at 2 Gy per fraction

over 30 daily fractions. In the concurrent chemoradiation arm, radiation was delivered to a total of 50 Gy in 25 fractions with concurrent cisplatin and 5-FU, followed by two cycles of cisplatin and 5-FU. Concurrent chemoradiation improved median survival (14.1 months vs. 9.3 months). Five-year overall survival with RT alone was 0 % versus 26 % with chemoRT. The study was stopped early due to the clear benefit of chemoradiation over radiation alone. Herskovic A. et al. Combined chemotherapy and radiotherapy compared with radiotherapy alone in patients with cancer of the esophagus. N Engl J Med. 1992;326(24):1593–8.

10. The correct answer is D. RTOG 8501 randomized 121 patients with unresectable esophageal cancer to chemoradiation (experimental arm) versus radiation alone (control arm). In the radiation alone arm, radiation was delivered to a total of 64 Gy at 2 Gy per fraction over 30 daily fractions. Concurrent chemoradiation improved median survival (14.1 months vs. 9.3 months). Five-year overall survival with RT alone was 0 % versus 26 % with chemoRT. The study was stopped early due to the clear benefit of chemoradiation over radiation alone. Herskovic A. et al. Combined chemotherapy and radiotherapy compared with radiotherapy alone in patients with cancer of the esophagus. N Engl J Med. 1992;326(24):1593–8.

11. The correct answer is D. RTOG 8501 randomized 121 patients with unresectable esophageal cancer to chemoradiation (experimental arm) versus radiation alone (control arm). In the radiation alone arm, radiation was delivered to a total of 64 Gy at 2 Gy per fraction over 30 daily fractions. Concurrent chemoradiation improved median survival (14.1 months vs. 9.3 months). Five-year overall survival with RT alone was 0 % versus 26 % with chemoRT. The study was stopped early due to the clear benefit of chemoradiation over radiation alone. Herskovic A. et al. Combined chemotherapy and radiotherapy compared with radiotherapy alone in patients with cancer of the esophagus. N Engl J Med. 1992;326(24):1593–8.

12. The correct answer is A. RTOG 94-05/INT0123 (Minsky et al.) randomized 236 patients with esophageal cancer to be treated with chemoradiation to receive either standard-dose RT (50 Gy) or high-dose RT (64.8 Gy). The chemotherapy employed was cisplatin and 5-FU. The radiation volume included an expansion of 5 cm superior and inferior to a total of 50.4 Gy, followed by a boost with a field reduction (GTV + 2 cm) to a total of 64.8 Gy. The high-dose RT arm showed higher treatment-related deaths and the study was closed after an interim analysis. Although there were 11 treatment-related deaths in the high-dose arm, seven of these occurred prior to reaching 50.4 Gy. Minsky BD et al. INT0123 (Radiation therapy oncology group 94-05) phase III trial of combined-modality therapy for esophageal cancer: high-dose versus standard-dose radiation therapy. J Clin Oncol. 2002;20:1167–74.

13. The correct answer is C. RTOG 94-05/INT0123 (Minsky et al.) randomized 236 patients with esophageal cancer to be treated with chemoradiation to receive either standard-dose RT (50 Gy) or high-dose RT (64.8 Gy). The chemotherapy employed was cisplatin and 5-FU. The radiation volume included an expansion of 5 cm superior and inferior to a total of 50.4 Gy, followed by a boost with a field reduction (GTV + 2 cm) to a total of 64.8 Gy. The high-dose RT arm showed higher treatment-related deaths and the study was closed after an interim analysis. Although there were 11 treatment-related deaths in the high-dose arm, seven of these occurred prior to reaching 50.4 Gy. Minsky BD et al. INT0123 (Radiation therapy oncology group 94-05) phase III trial of combined-modality therapy for esophageal cancer: high-dose versus standard-dose radiation therapy. J Clin Oncol. 2002;20:1167–74.

14. The correct answer is C. In the Walsh neoadjuvant trial, 190 patients with esophageal cancer (113 with adenocarcinoma) were randomized to surgery with or without neoadjuvant cisplatin (75 mg/m^2) and 5-FU (15 mg/kg days 1–5) + radiation (40 Gy/15 fractions). Pathological complete response rate in the neoadjuvant chemoRT arm was 25 %. With a median follow-up of 10 months, the addition of neoadjuvant therapy improved median survival, 16 months versus 11 months, and 3-year overall survival, 32 % versus 6 %, $p=0.01$. This interim survival benefit prompted early closure of the trial. However, the trial is criticized for its short follow-up time, as well as the poor outcome in the control arm. Walsh TN et al. A comparison of multimodal therapy and surgery for esophageal adenocarcinoma. N Engl J Med. 1996;335(7):462–7.

15. The correct answer is B. In the Walsh neoadjuvant trial, 190 patients with esophageal cancer (113 with adenocarcinoma) were randomized to surgery with or without neoadjuvant cisplatin (75 mg/m^2) and 5-FU (15 mg/kg days 1–5) + radiation (40 Gy/15 fractions). Walsh TN et al. A comparison of multimodal therapy and surgery for esophageal adenocarcinoma. N Engl J Med. 1996;335(7):462–7.

16. The correct answer is C. Pathological complete response rate in the neoadjuvant chemoRT arm was 22 % (13/58 patients). Walsh TN et al. A comparison of multimodal therapy and surgery for esophageal adenocarcinoma. N Engl J Med. 1996;335(7):462–7.

17. The correct answer is D. The CROSS study randomized 368 patients with resectable (T2-3N0-1) esophageal or GE junction cancers to receive surgery alone versus neoadjuvant chemoRT followed by surgery. Chemotherapy consisted of weekly carboplatin (AUC=2) and paclitaxel (50 mg/m^2). Concurrent radiotherapy was 41.4 Gy delivered in 23 fractions. Hagen et al. Preoperative chemoradiotherapy for esophageal or junctional cancer. N Engl J Med. 2012;366:2074–84.

18. The correct answer is A. Median overall survival was 49.4 months in the chemoradiotherapy–surgery group versus 24.0 months in the surgery-alone group. Complete resection (R0) was achieved in 92 % of patients who received neoadjuvant chemotherapy RT versus 69 % in the surgery-alone group. Pathological complete response rate was 29 % for patients receiving chemoradiotherapy. The majority of grade 3 toxicities were due to leukopenia. Postoperative mortality did not differ between the arms. Hagen et al. Preoperative chemoradiotherapy for esophageal or junctional cancer. N Engl J Med. 2012;366:2074–84.

19. The correct answer is C. The CROSS study randomized 368 patients with resectable (T2-3N0-1) esophageal or GE junction cancers to receive surgery alone versus neoadjuvant chemoRT followed by surgery. Median overall survival was 49.4 months in the chemoradiotherapy–surgery group versus 24.0 months in the surgery-alone group. Complete resection (R0) was achieved in 92 % of patients who received neoadjuvant chemotherapy RT versus 69 % in the surgery-alone group. Pathological complete response rate was 29 % for patients receiving chemoradiotherapy. Hagen et al. Preoperative chemoradiotherapy for esophageal or junctional cancer. N Engl J Med. 2012;366:2074–84.

20. The correct answer is C. The CROSS study randomized 368 patients with resectable (T2-3N0-1) esophageal or GE junction cancers to receive surgery alone versus neoadjuvant chemoRT followed by surgery. Median overall survival was 49.4 months in the chemoradiotherapy–surgery group versus 24.0 months in the surgery-alone group. The majority of grade 3 toxicities were due to leukopenia. Postoperative mortality did not differ between the arms. Hagen et al. Preoperative chemoradiotherapy for esophageal or junctional cancer. N Engl J Med. 2012;366:2074–84.

21. The correct answer is D. The cardia is the least common subsite of gastric cancer. The antrum is the most common, accounting for 40 % of cases. Gunderson LL, Tepper JE, Calvo FA, Callister MD. Gastric/GE junction cancer. In: Gunderson LL, Tepper JE, editors. Clinical radiation oncology. 3rd ed. Philadelphia: Elsevier Saunders; 2012.p. 903–33.

22. The correct answer is D. Only 25 % of patients with gastric cancer undergo potentially curative surgery. Gunderson LL, Tepper JE, Calvo FA, Callister MD.Gastric/GE junction cancer. In: Gunderson LL, Tepper JE, editors. Clinical radiation oncology. 3rd ed. Philadelphia: Elsevier Saunders;2012. p. 903–33

23. The correct answer is C. In the GITSG trial of locally advanced (node-positive or T4) gastric cancer, 90 patients were randomized to chemotherapy alone versus chemoradiation with concurrent 5-FU and then maintenance MeCCNU + 5-FU. Palliative resection of tumor was allowed, though the majority still had residual tumor. While the trial was closed early due to increased deaths in the chemoRT arm in the first 12 months, with longer follow-up, 5-year survival in

the combination therapy arm that had undergone resection was 18 % versus 7 % without RT. This provided the basis for subsequent adjuvant trials in gastric cancer. A comparison of combination chemotherapy and combined modality therapy for locally advanced gastric carcinoma. Cancer. 1982;49(9):1771–7.

24. The correct answer is C. The MAGIC trial (Cunningham et al.) randomized 503 patients to surgery alone versus surgery with perioperative chemotherapy. Perioperative chemotherapy consisted of epirubicin, cisplatin, and 5-FU (ECF). Cunningham D. et al. Perioperative chemotherapy versus surgery alone for resectable gastroesophageal cancer. N Eng J Med. 2006;355:11–20.

25. The correct answer is A. The MAGIC trial randomized 503 patients with adenocarcinoma of the stomach (74 %), gastroesophageal junction (11 %), or distal esophagus (15 %) to surgery versus surgery with perioperative chemotherapy (three cycles of epirubicin 50 mg/m^2, cisplatin 60 mg/m^2, and 5-FU 200 mg/m^2). The addition of perioperative chemotherapy improved 5-year overall survival, 36 % versus 23 %, and improved progression-free survival (HR 0.66; 95 % CI, 0.53–0.81, $p < 0.001$). The toxicity profile for the two groups was similar. The addition of perioperative chemotherapy also resulted in significantly increased tumor downstaging, with a median maximum diameter of 3 cm in the chemotherapy group versus 5 cm in the surgery-alone group ($p < 0.001$). Cunningham D et al. Perioperative chemotherapy versus surgery alone for resectable gastroesophageal cancer. N Eng J Med. 2006;355:11–20.

26. The correct answer is D. In order from most common to least common histologies of gastric cancer: adenocarcinoma (>90 %), lymphoma (4 %), carcinoid tumors (3 %), malignant stromal cell tumor (2 %), and squamous cell carcinoma (1 %). Gastric lymphoma, including MALT, is the second most common histology. Gunderson LL, Tepper JE, Calvo FA, Callister MD. Gastric/GE junction cancer. In: Gunderson LL, Tepper JE, editors. Clinical radiation oncology. 3rd ed. Philadelphia: Elsevier Saunders; 2012. p. 903–33

27. The correct answer is B. The INT 0116 trial randomized 582 patients with R0 resected gastric (≥T3 primaries or node-positive) or gastroesophageal junction tumors to observation versus postoperative chemoradiation. 10 % of patients underwent D2 resection; 50 % underwent D0 resection. After surgery, patients received one cycle of chemotherapy alone then concurrent chemotherapy RT starting at day 28 for two cycles followed by another two cycles of chemotherapy alone. Chemotherapy was 5-FU/leucovorin; radiation dose was 45 Gy in 25 daily fractions. The delay in starting radiotherapy was to allow for quality assurance of radiation portals. The addition of postoperative chemoradiation significantly improved median overall survival: 35 months versus 26 months, and 3-year overall survival: 50 % versus 41 %. The update of >10-year median follow-up shows a persistent overall and relapse-free survival benefit from postoperative chemoradiation. Macdonald JS et al. Chemoradiotherapy after surgery compared with surgery alone for adenocarcinoma of the stomach or

gastroesophageal junction. N Engl J Med. 2001;345:725–30. Smalley SR et al. Updated analysis of SWOG- directed intergroup study 0116: a phase III trial of adjuvant radiochemotherapy versus observation after curative gastric cancer resection. J Clin Oncol. 2012;30(19):2327–33.

28. The correct answer is A. The INT 0116 trial randomized 582 patients with R0 resected gastric (≥T3 primaries or node-positive) or gastroesophageal junction tumors to observation versus postoperative chemoradiation. 10 % of patients underwent D2 resection; 50 % underwent D0 resection. After surgery, patients received one cycle of chemotherapy alone then concurrent chemotherapy RT starting at day 28 for two cycles followed by another two cycles of chemotherapy alone. Macdonald JS. et al. Chemoradiotherapy after surgery compared with surgery alone for adenocarcinoma of the stomach or gastroesophageal junction. N Engl J Med. 2001;345:725–30.

29. The correct answer is C. The INT 0116 trial randomized 582 patients with R0 resected gastric (≥T3 primaries or node-positive) or gastroesophageal junction tumors to observation versus postoperative chemoradiation. After surgery, patients received one cycle of chemotherapy alone then concurrent chemotherapy RT starting at day 28 for two cycles followed by another two cycles of chemotherapy alone. Chemotherapy was 5-FU/leucovorin; radiation dose was 45 Gy in 25 daily fractions. The addition of postoperative chemoradiation significantly improved median overall survival: 35 months versus 26 months, and 3-year overall survival: 50 % versus 41 %. The 10-year update shows a persistent progression-free and overall survival benefit. Subset analyses showed a benefit for chemoRT in all groups except women and those with diffuse-type histology. On multivariate analysis, histology remained the only significant factor. Macdonald JS et al. Chemoradiotherapy after surgery compared with surgery alone for adenocarcinoma of the stomach or gastroesophageal junction. N Engl J Med. 2001;345:725–30. Smalley SR et al. Updated analysis of SWOG- directed intergroup study 0116: a phase III trial of adjuvant radiochemotherapy versus observation after curative gastric cancer resection. J Clin Oncol. 2012;30(19):2327–33.

30. The correct answer is C. Intestinal-type gastric cancer tends to occur in the older population, more commonly in older men, and in the body and distal stomach. Intestinal-type gastric cancer is often associated with *H. pylori* infection and is preceded by precancerous lesions. While it is more prone to develop subsequent hepatic metastases, overall, it is associated with a better prognosis. In comparison, diffuse-type gastric cancer occurs in a younger population and more commonly in women. It tends to occur in the proximal stomach and is often associated with hereditary factors. As it is prone to peritoneal metastases, diffuse-type is associated with a poorer prognosis. Gunderson LL, Tepper JE, Calvo FA, Callister MD. Gastric/GE junction cancer. In: Gunderson LL, Tepper JE, editors. Clinical radiation oncology. 3rd ed. Philadelphia: Elsevier Saunders; 2012. p. 903–33.

31. The correct answer is D. While GERD is a significant risk factor for esophageal adenocarcinoma, it is not considered a risk factor for gastric cancer. Diet is thought to be a primary risk factor, especially preserved, smoked foods and foods containing nitrites and nitrosamines. *H. pylori* infection is associated with a three- to six-fold increase in risk of developing gastric carcinoma. Individuals with genetic conditions such as Peutz–Jeghers syndrome, familial adenomatous polyposis, and HNPCC syndrome are also more prone to development of gastric cancer. Gunderson LL, Tepper JE, Calvo FA, Callister MD. Gastric/GE junction cancer. In: Gunderson LL, Tepper JE, editors., Clinical radiation oncology. 3rd ed. Philadelphia: Elsevier Saunders; 2012. p. 903–33.

32. The correct answer is D. Imatinib is a competitive inhibitor of mutant isoforms of *kit*. Heinrich MC et al. Inhibition of c-kit receptor tyrosine kinase activity by STI 571, a selective tyrosine kinase inhibitor. Blood. 2000;96:925–32.

33. The correct answer is B. In a phase II clinical study of imatinib in the treatment of metastatic gastrointestinal stromal tumors, most of the 127 enrolled patients had an exon 11 mutation ($n=85$). In those with the exon 11 mutation, the partial response rate (PR) was 83.5 % versus 47.8 % ($p=0.0006$) in those with the exon 9 or 0 % in those with no detectable *kit* mutation ($p<0.0001$). Patients with an exon 11 *kit* mutation had a longer event-free and overall survival than those with either exon 9 mutation or no *kit* mutation. Heinrich MC et al. Kinase mutations and imatinib response in patients with metastatic gastrointestinal stromal tumor. J Clin Oncol. 2003;21(23):4342–9.

34. The correct answer is D. Known risk factors include cigarette smoking, high-fat diet, exposure to ionizing radiation, history of chemotherapy, and exposure to aromatic chemicals. Other risk factors that are often cited but have no direct link are as follows: alcohol consumption, coffee consumption, chronic pancreatitis, and diabetes. In general, pancreatic cancer is usually diagnosed after the age of 65. A family history of pancreatic cancer also increases the risk of pancreatic cancer. Familial pancreatic cancer usually has a genetic predisposition with *Kras* activation, BRCA2 mutation, HNPCC syndrome, and Peutz–Jeghers polyposis. Shah AP, Abrams RA. Pancreatic cancer. In: Gunderson LL, Tepper JE, editors. Clinical radiation oncology. 3rd ed. Philadelphia: Elsevier Saunders; 2012. p. 935–57.

35. The correct answer is C. For most adults the pancreas lies between L1 and L2 vertebral bodies. The pancreas is a retroperitoneal organ and is divided into four regions: head, neck, body, and tail. Most of the cancers, 66 %, occur in the head of the pancreas, which often leads to common bile duct obstruction and jaundice. It is caudal to the celiac axis and cephalad to the superior mesenteric artery. On the right it abuts the duodenum and the tail of the pancreas lies close to the spleen. Kao GD et al. Anatomy of the superior mesenteric artery and its significance in radiation therapy. Int J Radiat Oncol Biol Phys. 1992;25: 131–4.

36. The correct answer is A. Pancreatic cells are divided into exocrine and endocrine cells based on their function. The exocrine pancreas consists of acinar and ductal cells. The endocrine pancreas consists of a, b, d, and PP cells. The most common malignant histology, greater than 75 %, is adenocarcinoma, which is of ductal origin. Ductal adenocarcinoma is aggressive and has poor survival. Other less common but aggressive histologies are acinar cell and giant cell cancers. Pancreatic cancers that are not aggressive and have an indolent course are cystadenocarcinomas, intraductal carcinomas, and solid and cystic papillary neoplasms (Hamoudi tumors). Shah AP, Abrams RA. Pancreatic cancer. In: Gunderson LL, Tepper JE, editors. Clinical radiation oncology. 3rd ed. Philadelphia: Elsevier Saunders; 2012. p. 935–57.

37. The correct answer is C. While migratory thrombophlebitis (Trousseau sign) and palpable gallbladder (Courvoisier's sign) can be seen in pancreatic cancer, they are fairly uncommon. The most common symptoms of pancreatic cancer are abdominal pain, jaundice, and weight loss. Abdominal pain radiating to the back is secondary to retroperitoneal invasion of the splanchnic nerve plexus. Tumors in the head of the pancreas usually have an earlier onset of symptoms and most commonly present with jaundice. Inflammation of the pancreas can lead to endocrine dysfunction causing diabetes. Nausea and anorexia are also common and lead to weight loss. Migratory thrombophlebitis is due to coagulopathy and is not specific to pancreatic cancer but is associated with other malignancies such as lung and ovarian. Other physical signs associated with pancreatic cancer are Virchow's node (supraclavicular lymphadenopathy) and Sister Mary Joseph node (periumbilical nodules). Shah AP, Abrams RA. Pancreatic cancer. In: Gunderson LL, Tepper JE, editors. Clinical radiation oncology. 3rd ed. Philadelphia: Elsevier Saunders; 2012. p. 935–57.

38. The correct answer is A. The *kras* mutation is seen in over 90 % of pancreatic cancer. The p16 tumor suppressor is also commonly seen (90 %). p53 mutation is seen in 70 % of pancreatic cancer cases. Shah AP, Abrams RA. Pancreatic cancer. In: Gunderson LL, Tepper JE, editors. Clinical radiation oncology. 3rd ed. Philadelphia: Elsevier Saunders; 2012. p. 935–57.

39. The correct answer is C. Only CA 19-9 (carbohydrate antigen 19-9) is known to have prognostic value in pancreatic cancer. However, it is nonspecific and is also associated with colon cancer. CEA-125 is associated with ovarian cancer and can be used for monitoring of treatment response. CEA is used to monitor recurrence of colorectal cancer. AFP is associated with hepatocellular carcinoma and nonseminomatous germ cell tumors. b-hCG is also used for nonseminomatous germ cell tumor or gestational trophoblastic disease. Steinberg W. The clinical utility of the CA 19-9 tumor-associated antigen. Am J Gastroenterol. 1990;85:350–5.

40. The correct answer is D. The minority (15–20 %) of cases of pancreatic cancer are resectable at diagnosis. This has fueled the investigation of neoadjuvant approaches, in the hopes of increasing tumor resectability. Shah AP, Abrams RA. Pancreatic cancer. In: Gunderson LL, Tepper JE, editors. Clinical radiation oncology. 3rd ed. Philadelphia: Elsevier Saunders; 2012.p. 935–57.

41. The correct answer is B. Unfortunately, approximately half of patients with pancreatic cancer present with distant metastases at diagnosis. Shah AP, Abrams RA.Pancreatic cancer. In: Gunderson LL, Tepper JE, editors. Clinical radiation oncology. 3rd ed. Philadelphia: Elsevier Saunders; 2012.p. 935–57.

42. The correct answer is B. The GITSG 9173 trial randomized patients after radical resection (R0) to either an observation arm or an adjuvant chemoradiation arm. Chemotherapy was 5-FU (500 mg/m^2) on days 1–3 of each split course. After completion of chemoRT, maintenance 5-FU was then given for 2 years or until tumor progression. Patients who received adjuvant chemoradiation had increased median survival: 20 months versus 11 months in the observation arm ($p = 0.03$). Two-year overall survival was 42 % versus 15 %. Kalser MH, Ellenberg SS. Pancreatic cancer. Adjuvant combined radiation and chemotherapy following curative resection. Arch Surg. 1985;120:899–903. Gastrointestinal tumor study group. Further evidence of effective adjuvant combined radiation and chemotherapy following curative resection of pancreatic cancer. Cancer. 1987;59:2006–10.

43. The correct answer is C. Radiation was given for a total of 40 Gy via two split courses of 20 Gy with an interposed 2-week rest period. Kalser MH, Ellenberg SS. Pancreatic cancer. Adjuvant combined radiation and chemotherapy following curative resection. Arch Surg. 1985;120:899–903. Gastrointestinal tumor study group. Further evidence of effective adjuvant combined radiation and chemotherapy following curative resection of pancreatic cancer. Cancer. 1987;59:2006–10.

44. The correct answer is D. RTOG 97-04 randomized 451 patients with resected adenocarcinoma of the pancreas to receive neoadjuvant (3 weeks) and adjuvant chemotherapy (12 weeks) with either 5-FU or gemcitabine. Concurrent chemoRT was delivered in both arms with 5-FU to 50.4 Gy. Regine WF et al. Fluorouracil vs. gemcitabine chemotherapy before and after fluorouracil-based chemoradiation following resection of pancreatic adenocarcinoma: a randomized controlled trial. JAMA. 2008;299:1019–26.

45. The correct answer is B. RTOG 97-04 randomized 451 patients with resected adenocarcinoma of the pancreas to receive neoadjuvant (3 weeks) and adjuvant chemotherapy (12 weeks) with either 5-FU or gemcitabine. Concurrent chemoRT was delivered with 5-FU to 50.4 Gy. In those patients with resected head of pancreas tumors ($n = 388$), those that received gemcitabine showed a

trend towards improved overall survival: 3-year OS, 31 % versus 22 % ($p = 0.09$). Median survival was 20.5 months versus 16.9 months, not statistically significant. There was no difference between the arms regarding the ability to complete the assigned treatment (>85 % in both groups). Regine WF et al. Fluorouracil vs. gemcitabine chemotherapy before and after fluorouracil-based chemoradiation following resection of pancreatic adenocarcinoma: a randomized controlled trial. JAMA. 2008;299:1019–26.

46. The correct answer is A. The CONKO-001 trial (Neuhaus 2008) randomized pancreatic cancer patients after gross total resection to chemotherapy only (gemcitabine) versus observation. Neuhaus P et al. CONKO-001: final results of the randomized, prospective, multicenter phase III trial of adjuvant chemotherapy with gemcitabine versus observation in patients with resected pancreatic cancer. J Clin Oncol. 2008;26 [Suppl]: Abstract 4504. Oettle H et al. Adjuvant chemotherapy with gemcitabine vs. observation in patients undergoing curative-intent resection of pancreatic cancer (CONKO-001). JAMA. 2007;297(3): 267–76.

47. The correct answer is A. The CONKO-001 trial (Neuhaus 2008) randomized pancreatic cancer patients after gross total resection to chemotherapy only (gemcitabine) versus observation. The addition of gemcitabine following surgery improved DFS but not overall survival. Median disease-free time significantly increased: 13.4 months versus 6.9 months favoring the gemcitabine arm. There was no significant median overall survival benefit (22.1 months versus 20.2 months). Neuhaus P et al. CONKO-001: final results of the randomized, prospective, multicenter phase III trial of adjuvant chemotherapy with gemcitabine versus observation in patients with resected pancreatic cancer. J Clin Oncol. 2008;26[Suppl]: Abstract 4504. Oettle H et al. Adjuvant chemotherapy with gemcitabine vs. observation in patients undergoing curative-intent resection of pancreatic cancer (CONKO-001). JAMA. 2007;297(3):267–76.

48. The correct answer is C. GITSG 9273 randomized 194 patients with locally unresectable pancreatic cancer to one of three arms: (1) 60 Gy/30 fractions by split course, (2) 40 Gy/20 fractions by split course with 5-FU, and (3) 60 Gy/30 fractions by split course with 5-FU. Maintenance 5-FU followed for 2 years. Median survival was statistically improved in the 60 Gy + 5-FU arm: 7.6 months versus 7.0 months (40 Gy + 5-FU) versus 2.9 months (40 Gy alone). One-year overall survival was highest in the 60 Gy + 5-FU arm: 46 % versus 35 % (40 Gy + 5-FU) versus 10 % (40 Gy alone). Moertel CG et al. Therapy of locally unresectable pancreatic carcinoma: a randomized comparison of high dose (6,000 rads) radiation alone, moderate dose radiation (4,000 rads + 5-fluorouracil), and high dose radiation + 5-fluorouracil: The gastrointestinal tumor study group. Cancer. 1981;48(8):1705–10.

49. The correct answer is A. The ESPAC trial of adjuvant therapy in resectable pancreatic cancer randomized 541 patients into a 2×2 factorial design: observation versus chemoradiotherapy versus chemotherapy alone versus chemoradiotherapy + chemotherapy. Chemoradiotherapy consisted of 20 Gy/10 fractions with 5-FU (500 mg/m² on D1-3, then repeated after 2 weeks). Chemotherapy alone consisted of 5-FU (425 mg/m² and folinic acid 20 mg/m² daily × 5 days, monthly × 6 months). An additional 68 patients were randomized to chemoradiotherapy versus no chemoradiotherapy and 188 were randomized to chemotherapy versus no chemotherapy. Median overall survival was 10 months. No benefit for adjuvant chemoradiotherapy was seen, but a survival benefit was seen for adjuvant chemotherapy – median survival of 19.7 months versus 14.0 months without chemotherapy. The poor radiation technique, low dose, and lack of quality control are criticisms of this study. Neoptolemos JP et al. Adjuvant chemoradiotherapy and chemotherapy in resectable pancreatic cancer: a randomised controlled trial. Lancet. 2001;358(9293):1576–85. Koshy MC et al. A challenge to the therapeutic nihilism of ESPAC-1. Int J Radiat Oncol Biol Phys. 2005;61(4):965–6.

50. The correct answer is D. The ESPAC trial of adjuvant therapy in resectable pancreatic cancer randomized 541 patients into a 2×2 factorial design: observation versus chemoradiotherapy versus chemotherapy alone versus chemoradiotherapy + chemotherapy. Chemoradiotherapy consisted of 20 Gy/10 fractions with 5-FU (500 mg/m² on D1-3, then repeated after 2 weeks). Chemotherapy alone consisted of 5-FU (425 mg/m² and folinic acid 20 mg/m² daily × 5 days, monthly × 6 months). An additional 68 patients were randomized to chemoradiotherapy versus no chemoradiotherapy and 188 were randomized to chemotherapy versus no chemotherapy. Median overall survival was 10 months. No benefit for adjuvant chemoradiotherapy was seen, but a survival benefit was seen for adjuvant chemotherapy – median survival of 19.7 months versus 14.0 months without chemotherapy. The poor radiation technique, low dose, and lack of quality control are criticisms of this study. Neoptolemos JP et al. Adjuvant chemoradiotherapy and chemotherapy in resectable pancreatic cancer: a randomised controlled trial. Lancet. 2001;358(9293):1576–85.

51. The correct answer is A. In treating a resected head of pancreas tumor, the splenic hilum does not need to be treated. Shah AP, Abrams RA. Pancreatic cancer. In: Gunderson LL, Tepper JE, editors. Clinical radiation oncology. 3rd ed. Philadelphia: Elsevier Saunders; 2012.p. 935–57.

52. The correct answer is B. In treating a resected tail of pancreas tumor, the duodenal bed does not need to be treated. Shah AP, Abrams RA. Pancreatic cancer. In: Gunderson LL, Tepper JE, editors. Clinical radiation oncology. 3rd ed. Philadelphia: Elsevier Saunders; 2012.p. 935–57.

53. The correct answer is C. Triple phase liver CT scan is part of workup of a liver mass and is not needed for screening. CT scan without contrast does not highlight early-stage hepatocellular carcinoma. A rising serum alpha-fetoprotein is proportional to burden of disease. A serum alpha-fetoprotein value of >400 ng/mL is diagnostic of HCC. Feng M, Lawrence TS.Hepatobiliary cancer. In: Gunderson LL, Tepper JE, editors. Clinical radiation oncology. 3rd ed. Philadelphia: Elsevier Saunders; 2012.p. 959–74.

54. The correct answer is C. Any node-positive liver disease is stage IV. A solitary tumor <5 cm with vascular invasion is T2. Patients with node-positive hepatocellular carcinoma, but no distant metastases, are stage IVA. Patients with distant metastatic disease are considered stage IVB. Edge SB, Byrd DR, Compton CC, et al. editors Liver. AJCC cancer staging handbook. 7th ed. New York, NY: Springer; 2010.

55. The correct answer is B. The Child–Pugh score is calculated based on encephalopathy, ascites, albumin, prothrombin time, and bilirubin. It is used to assess the prognosis of chronic liver disease. The MELD score (Model for End-Stage Liver Disease) is a more recently employed model. It uses serum bilirubin, creatinine, and INR to predict survival. A MELD score >20 is predictive of 50 % mortality in 30 days. Both the Child–Pugh score and the MELD score are used to predict surgical mortality. Teh SH et al. Risk factors for mortality after surgery in patients with cirrhosis. Gastroenterology. 2007;132 (4):1261–9.

56. The correct answer is A. In a retrospective analysis of gallbladder cancer from Memorial Sloan–Kettering Cancer Center, 47 % of cases of gallbladder cancer were incidentally diagnosed during laparoscopic cholecystectomy. Chronic cholelithiasis is the main risk factor for gallbladder cancer. Duffy A et al. Gallbladder cancer (GBC): 10-year experience at Memorial Sloan-Kettering Cancer Centre (MSKCC). J Surg Oncol. 2008;98(7):485–9.

57. The correct answer is D. A regression analysis of SEER data (Wang 2008) predicts that adjuvant RT provides a survival benefit in node-positive or T2 disease. Other factors that predict overall survival are age, sex, papillary histology, and stage. There is no role for neoadjuvant chemotherapy in *resectable* gallbladder cancer since this is primarily a surgical disease. Wang SJ et al. Prediction model for estimating the survival benefit of adjuvant RT for gallbladder cancer. J Clin Oncol. 2008;26:2112–7.

58. The correct answer is D. Cholecystectomy decreases the risk of cholangiocarcinoma. Risk factors associated with an increased risk of cholangiocarcinoma relate to chronic inflammation, such as choledochocyst, ulcerative colitis, PSC, and hepatitis B/C infections. It has been postulated that cholecystectomy decreases chronic inflammation from cholelithiasis, thereby reducing risk of cholangiocarcinoma. Anders E. et al. Risk of extrahepatic bile duct cancer after

cholecystectomy. The Lancet. 1993;342(8882):1262–5. Thomas CR Jr., Fuller CD, editors. Biliary tract and gallbladder cancer: diagnosis and therapy. 1st ed. New York: Demos Medical Publishing; 2009.

59. The correct answer is C. The most common location for extrahepatic cholangiocarcinoma is at the bifurcation of the common hepatic duct. These tumors are also known as Klatskin tumors. For extrahepatic cholangiocarcinoma, the location of the lesion determines prognosis. Proximal tumors are difficult to resect completely and have a more limited prognosis (6–12 months). Distal tumors are more likely to undergo complete resection and have a better prognosis. Alden ME et al. Cholangiocarcinoma: clinical significance of tumor location along the extrahepatic bile duct. Radiology. 1995;197(2):511–6. Thomas CR Jr., Fuller CD, editors. Biliary tract and gallbladder cancer: diagnosis and therapy. 1st ed. New York: Demos Medical Publishing; 2009.

60. The correct answer is C. Sclerosing adenocarcinoma is the most common subtype of bile duct adenocarcinoma, accounting for 90 % of cases. It is usually associated with extensive desmoplastic reaction and has low resectability. Nodular adenocarcinoma is highly invasive and has poor prognosis. Papillary adenocarcinoma is the least common subtype, but the most curable. Thomas CR Jr, Fuller CD, editors. Biliary tract and gallbladder cancer: diagnosis and therapy. 1st ed. New York: Demos Medical Publishing; 2009.

61. The correct answer is A. Carcinoid tumors stain for neuron-specific enolase, synaptophysin, and chromogranin. Fielding JR, Burke M, Jewells VS. Imaging in oncology. In: Gunderson LL, Tepper JE, editors. Clinical radiation oncology. 3rd ed. Philadelphia: Elsevier Saunders; 2012.p. 181–92.

62. The most site of carcinoid tumor is the appendix. The second most common site is the ileum. Fielding JR, Burke M, Jewells VS. Imaging in oncology. In: Gunderson LL, Tepper JE, editors. Clinical radiation oncology. 3rd ed. Philadelphia: Elsevier Saunders; 2012.p. 181–92.

63. The correct answer is D. Adenocarcinoma is the most common histology of tumors found in the small bowel. Neugut AI et al. Epidemiology of cancer of the small intestine. Cancer Epidemiol Biomarkers Prev. 1998;7:243–51.

Chapter 8
Lower Gastrointestinal Cancers

Sravana Chennupati, Celine Bicquart Ord, and Charles R. Thomas, Jr.

Questions

1. What percentage of anal canal cancer patients present with extrapelvic visceral metastasis?
   A. <5 %
   B. 10 %
   C. 20 %
   D. 25 %

2. Pelvic lymph node metastases are present in what percentage of anal cancer patients at time of diagnosis?
   A. 10 %
   B. 20 %
   C. 30 %
   D. 40 %

S. Chennupati, MD (✉)
Department of Radiation Medicine, Oregon Health & Science University,
3181 S.W. Sam Jackson Park Rd, Portland, OR 97239-3098, USA
e-mail: chennupa@ohsu.edu

C.B. Ord, MD
Department of Radiation Oncology, Scott & White Memorial Hospital,
Temple, TX 76508, USA
e-mail: cord@sw.org

C.R. Thomas Jr., MD
Department of Radiation Medicine, Knight Cancer Institute, Oregon Health &
Science University, 3181 SW Sam Jackson Park Road, KPV4, Portland, OR, USA
e-mail: thomasch@ohsu.edu; thomas@gmail.com

C.B. Ord et al. (eds.), *Radiation Oncology Study Guide*,
DOI 10.1007/978-1-4614-6400-6_8, © Springer Science+Business Media New York 2013

3. According to 7th edition of the AJCC Cancer Staging Manual, a patient with anal canal cancer with a metastasis in a R inguinal lymph node and a L internal iliac LN would be staged as:
   A. N1
   B. N2
   C. N3
   D. M1

4. What is the 5-year overall survival of a patient with stage I anal cancer?
   A. 95 %
   B. 85 %
   C. 80 %
   D. 75 %

5. According to the 7th edition of AJCC Cancer Staging Manual, a patient with anal canal cancer with a metastasis in a R inguinal lymph node and a perirectal lymph node would be staged as:
   A. N1
   B. N2
   C. N3
   D. M1

6. What was the pathological complete response rate seen in patients undergoing chemoRT, then surgery, as reported by Nigro et al.?
   A. <20 %
   B. 30–40 %
   C. 60–70 %
   D. >85 %

7. RTOG 98-11 compared mitomycin-C-based conventional chemoRT to induction 5-FU/cisplatin followed by chemoRT with 5-FU/cisplatin. It found a significant improvement in which of the following:
   A. Overall survival favoring the induction arm
   B. Progression-free survival favoring the mitomycin-C-based chemoRT arm
   C. Colostomy-free rate favoring the mitomycin-C-based chemoRT arm
   D. Local-regional failure rate favoring the induction arm

8. According to RTOG 05-29, what dose would be prescribed for a 3.0 cm anal canal primary and an involved inguinal lymph node measuring 3.5 cm?
   A. 54 Gy to the primary PTV and 54 Gy to the involved lymph node over 30 fractions
   B. 54 Gy to the primary PTV and 50.4 Gy to the involved lymph node over 30 fractions
   C. 50.4 Gy to the primary PTV and 50.4 Gy to the involved lymph node over 28 fractions
   D. 50.4 Gy to the primary PTV and 45 Gy to the involved lymph node over 28 fractions

9. According to 7th edition of the AJCC Cancer Staging Manual, a patient with a 4 cm rectal adenocarcinoma, 8 cm from the anal verge only invading into, but not through the muscularis propria, with one enlarged lymph node (1.5 cm) on endoscopic ultrasound, would be staged as:
   A. T1N1Mx
   B. T2N1Mx
   C. T2N2Mx
   D. Not enough information provided

10. The German Rectal Cancer Study (CAO/ARA/AIO-94) comparing preoperative versus postoperative chemoradiation for rectal cancer found:
    A. At a median f/u of 11 years, OS was improved for neoadjuvant chemoRT compared to adjuvant chemoRT.
    B. Long-term toxicity was worse in the neoadjuvant chemoRT arm compared to the adjuvant arm.
    C. At a median f/u of 11 years, there was no difference in local recurrence.
    D. More patients were converted to sphincter-preserving surgeries in the neoadjuvant chemoRT arm.

11. In the initial report of the German Rectal Cancer Study, what was the pathological complete response rate seen in those patients that underwent preoperative chemoRT?
    A. 5 %
    B. 8 %
    C. 12 %
    D. 15 %

12. In the initial report of the German Rectal Cancer Study, what percentage of patients initially thought to require abdominoperineal resection were able to undergo sphincter-preserving surgery?
    A. 19 %
    B. 26 %
    C. 39 %
    D. 45 %

13. Extending radially outwards from the lumen of the rectum, the correct order of tissue layers is:
    A. Lamina propria, submucosa, muscularis propria, serosa
    B. Lamina propria, muscularis propria, submucosa, serosa
    C. Serosa, lamina propria, submucosa, muscularis propria
    D. Muscularis propria, serosa, lamina propria, submucosa

14. A 65-year-old gentleman with good performance status is diagnosed with a pT2N1 rectal adenocarcinoma, 7 cm from the anal verge. He is set to start adjuvant chemoradiation. Which of the following is the most established systemic therapy option?
    A. Cisplatin and CI 5-FU
    B. Cisplatin and bolus 5-FU
    C. CI 5-FU
    D. CI 5-FU + irinotecan

15. In which of the following rectal cancer studies was total mesorectal excision (TME) required?
    A. Polish rectal cancer study
    B. MRC07
    C. Swedish rectal cancer trial
    D. Dutch CKVO trial

16. A 68-year-old woman with a 4 cm T3N1 rectal adenocarcinoma, 8 cm from the anal verge, presents for consideration of definitive treatment. According to results of the MRC CR07 trial:
    A. There is a survival advantage for preoperative chemotherapy and radiation versus adjuvant chemotherapy and radiation for patients with a positive margin.
    B. Preoperative chemotherapy and radiation reduces local recurrence and disease-free survival compared to selective adjuvant chemotherapy and radiation.
    C. Short-course preoperative radiation (25 Gy over 5 fractions) improves local recurrence rates and disease-free survival compared to selective adjuvant chemotherapy and radiation.
    D. Adjuvant chemotherapy and radiation was able to compensate for a positive margin with respect to local control and disease-free survival.

17. Late side effects of the short-course preoperative radiotherapy arm for rectal cancer compared to TME-alone arm as reported by the Dutch colorectal cancer group study found:
    A. Stoma function was worse in the radiated arm.
    B. Urinary function was worse in the radiated arm.
    C. Fecal incontinence was worse in the radiated arm.
    D. Satisfaction with bowel function was similar between both arms.

18. The UK ACT II trial for anal canal cancer was a randomization of:
    A. RT and two different chemotherapy regimens: MMC/5-FU versus CDDP/5-FU
    B. Observation after chemoRT versus maintenance CDDP/5-FU for 2 cycles
    C. IMRT + MMC/5-FU versus 3D RT + MMC/5-FU
    D. A and B

19. A 66-year-old man with a T2N1 anal canal cancer is being evaluated for defini-
    tive chemotherapy and radiation. The addition of mitomycin C to 5-FU for
    systemic therapy with concurrent radiation has been shown to decrease:
    A. Toxicity
    B. Colostomy rate
    C. Overall survival
    D. Colostomy free survival

20. Which of the following would be classified as an anal margin tumor?
    A. A lesion confined to within 5 cm of the anal verge, but not including the
       anal verge
    B. A circumferential lesion confined to the anal canal
    C. A lesion confined to 1 cm proximal to the anal verge
    D. A lesion at the same level as the dentate line

21. A 71-year-old woman with an ECOG 1 performance status presents with a 1 cm
    well-differentiated perianal squamous cell lesion within 1 cm of the anal verge.
    The lesion does not come into contact with the anal verge. Inguinal exam,
    gynecologic exam, and CT are negative for any other sites of disease. The recom-
    mended treatment of this lesion would be:
    A. Cisplatin-based chemotherapy +/− radiation
    B. MMC/5-FU-based chemoradiation
    C. Abdominoperineal resection
    D. Local excision

22. A 62-year-old woman was initially diagnosed with a T3N1 rectal adenocarci-
    noma 7 cm from the anal verge. She received preoperative chemoRT (CI 5-FU
    and 50.4 Gy to tumor), followed by a low anterior resection 6 weeks later. Upon
    final review of the pathology, the tumor was pT2N0. She has since recovered
    from this procedure and has a performance status of ECOG 1. What is the most
    appropriate next treatment step for this patient?
    A. Close observation with CT CAP and CEA annually for 3–5 years
    B. Adjuvant oxaliplatin for 6 months
    C. Adjuvant 5-FU and leucovorin for 6 months
    D. Adjuvant oxaliplatin for 6 months

23. A 68-year-old woman with a history of T2N1 rectal adenocarcinoma treated
    with neoadjuvant chemoradiotherapy (CI 5-FU and 50.4 Gy to the primary),
    LAR, and 6 months of adjuvant chemotherapy is found to have a recurrence
    at the anastomotic site at her 2-year follow-up. Performance status ECOG is 1.

Restaging studies identify this as the only site of disease. The gross area of disease is technically resectable. Which of the following is true regarding her treatment options at this time?
  A. Given the prior history of radiation, the risks of more radiation would outweigh the benefits.
  B. Given the prior history of radiation, the risks of surgery would outweigh the benefits.
  C. The only acceptable treatment at this time other than observation is chemotherapy.
  D. Repeat radiation or chemoradiation, followed by surgery, may result in long-term local control.

24. Approximately what percentage of patients with anal canal carcinoma present with rectal bleeding?
  A. 75 %
  B. 65 %
  C. 55 %
  D. 45 %

25. A 56-year-old man with an ECOG 1 performance status has a new diagnosis of T2N1 rectal adenocarcinoma and is found to have a liver mass on staging CT chest/abdomen/pelvis. Biopsy of this lesion is consistent with metastatic adenocarcinoma. This is the only site of distant disease found on staging studies. After evaluation by the surgery team, it is felt that the liver lesion is resectable. Which of the following is the most appropriate treatment approach?
  A. This patient has metastatic disease – chemotherapy alone.
  B. Resection of the liver lesion followed by neoadjuvant chemoRT to the primary followed by resection of the primary.
  C. Neoadjuvant chemoRT followed by resection of the primary and the liver lesion.
  D. Either B or C.

26. A 59-year-old man presents with a rectal mass, 10 cm from the anal verge. Biopsy shows moderately differentiated adenocarcinoma. It invades through the muscularis propria on EUS, and there is one enlarged perirectal lymph node on CT. CT liver is negative for metastatic disease. He is to be treated with neoadjuvant chemotherapy and radiation. Which of the following regions does not need to be included in the radiation treatment field?
  A. Internal iliac lymph nodes
  B. External iliac lymph nodes
  C. Presacral iliac lymph nodes
  D. Perirectal lymph nodes

27. A 68-year-old male with a newly diagnosed 3 cm anal cancer and a biopsy proven left inguinal lymph node presents to clinic. An HIV test returns positive and CD4$^+$ count returns 250/mm^3. The most appropriate treatment regimen for this patient is:
    A. Concurrent chemotherapy and radiation with MMC and 5-FU
    B. Treatment with chemotherapy only using a 5-FU-based regimen
    C. Radiation alone
    D. Optimization of CD4$^+$ count to greater than 400/mm^3 prior to starting chemotherapy and radiation with MMC and 5-FU

28. What percentage of clinically positive lymph nodes in patients with anal canal cancer are pathologically positive on biopsy?
    A. 100 %
    B. 75 %
    C. 50 %
    D. 25 %

29. 80 % of colon cancer has the following mutation:
    A. *1p19q*
    B. *4p*
    C. *9q*
    D. *17p, 18q*

30. Patients with familial adenomatous polyposis contain a mutation of which tumor suppressor gene?
    A. *p53*
    B. *APC*
    C. *FAP*
    D. *VHL*

31. What is the risk of developing colorectal cancer for a patient who is a carrier of a *5q21* mutation?
    A. 55 %
    B. 70 %
    C. 85 %
    D. 100 %

32. All of the following are cancers that can be seen in those with Lynch II syndrome, **except**:
    A. Endometrial cancer
    B. Breast cancer
    C. Gastric cancer
    D. Ovarian cancer

33. A 64-year-old woman with a performance status of ECOG 1 presents with a small rectal mass, approximately 7 cm from the anal verge. Biopsy reveals adenocarcinoma and EUS finds that the lesion is limited to the submucosa. She undergoes local excision. Which of the following pathologic findings would require consideration of adjuvant therapy?
    A. Moderately differentiated adenocarcinoma is found on final pathology.
    B. The margins are negative by 0.5 cm.
    C. The lesion is found to be 2.5 cm in greatest dimension.
    D. The specimen invades through the muscularis propria.

34. What colon cancer screening program is appropriate for a 48-year-old male with no personal or family history of colorectal cancer or polyps and no history of inflammatory bowel disease (ulcerative colitis or Crohn's disease)?
    A. Flexible sigmoidoscopy every 10 years starting at age 50
    B. Double-contrast barium enema every 5 years starting at age 50
    C. Colonoscopy every 10 years starting at age 60
    D. CT colonography every 10 years starting at age 50

35. The most common site of local recurrence for patients with rectal cancer is:
    A. Presacral space
    B. Perineum
    C. Posterior wall of the bladder
    D. Common iliac lymph nodes

36. What is the most common presenting symptom for patients with rectal cancer?
    A. Weight loss
    B. Rectal bleeding
    C. Urinary symptoms
    D. Sciatic pain

37. Which of the following parts of the large bowel is retroperitoneal?
    A. Transverse colon
    B. Sigmoid colon
    C. Appendix and cecum
    D. Ascending colon

38. Hereditary nonpolyposis colorectal cancer (HNPCC) is characterized by which of the following?
    A. It is characterized by an autosomal recessive inheritance.
    B. It results from a defect in p53.
    C. It leads to malignancy more common in the proximal/ascending colon.
    D. HNPCC-associated cancers present at an average age of 25.

39. For patients with metastatic rectal adenocarcinoma, mutations in codons 12 and 13 of the coding region of the *KRAS* gene predict:
    A. A lack of response to therapy with antibodies targeting the epidermal growth factor receptor
    B. An increased response to therapy with antibodies targeting the epidermal growth factor receptor
    C. A lack of response to therapy with antibodies targeting the vascular endothelial growth factor receptor
    D. An increased response to therapy with antibodies targeting the vascular endothelial growth factor receptor

40. A 51-year-old woman with a history of rectal adenocarcinoma treated with neoadjuvant chemotherapy, surgery, and adjuvant chemotherapy is found to have metastatic disease 6 months after completing therapy. *KRAS* and *BRAF V600E* mutation testing are requested. Which of the following is true concerning *BRAF* testing?
    A. A new specimen is required, as *BRAF* testing cannot be performed on fixed tissues.
    B. Allele-specific PCR is an acceptable method of detecting the *BRAF V600E* mutation.
    C. Patients with the *BRAF V600E* mutation have a better prognosis.
    D. Tissue specimens cannot be paraffin embedded as it degrades the DNA.

41. Which of the following is true regarding the accuracy of endoscopic ultrasound (EUS), MRI, and CT in preoperative staging of rectal cancer according to NCCN Guidelines?
    A. EUS and MRI have similarly high sensitivities for evaluating the depth of tumor penetration into the muscularis propria (~94 %).
    B. CT is an acceptable substation for EUS for determining T stage.
    C. EUS has >90 % sensitivity for detecting involved lymph nodes.
    D. The high degree of operator dependence of EUS makes it an unreliable option for determining T stage.

42. Vitamin D may contribute to colorectal cancer incidence in which way?
    A. Deficiency may contribute to increased incidence of colorectal cancer.
    B. Deficiency may contribute to decreased mortality in patients with stage III and IV disease.
    C. Supplementation has been shown to improve outcomes in patients with early stage disease.
    D. Excess vitamin D has been shown to contribute to incidence of colorectal cancer.

43. All are true regarding the GITSG 7175 trial to determine optimal adjuvant therapy for rectal cancer, except:
    A. No overall survival benefit has been seen.
    B. Time to recurrence was prolonged with combined adjuvant therapy.
    C. The control arm was observed after surgery.
    D. Chemotherapy consisted of 5-FU and MeCCNU.

44. Which statement is true regarding the MOSAIC trial of adjuvant chemotherapy for resected colon cancer?
    A. 5-FU alone was compared to FOLFOX.
    B. Disease-free survival improved with the addition of oxaliplatin.
    C. Only stage II patients experienced an overall survival benefit with the addition of oxaliplatin.
    D. Both stage II and III patients experienced an overall survival benefit with the addition of oxaliplatin.

45. By anatomical landmarks, which of the following structures marks the superior border of the anal canal?
    A. Levator ani
    B. Anal verge
    C. Upper border of the anal sphincter and puborectalis muscles of the anorectal ring
    D. Lowermost edge of the sphincter muscles

46. Which of the following pathologic features is useful in differentiating anal margin tumors from anal canal tumors?
    A. The lack of skin appendages (hair follicles or sweat glands) indicates an anal margin tumor.
    B. Non-keratinizing, large-cell-type squamous cell carcinomas are more likely to be anal margin tumors.
    C. Well-differentiated tumors are more likely to be anal margin tumors.
    D. There are no clear pathologic differences.

47. A 58-year-old HIV-negative man presents with a new diagnosis of T1Nx squamous cell carcinoma of the anal canal found on digital rectal exam. The lesion is located at the level of the anal verge, distal to the dentate line. The location of this primary, as opposed to a tumor above the dentate line, makes lymph node metastases to which site more likely?
    A. Internal iliac lymph nodes
    B. Perirectal lymph nodes
    C. Paravertebral lymph nodes
    D. Superficial inguinal lymph nodes

48. The phase III, UK ACT II trial was one of the largest trials for patients with anal cancer. Patients with newly diagnosed anal cancer were randomized to either 5-FU/MMC or 5-FU/cisplatin combined with radiation to a dose of 50.4 Gy. Following treatment, patients in each arm were randomized to receive 2 cycles of maintenance chemotherapy (5-FU/cisplatin) versus observation. Results were presented after a median follow-up of 3 years. Which of the following is a result from the trial?
   A. Recurrence-free survival was not impacted by maintenance therapy compared to observation.
   B. Colostomy-free survival was improved for patients in 5-FU/cisplatin arm compared to the 5-FU/MMC arm.
   C. Complete response rate was improved for patients receiving MMC.
   D. Overall survival was improved for patients receiving MMC.

49. A 75-year-old man with a history of a T2N1 anal canal SCCA treated with concurrent chemoRT 1 year ago presents for follow-up. Which of the following should be performed as routine follow-up?
   A. PET-CT
   B. Biopsy of the treatment site
   C. Digital rectal exam/anoscopy
   D. MRI pelvis

50. A 65-year-old woman recently completed chemoRT for treatment of a T1N2 anal carcinoma. Serial examinations after completion of treatment noted persistent disease. At the 3-month follow-up, the primary lesion was felt to be increasing in size. Which of the following is the most appropriate next step in management?
   A. Referral for salvage surgery
   B. Check CEA level
   C. Repeat examination in 4 weeks
   D. Biopsy of the lesion

51. When determining if a liver metastasis in a patient with colorectal cancer is resectable, which of the following is the most important criteria to determine resectability?
   A. Tumor size
   B. Ability to achieve at least an R1 resection while maintaining adequate liver reserve
   C. Ability to achieve an R0 resection while maintaining adequate liver reserve
   D. Ability to resect the lesion while minimizing tumor spillage into the peritoneum

52. Excluding hemorrhage, what is the most common fatal adverse event observed with the addition of bevacizumab to chemotherapy?
   A. Venous thromboembolism
   B. Gastrointestinal tract perforation
   C. Aneurysm
   D. Neutropenia

53. A 61-year-old man has recently completed definitive treatment for his T3N1 rectal adenocarcinoma (neoadjuvant chemoRT, surgery, adjuvant chemotherapy). The first posttreatment colonoscopy should be scheduled at what time interval?
    A. 1 year
    B. 2 years
    C. 5 years
    D. 10 years

54. Excluding cutaneous cancers, rectal cancer is the ___ most common cancer in the United States.
    A. First
    B. Second
    C. Third
    D. Fourth

55. A 51-year-old man is found to have a pedunculated polyp on routine colonoscopy. The site of the polyp was marked during the colonoscopy. Pathology revealed a single pedunculated polyp with grade 2 invasive cancer that was completely removed with no evidence of angiolymphatic invasion. What is the appropriate next step?
    A. Proceed on to LAR followed by adjuvant chemotherapy and radiation.
    B. Repeat colonoscopy in 3 years.
    C. Proceed to WLE of the marked region.
    D. Proceed with 6 months of adjuvant chemotherapy.

56. A 62-year-old woman is found to have a rectal mass measuring 4 cm. The pathology returns as moderately differentiated adenocarcinoma. On endoscopic ultrasound, the mass is found to invade through the muscularis propria into the perirectal fat. There are two enlarged regional lymph nodes. The remainder of the staging work-up is negative. What is the correct AJCC 7th edition TNM stage?
    A. yT3N2aM0
    B. uT2N2aM0
    C. uT3N1aM0
    D. uT3N1bM0

57. Which of the following is the standard chemotherapeutic option for patients with metastatic anal carcinoma?
    A. There is no standard; chemotherapy should be individualized.
    B. Bevacizumab
    C. Cetuximab
    D. Taxotere

Answers and Rationales

1. The correct answer is A. A minority of patients present with extrapelvic visceral metastases. When present, these lesions occur most commonly in the liver and lungs. Of note, involvement of para-aortic lymph nodes constitutes M1 disease. Minsky BD, Welton ML, Pineda CE, Fisher GA. Cancer of the anal canal. In: Hoppe RT, Phillips TL, Roach M, editors. Leibel and Phillips textbook of radiation oncology. 3rd ed. Philadelphia: Elsevier Saunders; 2010. p. 870–82.

2. The correct answer is C. Pelvic LNs are involved in 30 % of patients at presentation. Minsky BD, Welton ML, Pineda CE, Fisher GA. Cancer of the anal canal. In: Hoppe RT, Phillips TL, Roach M, editors. Leibel and Phillips textbook of radiation oncology. 3rd ed. Philadelphia: Elsevier Saunders; 2010. p. 870–82.

3. The correct answer is B. N2 disease is defined as "metastasis in unilateral internal iliac and/or inguinal lymph node(s)." Having bilateral internal iliac lymph node involvement or bilateral inguinal lymph node involvement would be defined as N3 disease. Edge SB, Byrd DR, Compton CC, et al., editors. Anus. AJCC cancer staging handbook. 7th ed. New York: Springer; 2010.

4. The correct answer is B. The 5-year overall survival of stage I anal cancer is 85 %. For stages II–IV, it is 75 %, 50 %, and 5 %, respectively. Minsky BD, Welton ML, Pineda CE, Fisher GA. Cancer of the anal canal. In: Hoppe RT, Phillips TL, Roach M, editors. Leibel and Phillips textbook of radiation oncology. 3rd ed. Philadelphia: Elsevier Saunders; 2010. p. 870–82.

5. The correct answer is C. N3 disease is defined as "metastasis in perirectal and inguinal lymph nodes and/or bilateral internal iliac and/or inguinal lymph nodes." Edge SB, Byrd DR, Compton CC, et al., editors. Anus. AJCC cancer staging handbook. 7th ed. New York: Springer; 2010.

6. The correct answer is D. Ten years after first publishing his protocol of 5-FU, mitomycin C, and radiation, follow-up data of 104 patients undergoing preoperative chemoRT, then surgery, showed pathological complete response in 97 of 104 patients (93 %). This high pathological complete response rate pioneered chemoRT as a viable treatment option, precluding the need for abdominoperineal resection. Nigro ND et al. An evaluation of combined therapy for squamous cell cancer of the anal canal. Dis Colon Rectum. 1984;27:763–6.

7. The correct answer is C. Six hundred eighty-two patients with anal cancer were randomized to receive either (1) concurrent fluorouracil and mitomycin with radiotherapy (45–59 Gy) or (2) induction fluorouracil and cisplatin with radiotherapy starting on day 57. With a median follow-up of 2.5 years, there was no

significant benefit in 5-year disease-free survival, overall survival, local-regional failure, or the distant metastasis rate. The cumulative rate of colostomy was significantly improved in the mitomycin-C arm (10 % vs. 19 %, $p=0.02$). There was increased severe hematologic toxicity in the mitomycin arm ($p<0.001$). Ajani JA et al. Fluorouracil, mitomycin, and radiotherapy vs. fluorouracil, cisplatin, and radiotherapy for carcinoma of the anal canal. JAMA. 2008;299(16): 1914–21.

8. The correct answer is A. This patient has a T2N2 primary. According to RTOG 0529, for N+ disease the primary lesion would be prescribed a dose of 54 Gy over 30 fractions. Because the involved lymph node is greater than 3 cm in size, it would also receive a dose of 54 Gy over 30 fractions. If the lymph node were less than 3 cm in size, it would be prescribed a dose of 50.4 Gy. Kachnic L et al. RTOG 0529: a phase II study of dose-painted IMRT (DP-IMRT), 5-Fluorouracil, and mitomycin-C for the reduction of acute morbidity in anal cancer. Int J Radiat Oncol Biol Phys. 2009;75:s5.

9. The correct answer is B. According to the 7th edition of AJCC staging, invasion *into* the muscularis propria constitutes T2 disease. Invasion *through* the muscularis propria and into pericolorectal tissues constitutes T3 disease. One enlarged lymph node would be N1 disease, which is defined as metastasis in 1–3 regional lymph nodes. Size of the primary is not part of the staging criteria for rectal cancer. Edge SB, Byrd DR, Compton CC, et al., editors. Colon and rectum. AJCC cancer staging handbook. 7th ed. New York: Springer; 2010.

10. The correct answer is D. The German Rectal Cancer Study randomized 823 patients with cT3–T4 or cN+ rectal cancers to surgery (TME) followed by chemoRT (55.8 Gy) and 4 cycles of additional bolus 5-FU versus preoperative chemoRT (50.4 Gy) followed by TME followed by an additional 4 cycles of bolus 5-FU. In the initial report (2004) with a median follow-up of 3.8 years, preoperative chemoRT was found to decrease local failure (6 % vs. 13 %, $p=0.006$). There was no difference in overall or disease-free survival. More patients were converted to sphincter-preserving surgeries in the neoadjuvant chemoRT arm (39 % vs. 19 %). The latest update published in 2012 reported results with a median follow-up of 11 years. Local recurrence was decreased in the neoadjuvant chemoRT arm (7.1 vs. 10.1 %, $p=0.048$). There was still no difference in overall survival between the arms. The overall rates of acute and long-term side effects were lower in the neoadjuvant arm, especially with respect to acute and chronic diarrhea and the development of strictures at the anastomotic site. Sauer et al. Preoperative versus postoperative chemoradiotherapy for rectal cancer. N Engl J Med. 2004 Oct 21;351(17):1731–40. Sauer et al. Preoperative versus postoperative chemoradiotherapy for locally advanced rectal cancer: results of the German CAO/ARO/AIO-94 randomized phase III trial after a median follow-up of 11 years. J Clin Oncol. 2012 Jun 1;30(16): 1926–33.

11. The correct answer is B. The German Rectal Cancer Study randomized 823 patients with cT3–T4 or cN+ rectal cancers to surgery (TME) followed by chemoRT (55.8 Gy) and 4 cycles of additional bolus 5-FU versus preoperative chemoRT (50.4 Gy) followed by TME, followed by an additional 4 cycles of bolus 5-FU. Of those patients that were randomized to preoperative chemoRT prior to total mesorectal excision for rectal cancer, 8 % experienced a pathological complete response. Sauer et al. Preoperative versus postoperative chemoradiotherapy for rectal cancer. N Engl J Med. 2004 Oct 21;351(17):1731–40.

12. The correct answer is C. The German Rectal Cancer Study randomized 823 patients with cT3–T4 or cN+ rectal cancers to surgery (TME) followed by chemoRT (55.8 Gy) and 4 cycles of additional bolus 5-FU versus preoperative chemoRT (50.4 Gy) followed by TME followed by an additional 4 cycles of bolus 5-FU. Of the 415 patients randomized to preoperative chemoRT, 116 were thought to require abdominoperineal resection. Preoperative chemoRT was able to decrease the need for APR, and 45 of these patients (39 %) were able to undergo sphincter-preserving surgery. Sauer et al. Preoperative versus postoperative chemoradiotherapy for rectal cancer. N Engl J Med. 2004 Oct 21;351(17):1731–40.

13. The correct answer is A. Depth of invasion corresponds to T stage. Invasion of the submucosa is T1, invasion into the muscularis propria is T2, and invasion through and beyond the muscularis propria is T3. The serosa is the outermost layer of the rectum. Unlike the esophagus, there is no adventitia in the rectum. Edge SB, Byrd DR, Compton CC, et al., editors. Colon and rectum. AJCC cancer staging handbook. 7th ed. New York: Springer; 2010.

14. The correct answer is C. Six hundred sixty patients with stage II–III rectal cancer received either bolus or protracted venous infusion of fluorouracil with concurrent postoperative radiation. After completing postoperative chemoRT, they were subsequently randomized to receive either higher-dose fluorouracil alone or fluorouracil + semustine. With a median follow-up of 46 months, those patients that received CI 5-FU had an increased time to relapse and improved survival (70 % vs. 60 %, $p = 0.005$). Tumor relapse and distant metastases were also decreased. The addition of semustine provided no additional benefit. O'Connell MJ et al. Improving adjuvant therapy for rectal cancer by combining protracted-infusion fluorouracil with radiation therapy after curative surgery. N Engl J Med. 1994;331(8):502–7.

15. The correct answer is D. In the Polish rectal cancer study, TME was required only for distal rectal tumors. Not all, but 92 % of patients underwent TME in the MRC CR 07 trial. In the Swedish rectal cancer trial, TME was not required. The Dutch CKVO trial randomized 1,861 patients with resectable rectal cancer to either preoperative RT (5Gy×5) followed by TME or TME alone. In the initial report, the rate of local recurrence at 2 years was 2.4 % in the RT+TME

arm versus 8.2 % in the TME-alone arm. Bujko et al. Long-term results of a randomized trial comparing preoperative short-course radiotherapy with preoperative conventionally fractionated chemoradiation for rectal cancer. Br J Surg. 2006 Oct;93(10):1215–1523. Kapiteijn et al. Preoperative radiotherapy combined with total mesorectal excision for resectable rectal cancer. N Engl J Med. 2001;30:345(9):638–46. Sebag-Montefiore D et al. Preoperative radiotherapy versus selective postoperative chemoradiotherapy in patients with rectal cancer (MRC CR07 and NCIC-CTG C0616): a multicentre, randomized trial. Lancet. 2009;373(9666):811–20.

16. The correct answer is C. MRC CR 07 compared short-course preoperative RT versus initial surgery with selective postoperative chemoRT for patients with a positive circumferential margin. TME was encouraged, but not required (92 % underwent TME). One thousand three hundred fifty patients were randomized. Preoperative RT consisted of 25 Gy over 5 fractions and adjuvant chemoRT was 45 Gy/25 fractions with concurrent 5-FU. With a median follow-up of 4 years, 3-year local recurrence was 4.4 % versus 10.6 % favoring the preoperative RT arm. Three-year disease-free survival was also improved (77.5 % vs. 71.5 %). There was no difference in overall survival. Sebag-Montefiore D et al. Preoperative radiotherapy versus selective postoperative chemoradiotherapy in patients with rectal cancer (MRC CR07 and NCIC-CTG C0616): a multicentre, randomized trial. Lancet. 2009;373(9666):811–20.

17. The correct answer is C. Late side effects from the Dutch colorectal study were reported with a median follow-up of 5.1 years. Stoma function, urinary function, and hospital treatment rates did not differ significantly between the treatment arms. However, irradiated patients, compared with nonirradiated patients, reported increased rates of fecal incontinence (62 % vs. 38 %, respectively; $p < 0.001$), pad wearing as a result of incontinence (56 % vs. 33 %, respectively; $p < 0.001$), anal blood loss (11 % vs. 3 %, respectively; $p = 0.004$), and mucus loss (27 % vs. 15 %, respectively; $p = .005$). Satisfaction with bowel function was significantly lower and the impact of bowel dysfunction on daily activities was greater in irradiated patients compared with patients who underwent TME alone. Peeters et al. Late side effects of short-course preoperative radiotherapy combined with total mesorectal excision for rectal cancer: increased bowel dysfunction in irradiated patients – a Dutch colorectal cancer group study. J Clin Oncol. 2005;23(25):6199–206.

18. The correct answer is D. The ACT II trial was a 2×2 randomization. Nine hundred and forty patients were randomized to either arm 1 (RT 50.4 Gy/28 fractions + 5-FU 1,000 mg/m^2 days 1–4 and days 29–32 + cisplatin 60 mg/m^2 day 1 and day 29) or arm 2 (same RT and 5-FU + mitomycin 12 mg/m$^{2\,day}$ 1). Patients were then randomized to +/− maintenance chemo: arm 1 (cisplatin + 5-FU × 2 cycles) versus arm 2 (observation). Complete response did not differ between those receiving MMC versus cisplatin (~95 %). Comparing observation after CRT versus maintenance chemotherapy, there was no difference in

recurrence-free or overall survival, or the number of pretreatment colostomies reversed. James R et al. Randomized trial of chemoradiation using mitomycin or cisplatin, with or without maintenance cisplatin/5-FU in squamous cell carcinoma of the anus (ACT II). J Clin Oncol. 2009;27:18s. (ASCO abstract).

19. The correct answer is B. RTOG 87-04 randomized approximately 300 patients to treatment with (1) RT (45–50.4 Gy) and 5-FU versus RT (45–50.4 Gy) and 5-FU+mitomycin. At 4 years of follow-up, colostomy rates were lower in the MMC arm (9 % vs. 22 %), as was local failure (16 % vs. 34 %). Colostomy-free survival was increased in the MMC arm (71 % vs. 59 %). Toxicity was increased in the MMC arm (23 % vs. 7 %). Overall survival was not significantly different between the two arms. Despite its increased toxicity, this trial showed that MMC cannot be eliminated without a corresponding increase in colostomy rates and local failure. Flam et al. Role of mitomycin in combination with fluorouracil and radiotherapy, and of salvage chemoradiation in the definitive nonsurgical treatment of epidermoid carcinoma of the anal canal: results of a phase III randomized intergroup study. J Clin Oncol. 1996;14(9):2527–39.

20. The correct answer is A. According to the NCCN Guidelines from 2012, the anal margin starts at the anal verge and includes the perianal skin over a 5–6 cm radius from the squamous mucocutaneous junction. Anal Cancer. NCCN Clinical Practice Guidelines in Oncology (NCCN Guidelines ®) Version 2.2012.

21. The correct answer is D. This is technically an anal margin tumor. NCCN Guidelines recommend that it should be treated as if it were a skin cancer, i.e., local excision. If the lesion had come into contact with the anal verge or was unresectable, chemoRT could be considered. Anal Cancer. NCCN Clinical Practice Guidelines in Oncology (NCCN Guidelines ®) Version 2.2012.

22. The correct answer is C. This patient should receive adjuvant chemotherapy for 6 months with any of the following regimens: 5-FU+/−leucovorin, FOLFOX, and capecitabine +/− oxaliplatin. Rectal Cancer. NCCN Clinical Practice Guidelines in Oncology (NCCN Guidelines ®) Version 3.2012.

23. The correct answer is D. Several studies have shown that if appropriately managed, patients with a local recurrence can have good long-term control. Das et al. Hyperfractionated accelerated radiotherapy for rectal cancer in patients with prior pelvic irradiation. Int J Radiat Oncol Biol Phys. 2010;77(1):60–5. Valentini et al. Preoperative hyperfractionated chemoradiation for locally recurrent rectal cancer in patients previously irradiated to the pelvis: a multicentric phase II study. Int J Radiat Oncol Biol Phys. 2006;64(4):1129–39.

24. The correct answer is D. 45 % of patients with anal carcinoma present with rectal bleeding. Approximately one third present with either pain or the sensation of a rectal mass. Ryan et al. Carcinoma of the anal canal. N Engl J Med. 2000;342(11):792–800.

25. The correct answer is D. Management of patients that present with oligometastatic disease is controversial. However, given 5-year survival rates of 30–70 % following resection, there is a good argument to be made for aggressive treatment in patients with good performance status. The sequencing of treatment of primary and metastatic lesion is variable and is often determined by patient symptoms. Expert Panel on Radiation Oncology. American College of Radiology: Rectal Cancer – Metastatic Disease at Presentation. American College of Radiology ACR Appropriateness Criteria® 2010.

26. The correct answer is B. The patient has a T3N1 rectal adenocarcinoma. The external iliac lymph nodes are not likely to be involved for this particular case. In T3 rectal carcinoma, the anterior border of the lateral fields is behind the pubic symphysis. For patients with T4 tumors invading anterior structures, the anterior block is often brought forward to cover a portion of the external iliac lymph nodes. Rectal Cancer. NCCN Clinical Practice Guidelines in Oncology (NCCN Guidelines ®) Version 3.2012.

27. The correct answer is A. Patients with HIV/AIDS have been reported to be at an increased risk of developing anal carcinoma. Numerous studies have found that patients with anal carcinoma as the first manifestation of HIV may be treated with the same regimen as non-HIV patients. Several retrospective series have found no difference with respect to treatment or 2-year survival when comparing HIV patients versus non-HIV patients. Chiao et al. Human immunodeficiency virus-associated squamous cell cancer of the anus: epidemiology and outcomes in the highly active antiretroviral therapy era. J Clin Oncol. 2008;26(3):474–9. Hoffman et al. The significance of pretreatment CD4 count on the outcome and treatment tolerance of HIV-positive patients with anal cancer. Int J Radiat Oncol Biol Phys. 1999;44(1):127–31. Fraunholz et al. Concurrent chemoradiotherapy with 5-fluorouracil and mitomycin C for invasive anal carcinoma in human immunodeficiency virus-positive patients receiving highly active antiretroviral therapy. Int J Radiat Oncol Biol Phys. 2010;76(5):1425–32.

28. The correct answer is C. This stresses the importance of sampling any clinically positive lymph nodes to accurately stage patients. This is increasingly important as many treatment protocols stratify treatment of patients with anal cancer based on N stage. Anal Cancer. NCCN Clinical Practice Guidelines in Oncology (NCCN Guidelines ®) Version 2.2012.

29. The correct answer is D. Colon cancer has a major genetic component. Approximately 80 % of these cancers contain *17p (p53)* or *18q* (DCC – deleted colon cancer) mutation. Lurje et al. Molecular prognostic markers in locally advanced colon cancer. Clin Colorectal Cancer. 2007;6(10):683–90.

30. The correct answer is B. Patients with FAP contain a mutation of the *APC* tumor suppressor gene – the most common of which is 5q21. O'Sullivan et al.

Familial adenomatous polyposis: from bedside to benchside. Am J Clin Pathol. 1998;109(5):521–6.

31. The correct answer is D. Familial adenomatous polyposis (5q21 mutation) has an autosomal dominant inheritance. There is a 100 % risk of developing colorectal cancer for these patients. Over 95 % of patients have cancer by age 45 if left untreated. Surveillance is recommended to start in the early teens per the American Cancer Society. Galiatsatos P, Foulkes WD. Familial adenomatous polyposis. Am J Gastroenterol. 2006;101(2):385–98.

32. The correct answer is B. Lynch II syndrome is a variant of hereditary nonpolyposis colorectal cancer (HNPCC), due to a DNA mismatch repair defect. It is autosomal dominantly inherited and tends to occur in younger individuals (mean age of 46 years). In addition to colon cancer, other associated cancers include endometrial, ovarian, gastric, and upper urinary tract cancers. Lynch HT et al. Hereditary factors in cancer. Study of two large midwestern kindreds. Arch Intern Med. 1966;117(2):206–12.

33. The correct answer is D. RTOG 89-02 was a phase II clinical trial in which patients with T1-3 rectal tumors were assigned transanal or trans-sacral excisions followed by observation or chemoRT. Local failure was 0 % for patients with T1 tumors versus 20 % for patients with T2 tumors. The current NCCN Guidelines recommend transanal excision alone only for T1N0 tumors that are less than 3 cm in size, mobile/nonfixed, negative surgical margins (>3 mm) with no PNI or LVSI, and not poorly differentiated. Russell et al. Anal sphincter conservation for patients with adenocarcinoma of the distal rectum: long-term results of Radiation Therapy Oncology Group protocol 89-02. Int J Radiat Oncol Biol Phys. 2000;46(2):313–22.

34. The correct answer is B. According to the American Cancer Society, patients with average risk (i.e., no personal or family history, no inflammatory bowel disease) should have screening starting age 50 with any of the following: flexible sigmoidoscopy every 5 years, colonoscopy every 10 years, double-contrast barium enema every 5 years, or CT colonography (virtual colonoscopy) every 5 years. American Cancer Society. American Cancer Society recommendations for colorectal early detection. Last revised 6/15/2012.

35. The correct answer is A. Multiple studies have reported the most common site of local recurrence is the presacral space. In patients from the Dutch TME trial, presacral recurrences were most common in both the RT+TME and the TME-alone arms. Local recurrences in this region can be extremely symptomatic and difficult to treat. This is the reason that the posterior border in both the initial and boost fields should extend just beyond the sacrum. Kusters et al. Patterns of local recurrence in rectal cancer a study of the Dutch TME trial. Eur J Surg Oncol. 2010;36(5):470–76.

36. The correct answer is B. The most common presenting symptom for patients with rectal cancer is frank rectal bleeding. Minsky BD, Welton ML, Venook AP. Cancer of the rectum. In: Hoppe RT, Phillips TL, Roach M, editors. Leibel and Phillips textbook of radiation oncology. 3rd ed. Philadelphia: Elsevier Saunders; 2010. p. 851–69.

37. The correct answer is D. The ascending colon and descending colon are retroperitoneal. Minsky BD, Welton ML, Venook AP. Cancer of the rectum. In: Hoppe RT, Phillips TL, Roach M, editors. Leibel and Phillips textbook of radiation oncology. 3rd ed. Philadelphia: Elsevier Saunders; 2010. p. 851–69.

38. The correct answer is C. Almost two thirds of these cancers occur in the proximal colon. HNPCC is an autosomal dominant trait characterized by a defect in mismatch repair. The average age of colorectal cancer diagnosis is around 45. These patients have an 80 % chance of developing a colorectal cancer. Minsky BD, Welton ML, Pineda CE, Venook AP. Cancer of the colon. In: Hoppe RT, Phillips TL, Roach M, editors. Leibel and Phillips textbook of radiation oncology. 3rd ed. Philadelphia: Elsevier Saunders; 2010. p. 842–50.

39. The correct answer is A. Antibodies targeting the epidermal growth factor receptor have been shown to be more effective in patients with an intact (i.e., wild type) *KRAS* gene. Cunningham et al. Cetuximab monotherapy and cetuximab plus irinotecan in irinotecan-refractory metastatic colorectal cancer. N Engl J Med. 2004;351(4):337–45. Amado et al. Wild-type KRAS is required for panitumumab efficacy in patients with metastatic colorectal cancer. Clin Oncol. 2008;26(10):1626–34.

40. The correct answer is B. Allele-specific PCR is an acceptable method of detecting this mutation. Other alternatives include PCR amplification and direct DNA sequence analysis. This can be done on formalin-fixed, paraffin-embedded tissues. Patients with a *BRAF V600E* mutation have a poorer prognosis. Bokemeyer et al. Cetuximab with chemotherapy (CT) as first-line treatment for metastatic colorectal cancer (mCRC): analysis of the CRYSTAL and OPUS studies according to KRAS and BRAF mutation status. J Clin Oncol. 2010;28(Suppl):3506.

41. The correct answer is A. MRI and EUS are similarly sensitive for evaluating depth of tumor penetration into the muscularis propria (~94 %). CT is not considered to be an optimal method for staging the extent of tumor penetration. A meta-analysis reported the sensitivity of EUS for detecting lymph node involvement to be approximately 67 %. While the degree of operator dependence of EUS is a disadvantage, it is still the most commonly used staging method for determining depth of invasion. Bipat et al. Rectal cancer: local staging and assessment of lymph node involvement with endoluminal US, CT, and MR imaging – a meta-analysis. Radiology. 2004;232:773–83. Rectal Cancer. NCCN Clinical Practice Guidelines in Oncology (NCCN Guidelines ®) Version 3.2012.

42. The correct answer is A. Prospective studies have suggested that vitamin D deficiency may increase the incidence of colorectal cancer. Two prospective trials have shown that colorectal cancer patients with low vitamin D levels had increased mortality, especially those with stage III–IV disease. There is still no clear evidence to suggest that supplementation would improve outcomes. Ng K et al. Circulating 25-hydroxyvitamin d levels and survival in patients with colorectal cancer. J Clin Oncol. 2008;26:2984–91. Lappe JM et al. Vitamin D and calcium supplementation reduces cancer risk: results of a randomized trial. Am J Clin Nutr. 2007;85:1586–91.

43. The correct answer is A. GITSG 7175 was a 4-arm study to determine the optimal adjuvant therapy. Two hundred twenty-seven patients with locally advanced rectal cancer were randomized to one of four arms: (1) surgery alone, (2) surgery + radiation alone (40 or 48 Gy), (3) surgery + chemotherapy alone, and (4) surgery + chemoradiation. Chemotherapy consisted of 5-FU and MeCCNU. The initial report in 1985 with a median follow-up of 80 months showed the lowest recurrence rate in those receiving adjuvant chemoRT (33 %) and the highest in those receiving no adjuvant therapy (55 %). Time to tumor recurrence was also the longest in the chemoRT arm versus observation ($p < 0.009$). In the initial report, there was no overall survival benefit. The latest update in 1988 did show an overall survival benefit for chemoRT versus observation (45 % vs. 27 %, $p = 0.01$), in addition to prolonged time to recurrence. Prolongation of the disease-free interval in surgically treated rectal carcinoma. N Engl J Med. 1985;312:1265–472. Thomas PR et al. Adjuvant postoperative radiotherapy and chemotherapy in rectal carcinoma: a review of the Gastrointestinal Tumor Study Group experience. Radiother Oncol. 1988;13(4):245–52.

44. The correct answer is B. The MOSAIC trial randomized 2,246 patients with stage II/II colon cancer s/p curative resection to receive either bolus + continuous infusion 5-FU + leucovorin or bolus + continuous infusion 5-FU + leucovorin + oxaliplatin (FOLFOX). Final results of the study reported improved in 6-year overall survival in stage III patients (72.9 % vs. 68.7 %, $p = 0.023$) and improved 5-year disease-free survival (73.3 % vs. 67.4 %, $p = 0.003$) in all patients with the addition of oxaliplatin. No overall survival benefit was seen in stage II patients. André T et al. Improved overall survival with oxaliplatin, fluorouracil, and leucovorin as adjuvant treatment in stage II or III colon cancer in the MOSAIC trial. J Clin Oncol. 2009;27(19):3109–16.

45. The correct answer is C. The superior border is defined as the upper border of the anal sphincter and puborectalis muscles of the anorectal ring. This functional definition is used primarily in the radical surgical treatment of anal cancer. Cummings BJ, Ajani JA, Swallow CJ. Cancer of the anal region. In: DeVita Jr VT, Lawrence TS, Rosenberg SA, et al., editors. Cancer: principles and practice of oncology. 8th ed. Philadelphia: Lippincott, Williams & Wilkins; 2008.

46. The correct answer is C. Squamous cell carcinomas of the anal margin are more likely to be well differentiated and contain skin appendages (hair follicles or sweat glands). Keratinizing large-cell-type squamous cell carcinomas are more likely to be anal margin tumors. It is not always possible to distinguish between anal margin and anal canal tumors since these lesions can involve both areas. Cummings BJ, Ajani JA, Swallow CJ. Cancer of the anal region. In: DeVita Jr VT, Lawrence TS, Rosenberg SA, et al., editors. Cancer: principles n practice of oncology. 8th ed. Philadelphia: Lippincott, Williams & Wilkins; 2008.

47. The correct answer is D. A distal anal cancer has a higher incidence of metastasizing to the inguinal lymph nodes, compared to a more proximal cancer. Drainage of lesions proximal to the dentate line is towards the anorectal, perirectal, paravertebral, and internal iliac lymph nodes. It is important to note that the drainage of each site is not isolated and a proper staging work-up is always warranted. Rectal Cancer. NCCN Clinical Practice Guidelines in Oncology (NCCN Guidelines ®) Version 3.2012.

48. The correct answer is A. The ACT II trial was a 2×2 randomization. Nine hundred and forty patients were randomized to either arm 1 (RT 50.4 Gy/28 fractions + 5-FU 1,000 mg/m^2 days 1–4 and days 29–32 + cisplatin 60 mg/m^2 day 1 and day 29) or arm 2 (same RT and 5-FU + mitomycin 12 mg/m^2 day 1). Patients were then randomized to +/– maintenance chemo: arm 1 (cisplatin + 5-FU $\times$ 2 cycles) versus arm 2 (observation). At a median follow-up of 3 years, complete response did not differ between those receiving MMC versus cisplatin (~95 %). Comparing observation after CRT versus maintenance chemotherapy, there was no difference in recurrence-free or overall survival, or the number of pretreatment colostomies reversed. Longer follow-up of this trial is still pending. James R et al. Randomized trial of chemoradiation using mitomycin or cisplatin, with or without maintenance cisplatin/5-FU in squamous cell carcinoma of the anus (ACT II). J Clin Oncol. 2009;27:18s. (ASCO abstract).

49. The correct answer is C. Digital rectal exam/anoscopy is recommended every 3–6 months following treatment. Exam should also include inguinal lymph node palpation. Annual CT of the chest, abdomen, and pelvis is recommended for 3 years in patients with initially locally advanced disease (T3/T4) tumors or LN + tumors. Anal Cancer. NCCN Clinical Practice Guidelines in Oncology (NCCN Guidelines ®) Version 2.2012.

50. The correct answer is D. Following treatment, patients should be monitored closely with repeat DREs. They should be classified according to whether they have a complete remission, persistent disease, or progressive disease. At sign of progression, biopsy and restaging CT or PET should be performed. If the biopsy is positive, they should be evaluated for radical salvage surgery with an APR. Anal Cancer. NCCN Clinical Practice Guidelines in Oncology (NCCN Guidelines ®) Version 2.2012.

51. The correct answer is C. The most important criterion in determining resect-ability is the likelihood of achieving a complete (R0) resection while maintaining adequate liver reserve. Incomplete resection and debulking have not been shown to be beneficial unless the lesion is symptomatic. Yoo et al. Liver resection for metastatic colorectal cancer in the age of neoadjuvant chemotherapy and bevacizumab. Clin Clin Colorectal Cancer. 2006;6(3):202–7.

52. The correct answer is D. Based on a recent meta-analysis of randomized controlled trials to assess the role of bevacizumab in treatment-related mortality, the most common causes of fatal adverse events were hemorrhage (23.5 %), neutropenia (12.2 %), and gastrointestinal tract perforation (7.1 %). Ranpura et al. Treatment-related mortality with bevacizumab in cancer patients – a meta-analysis. JAMA. 2011;305(5):487–94.

53. The correct answer is A. NCCN Guidelines recommend the first colonoscopy at approximately 1 year following resection. If no preoperative colonoscopy was done due to an obstructive lesion, the first colonoscopy can be done at 3–6 months. Proctoscopy should be considered every 6 months for 5 years to evaluate for local recurrence at the rectal anastomosis in patients that underwent a LAR. Rectal Cancer. NCCN Clinical Practice Guidelines in Oncology (NCCN Guidelines ®) Version 3.2012.

54. The correct answer is C. Rectal cancer is the third most common cancer in the United States. In 2012, 40,290 cases of rectal cancer are expected to occur, though the incidence of colorectal cancer has been decreasing, presumably due to increases in the use of colorectal cancer screening tests. American Cancer Society. Cancer facts and figures. 2012. http://www.cancer.org/research/cancer-factsfigures/cancer-facts-figures-2012

55. The correct answer is B. According to the American Cancer Society guidelines, this patient should have a repeat colonoscopy in 3 years.

56. The correct answer is D. The correct 7th edition AJCC stage is uT3N1bM0. "u" denotes staging of the primary was done with EUS. "y" denotes pathologic review after surgical resection. N1b denotes 2–3 involved lymph nodes; N1a denotes 1 involved lymph node. Edge SB, Byrd DR, Compton CC, et al., editors. Colon and rectum. AJCC cancer staging handbook. 7th ed. New York: Springer; 2010.

57. The correct answer is A. There is no clear consensus on the most appropriate chemotherapy in this setting. Treatment should be individualized and is often comprised of cisplatin-based chemotherapy. Enrollment on a clinical trial could also be considered. Ajani et al. Combination of cisplatin plus fluoropyrimidine chemotherapy effective against liver metastases from carcinoma of the anal canal. Am J Med. 1989;87(2):221–4. Cummings et al. Metastatic anal cancer: the search for cure. Onkologie. 2006;29(1–2):5–6.

Chapter 9
Urinary System Cancers

Celine Bicquart Ord and Eric K. Hansen

Questions

1. A 9.5 cm renal cell carcinoma that is limited to the kidney with no regional lymph node metastases is classified as 7th edition AJCC TNM stage:
   A. T1bN0
   B. T2aN0
   C. T2bN0
   D. T3N0

2. Renal cell carcinoma that extends into the vena cava below the diaphragm is classified as 7th edition AJCC T stage:
   A. T2b
   B. T3a
   C. T3b
   D. T3c

3. A 5 cm tumor in the kidney, limited to the kidney, is classified as AJCC stage:
   A. T1a
   B. T1b
   C. T2a
   D. T2b

C.B. Ord, MD (✉)
Department of Radiation Oncology, Scott & White Memorial Hospital, Temple, TX 76508, USA
e-mail: cord@sw.org

E.K. Hansen, MD
Department of Radiation Oncology, The Oregon Clinic, Providence St.
Vincent Medical Center, Portland, OR 97225, USA
e-mail: ehansen@orclinic.com

C.B. Ord et al. (eds.), *Radiation Oncology Study Guide*,
DOI 10.1007/978-1-4614-6400-6_9, © Springer Science+Business Media New York 2013

4. Renal cell carcinoma accounts for what percentage of kidney cancers?
   A. 95 %
   B. 90 %
   C. 85 %
   D. 80 %

5. The most common hereditary type of renal cell carcinoma is associated with:
   A. Von Hippel-Lindau syndrome
   B. Ataxia telangiectasia
   C. Cockayne syndrome
   D. Xeroderma pigmentosum

6. One possible explanation for the increased incidence of renal cell carcinoma is:
   A. Increased genetic mutation rate.
   B. Increased use of computed tomography.
   C. Unknown.
   D. The incidence of renal carcinoma is actually decreasing.

7. If a mass is centrally located, as opposed to on either pole of the kidney, what type of carcinoma should be suspected?
   A. Renal cell carcinoma
   B. Papillary carcinoma
   C. Chromophobe carcinoma
   D. Urothelial carcinoma

8. What is the approximate expected 5-year survival of stage IV renal cell carcinoma?
   A. 45 %
   B. 25 %
   C. 15 %
   D. 10 %

9. According to the EORTC 30881 phase three trial comparing radical nephrectomy with or without lymph node dissection, which outcome was demonstrated?
   A. No difference in progression-free survival or overall survival
   B. Improvement in progression-free survival without an overall survival improvement
   C. No improvement in progression-free survival, but an overall survival benefit
   D. An improvement in both progression-free and overall survival

10. Which is the most common site of distant metastasis for renal cell carcinoma?
    A. Bone
    B. Brain
    C. Liver
    D. Lung

11. According to a SWOG study looking at the value of interferon alfa-2b with or without cytoreductive nephrectomy in stage IV renal cell carcinoma:
    A. There was a trend toward improved median survival in those that received interferon alfa-2b therapy in addition to nephrectomy.
    B. There was a statistically significant improvement in median survival in those that received interferon alfa-2b therapy in addition to nephrectomy.
    C. There was a statistically significant improvement in median survival in those that received interferon alfa-2b therapy alone, without nephrectomy.
    D. There was a statistically significant improvement in median survival in those that received cytoreductive nephrectomy alone.

12. The targets of temsirolimus and sunitinib are respectively:
    A. PDGFR and EGFR
    B. EGFR and PDGFR
    C. mTor and PDGFR
    D. PDGFR and mTor

13. Which of the following is the most common presentation of renal cell carcinoma?
    A. Hematuria
    B. Flank pain
    C. Asymptomatic
    D. Palpable mass

14. All of the following are histologic subtypes of renal cell carcinoma except:
    A. Granular cell
    B. Clear cell
    C. Papillary
    D. Chromophobe

15. Which of the following is the most common presenting symptom of renal pelvis or ureteral cancer?
    A. Hematuria
    B. Dysuria
    C. Flank pain
    D. Palpable mass

16. All of the following have been found to be risk factors for distant metastasis in resected renal cell carcinoma except:
    A. Lymph node involvement
    B. Primary tumor size
    C. Pathologic tumor type
    D. Renal vein involvement

17. Which one of the following is not an acceptable indication for partial nephrectomy, as opposed to radical nephrectomy?
    A. Presence of bilateral tumors
    B. Cancer involving a solitary kidney
    C. Tumor measuring 2.5 cm
    D. Tumor involving the renal hilum

18. What is the risk of local failure following gross total resection of a renal cell
carcinoma?
    A. 20 %
    B. 15 %
    C. 10 %
    D. 5 %

19. All of the following are true regarding the surgical management of renal pelvis
or ureteral cancers except:
    A. The standard surgery is nephroureterectomy with removal of the bladder cuff.
    B. Laparoscopic nephroureterectomy has been shown to have no decreased
       cancer effectiveness with decreased anesthesia time, recovery time, and
       hospital stay.
    C. Partial ureterectomy can be performed for tumors <3 cm.
    D. Locoregional failure develops in up to 15 % of low-grade, low-stage disease.

20. All of the following are true regarding patterns of failure in renal pelvis and
ureteral cancers after surgery as reported by Cozad et al. except:
    A. Risk of local relapse correlates with stage and grade of tumor.
    B. Half of local relapses manifest as an isolated site of local recurrence.
    C. Five-year local control of grade 3 and 4 tumors treated with surgery alone is
       >75 %.
    D. Overall, local recurrence occurs in almost half of patients treated with sur-
       gery alone.

21. All of the following are true regarding urethral cancer except:
    A. There is a 4:1 incidence in women to men.
    B. The most common site in men is the bulbomembranous urethra.
    C. Anterior urethral tumors drain to the inguinal lymph nodes.
    D. Posterior urethral tumors drain to internal but not external iliac lymph nodes.

22. What is the correct 7th edition AJCC TNM stage for a urethral cancer that
invades into the corpus spongiosum with a single 2.0 cm lymph node
metastasis?
    A. T2N1
    B. T2N2
    C. T3N1
    D. T3N2

23. Which of the following statements regarding urethral carcinoma is false?
    A. Most bulbomembranous urethral cancers are squamous cell carcinoma type.
    B. Most prostatic urethral cancers are squamous cell carcinoma type.
    C. Proximal tumors have a worst prognosis than distal tumors.
    D. The prostatic urethra is the least common site of urethral cancer in men.

24. A woman is found to have a urethral cancer that invades the anterior vagina with multiple involved lymph nodes. What is the correct AJCC TNM stage?
    A. T3N1
    B. T3N2
    C. T4N1
    D. T4N2

25. A 67-year-old man is found to have a urethral cancer that invades into the corpus cavernosum, with a single 5 mm lymph node metastasis. What is the correct 7th edition AJCC TNM stage?
    A. T2N1
    B. T3N1
    C. T2N2
    D. T3N2

26. All of the following are true regarding bladder cancer except:
    A. The majority of diagnosed bladder cancer is not muscle invasive.
    B. The incidence of bladder cancer is increasing.
    C. Bladder cancer is more common in women than men.
    D. The most common histology is transitional cell.

27. What percentage of those with an upper tract urinary cancer develops bladder cancer?
    A. 5 %
    B. 15 %
    C. 40 %
    D. 60 %

28. All of the following are risk factors for developing transitional cell carcinoma of the bladder except:
    A. Tobacco use
    B. *Schistosoma haematobium* infection
    C. Aniline dye exposure
    D. Aromatic amine exposure

29. What percentage of bladder cancers are superficial at diagnosis?
    A. 5 %
    B. 25 %
    C. 50 %
    D. 75 %

30. Regarding prognosis of bladder transitional cell carcinoma, which of the following is true?
    A. Grade is the most important predictor of outcome for non-muscle-invasive tumors, while depth of invasion is the most important predictor of outcome for muscle-invasive tumors.
    B. Depth of invasion is the most important predictor of outcome for non-muscle-invasive tumors, while grade is the most important predictor of outcome for muscle-invasive tumors.
    C. Grade is the most important predictor of outcome for both non-muscle-invasive and muscle-invasive tumors.
    D. Depth of invasion is the most important predictor of outcome for both non-muscle-invasive and muscle-invasive tumors.

31. Which of the following lymph node regions is considered second echelon for bladder cancer?
    A. Internal iliac
    B. External iliac
    C. Perivesical
    D. Paracaval

32. What is the most common presentation of bladder cancer?
    A. Asymptomatic
    B. Painless hematuria
    C. Dysuria
    D. Pyuria

33. A bladder tumor is found to invade into the superficial muscle with metastasis to a single 2.5 cm pelvic lymph node. What is the current AJCC TNM stage?
    A. T2aN1
    B. T2aN2
    C. T2bN1
    D. T2bN2

34. A bladder tumor is found to involve a single external iliac lymph node. What is the correct 7th edition AJCC stage?
    A. Stage I
    B. Stage II
    C. Stage III
    D. Stage IV

35. What is the most appropriate therapy for a noninvasive bladder tumor?
    A. Neoadjuvant chemotherapy, followed by TURBT
    B. Neoadjuvant chemoradiation, followed by TURBT
    C. TURBT followed by intravesicular chemotherapy
    D. TURBT followed by chemoradiation

36. All are true regarding the use of Bacille Calmette-Guérin in bladder cancer except:
    A. Addition of BCG to TURBT has been shown to reduce disease progression.
    B. Addition of BCG to TURBT has been shown to reduce disease recurrence.
    C. Addition of BCG to TURBT has not been shown to increase extravesical relapse.
    D. Addition of BCG to TURBT has been shown to improve survival.

37. What is the 5-year overall survival rate after radical cystectomy alone for muscle-invasive bladder cancer?
    A. 20–30 %
    B. 30–40 %
    C. 40–50 %
    D. 50–60 %

38. In a retrospective review from MD Anderson Cancer Center of radiation given preoperatively for cT3b tumors reported by Cole et al., all of the following are true except:
    A. The addition of radiation therapy reduced pelvic recurrence by more than half.
    B. Preoperative radiation consisted of 50 Gy.
    C. Actuarial pelvic control at 5 years was over 90 %
    D. Discontinuation of pelvic radiotherapy did not affect survival.

39. In the University of Paris study of multimodality therapy (TURBT followed by cisplatin/5-FU with concurrent accelerated RT, followed by cystectomy), what was the pathological complete response rate of the initial 18 patients enrolled?
    A. 100 %
    B. 50 %
    C. 25 %
    D. <5 %

40. In the RTOG 89-03 trial assessing the benefit of neoadjuvant MCV chemotherapy prior to consolidation therapy, which of the following is not true?
    A. Fewer patients were able to complete the protocol on the neoadjuvant arm.
    B. Complete response rate was improved with neoadjuvant MCV.
    C. Five-year bladder preservation was not improved with neoadjuvant MCV.
    D. Five-year overall survival was not improved with neoadjuvant MCV.

41. All of the following were chemotherapy agents included in RTOG 89-03 except:
    A. Methotrexate
    B. Cyclophosphamide
    C. Cisplatin
    D. Vinblastine

42. What was the reported bladder preservation rate in RTOG 89-03 as reported by Shipley et al.?
    A. 35 %
    B. 45 %
    C. 55 %
    D. 65 %

43. Which one of the following characteristics is unsuitable for bladder preservation?
    A. Unifocal T2-T3a tumor
    B. Tumor size < 5 cm in maximum diameter
    C. Ureteral obstruction requiring intervention
    D. Good bladder capacity and function

44. What was the most common urinary symptom reported by a quality-of-life questionnaire at the Massachusetts General Hospital for patients undergoing bladder-preserving TURBT, chemotherapy, and radiation?
    A. Urinary control problems
    B. Dysuria
    C. Hematuria
    D. Urinary obstruction

45. All of the following are true regarding the recently published (NEJM 2012) randomized trial of radiotherapy with or without chemotherapy in muscle-invasive bladder cancer, as reported by James et al. except:
    A. Locoregional disease-free survival was improved in those receiving whole bladder radiotherapy.
    B. Concurrent chemotherapy was mitomycin C and 5-FU.
    C. Locoregional disease-free survival was improved with the addition of chemotherapy.
    D. There was no increased grade 3 or 4 toxicity with the addition of chemotherapy.

Answers and Rationales

1. The correct answer is B. A 9.5 cm renal carcinoma that is limited to the kidney with no regional lymph node metastases is classified as AJCC stage T2aN0. Edge SB, Byrd DR, Compton CC, et al., editors. Kidney. AJCC cancer staging handbook. 7th ed. New York: Springer; 2010.

2. The correct answer is C. Renal cell carcinoma that extends into the vena cava below the diaphragm is classified as AJCC T stage T3b. Edge SB, Byrd DR, Compton CC, et al., editors. Kidney. AJCC cancer staging handbook. 7th ed. New York: Springer; 2010.

3. The correct answer is B. A 5 cm tumor in the kidney, limited to the kidney, is classified as AJCC T stage T1b. Edge SB, Byrd DR, Compton CC, et al., editors. Kidney. AJCC cancer staging handbook. 7th ed. New York: Springer; 2010.

4. The correct answer is B. Renal cell carcinoma accounts for 90 % of kidney cancers. Wong WW, Buskirk SJ, Tan WW, Peterson JL, Haddock MG, Parker AS, Wehle MJ. Kidney and ureteral cancer. In: Gunderson LL, Tepper JE, editors. Clinical radiation oncology. 3rd ed. Philadelphia: Elsevier Saunders; 2012. p. 1145–65.

5. The correct answer is A. The most common hereditary type of renal cell carcinoma is associated with Von Hippel-Lindau syndrome. Wong WW, Buskirk SJ, Tan WW, Peterson JL, Haddock MG, Parker AS, Wehle MJ. Kidney and ureteral cancer. In: Gunderson LL, Tepper JE, editors. Clinical radiation oncology. 3rd ed. Philadelphia: Elsevier Saunders; 2012. p. 1145–65.

6. The correct answer is B. The increased use of computed tomography is one possible explanation for the increased incidence of renal cell carcinoma (early detection). Wong WW, Buskirk SJ, Tan WW, Peterson JL, Haddock MG, Parker AS, Wehle MJ. Kidney and ureteral cancer. In: Gunderson LL, Tepper JE, editors. Clinical radiation oncology. 3rd ed. Philadelphia: Elsevier Saunders; 2012. p. 1145–65.

7. The correct answer is D. If a mass is centrally located, as opposed to on either pole of the kidney, urothelial carcinoma should be suspected, as opposed to renal cell carcinoma. Wong WW, Buskirk SJ, Tan WW, Peterson JL, Haddock MG, Parker AS, Wehle MJ. Kidney and ureteral cancer. In: Gunderson LL, Tepper JE, editors. Clinical radiation oncology. 3rd ed. Philadelphia: Elsevier Saunders; 2012. p. 1145–65.

8. The correct answer is B. The expected 5-year OS of stage IV RCC is 25 %. Wong WW, Buskirk SJ, Tan WW, Peterson JL, Haddock MG, Parker AS, Wehle MJ. Kidney and ureteral cancer. In: Gunderson LL, Tepper JE, editors. Clinical radiation oncology. 3rd ed. Philadelphia: Elsevier Saunders; 2012. p. 1145–65.

9. The correct answer is A. According to the EORTC 30881 phase 3 trial comparing radical nephrectomy with or without lymph node dissection, no improvement in progression-free survival or overall survival was seen with the addition of lymph node dissection. Blom JH et al. EORTC Genitourinary Tract Cancer Group. Radical nephrectomy with and without lymph-node dissection: final results of European Organization for Research and Treatment of Cancer (EORTC) randomized phase 3 trial 30881. Eur Urol. 2009;55(1):28–34.

10. The correct answer is D. The most site of distant metastasis for renal cell carcinoma is the lung. Wong WW, Buskirk SJ, Tan WW, Peterson JL, Haddock MG, Parker AS, Wehle MJ. Kidney and ureteral cancer. In: Gunderson LL, Tepper JE, editors. Clinical radiation oncology. 3rd ed. Philadelphia: Elsevier Saunders; 2012. p. 1145–65.

11. The correct answer is B. According to a SWOG study looking at the value of interferon alfa-2b without or without cytoreductive nephrectomy in stage IV renal cell carcinoma, there was a statistically significant improvement in median survival in those that received interferon alfa-2b therapy in addition to nephrectomy. Flanigan RC et al. Nephrectomy followed by interferon alfa-2b compared with interferon alfa-2b alone for metastatic renal-cell cancer. N Engl J Med. 2001;345(23):1655–59.

12. The correct answer is C. The targets of temsirolimus and sunitinib are respectively –mTor and PDGFR. Motzer et al. Activity of SU11248, a multitargeted inhibitor of vascular endothelial growth factor receptor and platelet-derived growth factor receptor, in patients with metastatic RCC. JCO. 2006;24(1): 16–24.

13. The correct answer is C. The majority of patients are asymptomatic when diagnosed with renal cell carcinoma. This is in part due to increased use of computed tomography and ultrasound, with which tumors are being discovered at earlier stages. Less than 10 % of patients present with the classic triad of flank pain, hematuria, and a palpable mass. Curti BD. Renal cell carcinoma. JAMA. 2004;292:97–100. Sokoloff MH et al. Current management of renal cell carcinoma. CA Cancer J Clin. 1996;46:284–302.

14. The correct answer is A. Of the listed histologic subtypes, granular cell is not a subtype of renal cell carcinoma. Wong WW, Buskirk SJ, Tan WW, Peterson JL, Haddock MG, Parker AS, Wehle MJ. Kidney and ureteral cancer. In: Gunderson LL, Tepper JE, editors. Clinical radiation oncology. 3rd ed. Philadelphia: Elsevier Saunders; 2012. p. 1145–65.

15. The correct answer is A. Renal pelvis and ureteral carcinomas typically present with gross or microscopic hematuria (75–80 %). Thirty-five to forty-five percent of patients present with flank pain. Urinary symptoms, such as dysuria or

frequency, present in 25 % of patients. A palpable mass is the least common presenting symptom (10 %). Batata MA et al. Primary carcinoma of the ureter: a prognostic study. Cancer. 1975;1626–2632. Abeshouse BS. Primary benign and malignant tumors of the ureter. Am J Surg. 1956;91:237. Bloom NA et al. Primary carcinoma of the ureter: a report of 102 new cases. J Urol. 1970;103:590–8.

16. The correct answer is B. Rabinovitch et al. reported on the patterns of failure of RCC after nephrectomy. Factors that significantly predicted for distant metastasis included lymph node involvement, pathologic subtype, and renal vein involvement. Rabinovitch RA et al. Patterns of failure following surgical resection of renal cell carcinoma: implications for adjuvant local and systemic therapy. J Clin Oncol. 1994;12:206–12.

17. The correct answer is D. Partial (nephron-sparing) nephrectomy is indicated in cases of bilateral renal tumors, cancer of a solitary kidney, or in a small <4 cm tumor. Use of partial nephrectomy has been found to result in low incidences of local recurrence in tumors <4 cm. Tumors involving the renal hilum should undergo radical nephrectomy if possible. Sokoloff MH et al. Current management of renal cell carcinoma. CA Cancer J Clin. 1996;46:284–302. Lerner SE. et al. Disease outcome in patients with low stage renal cell carcinoma treated with nephron sparing or radical surgery. J Urol. 1994;155:1868–73.

18. The correct answer is D. The risk of local failure following gross total resection of a renal cell carcinoma is 5 %. As such, the routine use of adjuvant therapy has not been established. Radical nephrectomy is the cornerstone of management of these tumors. Lerner SE et al. Disease outcome in patients with low stage renal cell carcinoma treated with nephron sparing or radical surgery. J Urol. 1994;155:1868–73.

19. The correct answer is C. Standard surgery for renal pelvis or ureteral cancers is nephroureterectomy with removal of the bladder cuff. However, laparoscopic nephroureterectomy has been shown to have no decreased cancer effectiveness with decreased anesthesia time, recovery time, and hospital stay, compared to standard nephroureterectomy. Partial ureterectomy (nephron-sparing) is an option for patients with a solitary kidney, bilateral disease, or a small (<1.5 cm) low-grade tumor. After nephroureterectomy, locoregional failure develops in up to 15 % of low-grade, low-stage disease and in 30–50 % of patients with high-stage, high-grade disease. Cozad SC et al. Transitional cell carcinoma of the renal pelvis or ureter: patterns of failure. Urology. 1995;46:796–800. Zincke H et al. Feasibility of conservative surgery for transitional cell cancer of the upper urinary tract. Urol Clin North Am. 1984;11:717–24. McDougall EM et al. Laparoscopic nephroureterectomy for upper tract transitional cell cancer: the Washington University Experience. J Urol. 1995;154:975–9. Pohar KS et al. When is partial ureterectomy acceptable for transitional-cell carcinoma of the ureter? J Endourol. 2001;15:405–8.

20. The correct answer is C. Cozad et al. described patterns of failure of renal pelvis and ureteral cancers after surgery alone, showing that the risk of local relapse correlates with tumor stage and tumor grade. Overall, half of patients will locally relapse after surgery alone. In those with grade 1 or 2 tumors, 5-year local control is 90 %; in those with grade 3 or 4 tumors, 5-year local control drops to 41 %. Half of local relapses were in an isolated local site, whereas the other half occurred in combination with distant recurrence. Cozad SC et al. Transitional cell carcinoma of the renal pelvis or ureter: patterns of failure. Urology. 1995;46:796–800.

21. The correct answer is D. Urethral cancer has a 4:1 female predilection. The most common site of urethral cancer in men is the bulbomembranous urethra versus near the meatus in women. Anterior urethral drainage is to the superficial and deep inguinal lymph nodes. Posterior urethral drainage is to the internal iliac, external iliac, and obturator lymph nodes.

22. The correct answer is A. Correct staging for a urethral cancer that invades into the corpus spongiosum with a single 2.0 cm lymph node metastasis is T2N1. Invasion of the corpus cavernosum is T3. A single lymph node 2.0 cm or less is N1. A single lymph node >2 cm or multiple lymph nodes are staged as N2. Edge SB, Byrd DR, Compton CC, et al., editors. Urethra. AJCC cancer staging handbook. 7th ed. New York: Springer; 2010.

23. The correct answer is B. While bulbomembranous urethral tumors are squamous cell in histology, prostatic urethral tumors are transitional cell in histology. Prostatic urethral tumors are the least common site of urethral cancer in men. Proximal tumors have a worse prognosis than distal tumors.

24. The correct answer is B. Invasion of the anterior vagina in urethral staging is 7th edition AJCC T3. Multiple lymph nodes are N stage – N2. Edge SB, Byrd DR, Compton CC, et al., editors.Urethra. AJCC cancer staging handbook. 7th ed. New York: Springer; 2010.

25. The correct answer is B. Whereas invasion of the corpus cavernosum is T2 in penile cancer, it is AJCC T stage-T3 in urethral cancer. Involvement of a single lymph node <2 cm is N1. Edge SB, Byrd DR, Compton CC, et al., editors. Urethra. AJCC cancer staging handbook. 7th ed. New York: Springer; 2010.

26. The correct answer is C. The incidence of bladder cancer has been increasing over the last 20 years. There is a 3:1 male predominance, with a peak incidence in the fifth to seventh decades. The majority of diagnosed bladder cancers are superficial and of transitional cell histology. Cohen SM. et al. Epidemiology and etiology of bladder cancer. Urol Clin North Am. 1992;19:421–8.

27. The correct answer is C. While 40 % of those with an upper urinary tract cancer develop bladder cancer, only 3 % with bladder cancer develop an upper urinary

tract cancer. Efstathiou JA, Zietman AL, Coen JJ, Shipley WU. Bladder cancer. In: Gunderson LL, Tepper JE, editors. Clinical radiation oncology. 3rd ed. Philadelphia: Elsevier Saunders; 2012. p. 1099–123.

28. The correct answer is B. Tobacco, chemical exposure (aniline dyes, aromatic amines, and nitrates), cyclophosphamide, *Schistosoma haematobium*, and chronic irritation (indwelling foley catheter) are all risk factors for development of bladder cancer. *Schistosoma haematobium* and chronic irritation (indwelling foley catheter) are more commonly associated with the development of squamous cell rather than transitional cell carcinoma. Nomura A et al. Smoking, alcohol, occupation and hair dye use in cancer of the lower urinary tract. Am J Epidemiol. 1989;130:1159–63. Bhagwandeen SB et al. Schistosomiasis and carcinoma of the bladder in Zambia. S Afr Med J. 1976;50:1616–20. Levine LA et al. Urological complications of cyclophosphamide. J Urol. 1989;141:1063–9.

29. The correct answer is D. The vast majority (75 %) of cases of bladder cancer are superficial at diagnosis. Efstathiou JA, Zietman AL, Coen JJ, Shipley WU. Bladder cancer. In: Gunderson LL, Tepper JE, editors. Clinical radiation oncology. 3rd ed. Philadelphia: Elsevier Saunders; 2012. p. 1099–123.

30. The correct answer is A. Grade is the most important predictor of outcome for non-muscle-invasive tumors, while depth of invasion is the most important predictor of outcome for muscle-invasive tumors. Efstathiou JA, Zietman AL, Coen JJ, Shipley WU. Bladder cancer. In: Gunderson LL, Tepper JE, editors. Clinical radiation oncology. 3rd ed. Philadelphia: Elsevier Saunders; 2012. p. 1099–123.

31. The correct answer is D. First-echelon draining lymph nodes for bladder cancer are the external iliac, internal iliac, and perivesical nodes. Paracaval, para-aortic, and common iliac are second-echelon lymph nodes. Efstathiou JA, Zietman AL, Coen JJ, Shipley WU. Bladder cancer. In: Gunderson LL, Tepper JE, editors. Clinical radiation oncology. 3rd ed. Philadelphia: Elsevier Saunders; 2012. p. 1099–123.

32. The correct answer is B. Painless hematuria is the most common presenting symptom of bladder cancer (80 % of cases). Efstathiou JA, Zietman AL, Coen JJ, Shipley WU. Bladder cancer. In: Gunderson LL, Tepper JE, editors. Clinical radiation oncology. 3rd ed. Philadelphia: Elsevier Saunders; 2012. p. 1099–123.

33. The correct answer is A. A superficially muscle-invasive tumor with a single 2.5 cm lymph node metastasis is 7th edition AJCC stage T2aN1. Deep muscle invasion is T2b. N1 describes a single lymph node in the true pelvis. N2 describes multiple lymph nodes in the true pelvis (hypogastric, external iliac, presacral, obturator lymph nodes). N3 describes metastases to the common iliac lymph nodes. Edge SB, Byrd DR, Compton CC, et al., editors. Urinary bladder. AJCC cancer staging handbook. 7th ed. New York: Springer; 2010.

34. The correct answer is D. Any lymph node positive bladder cancer is AJCC stage IV. Edge SB, Byrd DR, Compton CC, et al., editors. Urinary bladder. AJCC cancer staging handbook. 7th ed. New York: Springer; 2010.

35. The correct answer is C. For non-muscle-invasive bladder tumors, the most appropriate treatment is TURBT +/– intravesicular chemotherapy. The decision to add intravesicular chemotherapy is based on the risk of progression, not the risk of recurrence, as most superficial tumors recur. Intravesicular chemotherapy is added to prevent progression to invasive disease. Heney NH et al. Superficial bladder cancer: progression and recurrence. J Urol. 1983;1083–6.

36. The correct answer is C. The addition of BCG has been shown in randomized trials to reduce the rates of progression in patients with Ta G2-3 and T1 disease. This reduction in disease progression was shown to result in a survival advantage, 88 % versus 63 %. BCG has also been shown in six randomized trials comparing TURBT + BCG versus TURBT alone to decrease tumor recurrence in approximately half of patients. In improving bladder control of transitional cell carcinoma, the use of BCG has resulted in an increase in extravesical relapse of disease. Herr HW et al. Experience with intravesical *Bacillus Calmette-Guérin* therapy of superficial bladder tumors. Urology. 1985;25:119–23. Melekos MD et al. Intravesical *Bacillus Calmette-Guérin* immunoprophylaxis of superficial bladder cancer: results of a controlled prospective trial with modified treatment schedule. J Urol. 1993;149:744–8. Davis JW et al. Superficial bladder carcinoma treated with *Bacillus Calmette-Guérin*: progression-free and disease-specific survival with minimum 10-year follow-up. J Urol. 2002;167(2 Part 1):494–500.

37. The correct answer is C. The University of Southern California reported outcomes on 633 patients with pT2-4 bladder cancer with a 5-year actuarial survival rate of 48 %. A series from Memorial Sloan-Kettering Cancer Center reported a 5-year actuarial survival of 36 % in 184 patients with pT2-4 bladder cancer. Stein JP et al. Radical cystectomy in the treatment of invasive bladder cancer: long-term results in 1054 patients. J Clin Oncol. 2001;165:666–75. Dalbagni G et al. Cystectomy for bladder cancer: a contemporary series. J Urol. 1993;149:758–65.

38. The correct answer is D. In a retrospective review of 133 patients with T3b disease treated with preoperative radiation (50 Gy) followed by cystectomy 4 weeks later at MDACC, the pelvic recurrence rate was found to drop from 28 % to 10 %. Actuarial 5-year pelvic control was 91 %. After 1983, the preoperative radiation was discontinued, and pelvic control rates dropped to 73 %, with a subsequent decrement in survival (52–42 %). Skinner D et al. Contemporary cystectomy with pelvic node dissection compared to preoperative radiation plus cystectomy in management of invasive bladder cancer. J Urol. 1984;131:1069–72.

39. The correct answer is A. In this University of Paris study, patients underwent TURBT followed by cisplatin/5-FU with concurrent accelerated RT followed by planned cystectomy. After the concurrent chemoradiation, restaging showed no residual tumor on cystoscopy or repeat biopsy. In the pathological cystectomy specimens, all 18 patients (100 %) had a complete response. This prompted a protocol change to cystectomy only if there was evidence of disease on restaging. Five-year survival of all patients on the protocol was 63 %. Housset M et al. Combined radiation and chemotherapy for invasive transitional-cell carcinoma of the bladder: a prospective study. J Clin Oncol. 1993;11:2150–57.

40. The correct answer is B. To assess the benefit of neoadjuvant chemotherapy before consolidative treatment for bladder cancer, RTOG 89-03 randomized 123 patients with T2-T4a muscle-invasive bladder cancer to receive neoadjuvant MCV × 2 cycles (methotrexate, cisplatin, vinblastine) or not, followed by selective bladder preservation (combined chemoradiation with cisplatin), followed by either cystectomy or consolidation chemoradiation depending on response. Cyclophosphamide was not included. Shipley WU et al. Phase III trial of neoadjuvant chemotherapy in patients with invasive bladder cancer treated with selective bladder preservation by combined radiation therapy and chemotherapy: initial results of Radiation Therapy Oncology Group 89-03. J Clin Oncol. 1998;16(11):3576–83.

41. The correct answer is B. To assess the benefit of neoadjuvant chemotherapy before consolidative treatment for bladder cancer, RTOG 89-03 randomized 123 patients with T2-T4a muscle-invasive bladder cancer to receive neoadjuvant MCV × 2 cycles (methotrexate, cisplatin, vinblastine) or not, followed by selective bladder preservation (combined chemoradiation with cisplatin), followed by either cystectomy or consolidation chemoradiation depending on response. Those with a complete response after 39.6 Gy continued with chemoRT to a total of 64.8 Gy. Only 67 % of patients in the neoadjuvant arm completed the protocol, compared to the 81 % of the other arm. There were no differences in response rate, actuarial 5-year survival, 5-year survival with preserved bladder, or distant metastasis. Bladder preservation rate was 65 %. The most important predictor of bladder preservation was the extent of TURBT. Not surprisingly, morbidity was worse in the neoadjuvant chemotherapy arm with 14 % of patients dying of treatment-related causes, stopping the trial prematurely. Shipley WU et al. Phase III trial of neoadjuvant chemotherapy in patients with invasive bladder cancer treated with selective bladder preservation by combined radiation therapy and chemotherapy: initial results of Radiation Therapy Oncology Group 89-03. J Clin Oncol. 1998;16(11):3576–83.

42. The correct answer is D. To assess the benefit of neoadjuvant chemotherapy before consolidative treatment for bladder cancer, RTOG 89-03 randomized 123 patients with T2-T4a muscle-invasive bladder cancer to receive neoadjuvant MCV × 2 cycles (methotrexate, cisplatin, vinblastine) or not, followed by

selective bladder preservation (combined chemoradiation with cisplatin), followed by either cystectomy or consolidation chemoradiation depending on response. Those with a complete response after 39.6 Gy continued with chemoRT to a total of 64.8 Gy. Only 67 % of patients in the neoadjuvant arm completed the protocol, compared to the 81 % of the other arm. Bladder preservation rate was 65 %. Shipley WU et al. Phase III trial of neoadjuvant chemotherapy in patients with invasive bladder cancer treated with selective bladder preservation by combined radiation therapy and chemotherapy: initial results of Radiation Therapy Oncology Group 89-03. J Clin Oncol. 1998;16(11):3576–83.

43. The correct answer is C. To be considered a good candidate for bladder preservation, the primary tumor should be T2-3a and unifocal, <5 cm in maximum diameter, and have had visibly complete TURBT. The candidate must have good bladder capacity and function, with no ureteral obstruction. Efstathiou JA, Zietman AL, Coen JJ, Shipley WU. Bladder cancer. In: Gunderson LL, Tepper JE, editors. Clinical radiation oncology. 3rd ed. Philadelphia: Elsevier Saunders; 2012. p. 1099–123.

44. The correct answer is A. Zietman et al. reported quality-of-life outcomes on 221 patients with cT2-4a cancer of the bladder that underwent TURBT, chemotherapy, and radiation. All patients were asked to undergo urodynamic study and completed a QOL questionnaire. Median follow-up was 6.3 years. On urodynamic study, the majority of patients (75 %) had a normally functioning bladder. While reduced bladder compliance was seen in 22 %, it was only reported as distressing in one third of these patients. The most commonly reported urinary symptom was urinary control problems (19 %) with 11 % wearing pads; distress was reported on the QOL questionnaire in only half of these patients. Bowel symptoms were reported in 22 % of patients, but causing distress in only 14 %. Zietman AL et al. Organ-conservation in invasive bladder cancer treated by trans-urethral resection, chemotherapy, and radiation: results of a urodynamic and quality of life study on long-term survivors. J Urol. 2003;170(5):1772–6.

45. The correct answer is A. A multicenter trial in the UK randomized 360 patients with muscle-invasive bladder cancer in a 2×2 design. The first randomization was for radiotherapy with or without chemotherapy, 5-FU (500 mg/m^2) on days 1–5 and 16–20 and mitomycin C (12 mg/m^2) on day 1. The subsequent randomization (results not yet reported) assigned whole bladder radiation versus modified volume radiation (reduction in volume of bladder receiving full dose). The 2-year rates of locoregional disease-free survival favored the chemoradiotherapy group, 67 % (95 % CI 59–74) versus 54 % in the radiotherapy group (95 % CI 46–62). The addition of chemotherapy did not increase grade 3 or 4 toxicity, $p=0.07$. James ND, Hussain SA, Hall E, Jenkins P, Tremlett J, Rawlings C, Crundwell M, Sizer B, Sreenivasan T, Hendron C, Lewis R, Waters R, Huddart RA; BC2001 Investigators. N Engl J Med. 2012 Apr 19;366(16):1477–88.

Chapter 10
Male Genitourinary Cancer

Celine Bicquart Ord and Eric K. Hansen

Questions

1. What is the lifetime risk for the development of prostate cancer in men?
   A. One in four men will develop prostate cancer during his lifetime.
   B. One in five men will develop prostate cancer during his lifetime.
   C. One in six men will develop prostate cancer during his lifetime.
   D. One in seven men will develop prostate cancer during his lifetime.

2. Which is the most common subtype of prostate adenocarcinoma?
   A. Ductal
   B. Acinar
   C. Small cell
   D. Rhabomyosarcoma

3. Which of the following is a luteinizing hormone-releasing hormone analogue?
   A. Goserelin
   B. Bicalutamide
   C. Finasteride
   D. Flutamide

C.B. Ord, MD (✉)
Department of Radiation Oncology, Scott & White Memorial Hospital, Temple, TX 76508, USA
e-mail: cord@sw.org

E.K. Hansen, MD
Department of Radiation Oncology, The Oregon Clinic, Providence St. Vincent Medical Center,
9205 SW Barnes Rd, Portland, OR 97225, USA
e-mail: ehansen@orclinic.com

C.B. Ord et al. (eds.), *Radiation Oncology Study Guide*,
DOI 10.1007/978-1-4614-6400-6_10, © Springer Science+Business Media New York 2013

4. What type of drug is finasteride?
   A. Luteinizing hormone-releasing hormone analogue
   B. Anti-luteinizing hormone-releasing hormone analogue
   C. 5α-reductase inhibitor
   D. Nonsteroidal antiandrogen

5. All of the following are true regarding the Prostate Cancer Prevention Trial with finasteride except:
   A. Men were randomized to placebo versus daily 5 mg finasteride for 7 years.
   B. Sexual side effects were more common in men receiving placebo.
   C. Development of prostate cancer was decreased in the finasteride group.
   D. Higher-grade tumors developed in the finasteride group.

6. Which PSA velocity (rate of change of PSA/year) was shown to be significantly greater in subjects with prostate cancer compared to control subjects in a case–control study by Carter et al. at Johns Hopkins?
   A. 0.50 µg/L per year
   B. 0.75 µg/L per year
   C. 1.0 µg/L per year
   D. 1.25 µg/L per year

7. According to results of a multicenter clinical performance study published by Thiel et al., what free-to-total PSA ratio was highly suspicious for cancer?
   A. <5 %
   B. <6 %
   C. <7 %
   D. <8 %

8. What is the half-life of PSA?
   A. 0.9 days
   B. 1.6 days
   C. 2.2 days
   D. 4.3 days

9. Which is the current definition of post-radiotherapy PSA failure?
   A. Three consecutive rises after nadir with failure at halfway point between nadir and first rise or a rise that provoked initiation of salvage therapy
   B. Nadir PSA + 3 ng/mL with date of failure "at call"/not backdated
   C. PSA nadir > 0.5 ng/mL
   D. Nadir PSA + 2 ng/mL with date of failure "at call"/not backdated

10. As the percent-free PSA _____, the risk of prostate cancer _____.
    A. Increases, increases
    B. Increases, decreases
    C. Decreases, decreases
    D. Decreases, increases

11. Which of the following is the AUA definition of failure post-prostatectomy?
    A. Single value of >0.3 ng/mL
    B. Initial PSA value ≥0.2 ng/mL followed by a subsequent confirmatory PSA value ≥0.2 ng/mL
    C. Two successive values of >0.1 ng/mL
    D. Single value of >0.2 ng/mL

12. Which zone of the prostate is the most common site of carcinoma?
    A. Transition zone
    B. Peripheral zone
    C. Central zone
    D. Superior zone

13. Where do the paired neurovascular bundles run along the prostate?
    A. Posterolaterally
    B. Anterolaterally
    C. Posteromedially
    D. Anteriomedially

14. Which is the correct primary blood supply/venous drainage of the prostate?
    A. External iliac artery/external iliac vein
    B. Internal iliac artery/external iliac vein
    C. Internal iliac artery/internal iliac vein
    D. External iliac artery/internal iliac vein

15. Which 7th edition AJCC T stage would be most appropriate for prostate adeno-carcinoma incidentally detected in <5 % of resected tissue?
    A. T0
    B. T1a
    C. T1b
    D. T1c

16. Which is the appropriate 7th edition AJCC TNM stage for a prostate adenocar-cinoma found at prostatectomy to invade into the seminal vesicles, without evidence of lymph node metastases?
    A. cT3aN0
    B. pT3aN0
    C. cT3aN0
    D. pT3bN0

17. Which is the correct N stage (by TNM stage) and overall AJCC 7th edition stage for a prostate cancer that has spread to the regional lymph nodes, respectively?
    A. N1, Stage III
    B. N2, Stage III
    C. N1, Stage IV
    D. N2, Stage IV

18. Which of the following correctly describes microscopic invasion into the bladder neck according to the 7th edition AJCC staging?
    A. pT3a
    B. pT3b
    C. pT3c
    D. pT4

19. Which is the prediction equation as developed by Roach et al. that estimates lymph node involvement for prostate cancer?
    A. $\{3/2 \, PSA + [\text{Gleason score} - 6] \times 10\}$
    B. $\{2/3 \, PSA + [\text{Gleason score} - 6] \times 10\}$
    C. $\{3/2 \, PSA + [10 - \text{Gleason score}] \times 10\}$
    D. $\{2/3 \, PSA + [10 - \text{Gleason score}] \times 10\}$

20. Which is the prediction equation as developed by Roach et al. that estimates extracapsular extension for prostate cancer?
    A. $\{3/2 \, PSA + [\text{Gleason score} - 3] \times 10\}$
    B. $\{2/3 \, PSA + [\text{Gleason score} - 6] \times 10\}$
    C. $\{3/2 \, PSA + [\text{Gleason score} - 6] \times 10\}$
    D. $\{2/3 \, PSA + [\text{Gleason score} - 3] \times 10\}$

21. Which is the prediction equation as developed by Diaz et al. that estimates seminal vesicle involvement in prostate cancer?
    A. $\{PSA + [\text{Gleason score} - 3] \times 10\}$
    B. $\{PSA + [\text{Gleason score} - 6] \times 10\}$
    C. $\{2/3 \, PSA + [\text{Gleason score} - 6] \times 10\}$
    D. $\{2/3 \, PSA + [\text{Gleason score} - 3] \times 10\}$

22. All of the following regarding the randomized trial comparing radical prostatectomy versus watchful waiting in early prostate cancer as reported in the initial report by Bill-Axelson et al. in the NEJM are correct, except:
    A. Radical prostatectomy reduced disease-specific mortality and the risk of distant metastasis, but did not result in a reduction in overall mortality.
    B. Eligible patients had to have a negative bone scan and a PSA < 50 ng/mL.
    C. Men were allowed to begin hormonal therapy in either group if advised by a physician.
    D. Most patients had T2 tumors.

23. In the updated results of the randomized trial comparing radical prostatectomy versus watchful waiting in early prostate cancer as reported by Bill-Axelson et al. (NEJM 2011), what was the number needed to treat to avert one death in men < 65 years of age?
    A. 7
    B. 8
    C. 13
    D. 15

24. In the updated results of the randomized trial comparing radical prostatectomy versus watchful waiting in early prostate cancer as reported by Bill-Axelson et al. (NEJM 2011), the presence of extracapsular extension (as compared to the lack of extracapsular extension) was found to increase the risk of death from prostate cancer by:
    A. Two times
    B. Three times
    C. Five times
    D. Seven times

25. Each of the following is a viable indication for brachytherapy as monotherapy, deemed by ASTRO/ACR practice guidelines, except:
    A. Gleason 6 or less
    B. PSA 10 ng/mL or less
    C. Only clinical stage T1 or less
    D. Clinical stage T1-T2a

26. All of the following are isotopes used for prostate low-dose brachytherapy except:
    A. Pd^{103}
    B. I^{125}
    C. Ir^{192}
    D. Au^{89}

27. What is the half-life and average energy of I^{125}, respectively?
    A. 8 days, 28 keV
    B. 60 days, 28 keV
    C. 8 days, 21 keV
    D. 60 days, 21 keV

28. What is the half-life and average energy of Pd^{103}, respectively?
    A. 17 days, 28 keV
    B. 74 days, 28 keV
    C. 17 days, 21 keV
    D. 74 days, 21 keV

29. What is the usual prescription dose for brachytherapy using Pd^{103} as monotherapy for prostate cancer?
    A. 90 Gy
    B. 110 Gy
    C. 125 Gy
    D. 145 Gy

30. What is the usual prescription dose for brachytherapy using I^{125} as monotherapy for prostate cancer?
    A. 90 Gy
    B. 110 Gy
    C. 125 Gy
    D. 145 Gy

31. All of the following are true regarding brachytherapy as monotherapy for prostate cancer, as reported by Zelefsky et al., except:
    A. Biochemical control at 8 years was greater than 90 % with a D90 $\geq$130 Gy.
    B. Median PSA nadir level was 0.1 ng/mL in those patients free of biochemical relapse at 8 years.
    C. Gleason score was found on multivariate analysis to be associated with PSA relapse-free survival.
    D. I^{125} was the isotope employed for monotherapy.

32. Which of the following would be the best time to obtain a postimplantation CT study after prostate brachytherapy?
    A. 15 days postimplantation
    B. 30 days postimplantation
    C. 45 days postimplantation
    D. 60 days postimplantation

33. Which D90 (minimum dose to 90 % of the prostate volume), as described by Stock et al., predicts for PSA-RFS of >90 % at 4 years after completion of brachytherapy?
    A. 120 Gy
    B. 130 Gy
    C. 140 Gy
    D. 150 Gy

34. All of the following are contraindications to low-dose rate brachytherapy except:
    A. Prostate volume of 75 cc
    B. Gross seminal vesicle invasion
    C. Presence of lymph node metastases
    D. AUA score of seven preimplantation

35. In the dose escalation trial for prostate cancer as reported by Pollack et al., all of the following are true except:
    A. There was a statistically significant increase in both gastrointestinal and genitourinary grade 2 or higher toxicity in the high-dose arm.
    B. An improvement in PSA disease-free survival with higher dose was not seen in the low-risk group with an initial PSA of 10 ng/mL.
    C. In this trial, 70 Gy was compared to 78 Gy.
    D. The benefit in PSA disease-free survival in those with an initial PSA over 10 ng/mL was almost 20 % at 6 years.

36. In the combined photon and proton dose escalation trial for prostate cancer as reported by Zietman et al., all of the following are true except:
    A. Patients were randomized to receive 70.2GYE versus 79.2GYE.
    B. The first 45 Gy was given with photons.
    C. Patients had T1b-T2b disease.
    D. Patients had PSA < 15 ng/mL.

37. In the combined photon and proton dose escalation trial for prostate cancer as reported by Zietman et al., all of the following are false except:
    A. There was an improvement of PSA disease-free survival with higher dose in the intermediate-risk group alone.
    B. There was an improvement of PSA disease-free survival with higher dose in the low-risk group alone.
    C. There was no improvement of PSA disease-free survival in either group.
    D. There was improved PSA disease-free survival in both the low- and intermediate-risk groups.

38. All are true about the findings of hypofractionation (70 Gy in 28 fractions) for prostate cancer as reported by Kupelian et al. except:
    A. A hypofractionated course of 70 Gy in 28 fractions was compared to 78 Gy in 39 fractions.
    B. Radiation was delivered with intensity-modulated radiation therapy.
    C. There were no grade 3 acute rectal toxicities.
    D. Overall 5-year biochemical relapse-free survival was >80 %.

39. What is the time point that defines a late morbidity from radiation, as defined by RTOG?
    A. 30 days
    B. 60 days
    C. 90 days
    D. 120 days

40. Using data from the M.D. Anderson prostate dose escalation study (70 Gy vs. 78 Gy), what rectal V70 was found to predict for increased grade 2 or 3 GI toxicity, as described by Storey et al.?
    A. V70 > 20 %
    B. V70 > 25 %
    C. V70 > 30 %
    D. V70 > 35 %

41. Which of the following is the least likely secondary malignancy to result from prostate irradiation?
    A. In-field sarcoma
    B. Small bowel cancer
    C. Bladder cancer
    D. Rectal cancer

42. All are true regarding RTOG 86-10 (radiation +/− neoadjuvant and concurrent androgen deprivation therapy) except:
    A. Total duration of goserelin was 4 months.
    B. Eligible patients had bulky (≥25 cm²) T2-T4 tumors.
    C. Pelvic LNs were not treated.
    D. In all comers, there was no overall survival benefit with the addition of androgen deprivation therapy.

43. All are true regarding RTOG 85-31 (radiation +/− adjuvant androgen deprivation therapy) except:
    A. Patients who had prostatectomy were not excluded.
    B. Goserelin was administered monthly, indefinitely.
    C. Node-positive patients were excluded.
    D. The addition of androgen deprivation therapy improved overall survival.

44. All are true regarding the addition of long-term ADT to radiotherapy for locally advanced prostate cancer, as reported in EORTC 22863 by Bolla et al., except:
    A. With continued follow-up, there is a continued overall survival benefit.
    B. Goserelin was given monthly for 2 years.
    C. Radiotherapy was delivered to the pelvic LNs to a total 50 Gy, followed by a 20 Gy boost to the prostate.
    D. There was no increased risk of cardiovascular mortality associated with long-term ADT.

45. All are true regarding the continuation of long-term androgen deprivation for locally advanced prostate cancer, as reported in RTOG 92-02 by Hanks et al., except:
    A. Patients with PSA values up to 150 ng/mL were eligible for enrollment.
    B. Patients were randomized to continuation or not of long-term ADT after neoadjuvant and concurrent ADT during radiotherapy.
    C. Total duration of long-term androgen deprivation was 24 months in the long-term arm.
    D. Androgen deprivation consisted of flutamide and goserelin.

46. In which subgroup of RTOG 92-02 did the addition of long-term androgen deprivation for locally advanced prostate cancer improve overall survival?
    A. Gleason 2-6
    B. Gleason 6
    C. Gleason 7
    D. Gleason 8-10

47. Regarding the addition of short-term androgen deprivation therapy to prostate radiotherapy for intermediate-/high-risk prostate cancer as reported by D'Amico et al., all of the following are true except:
   A. The addition of ADT improved overall survival in those with minimal comorbidities.
   B. Androgen deprivation therapy started on day 1 of radiotherapy.
   C. Pelvic lymph nodes were not treated with radiotherapy.
   D. Duration of androgen deprivation therapy was 6 months.

48. All are true regarding RTOG 94-13, a four-arm study looking at volume of irradiation and timing of androgen deprivation therapy for prostate cancer, except:
   A. ADT consisted of 4 months of a LHRH agonist and antiandrogen.
   B. Eligible patients had a PSA up to 100 ng/mL.
   C. Progression-free survival was statistically significantly improved in the whole-pelvis versus prostate-only arms in the 7-year update.
   D. Progression-free survival did not differ between the neoadjuvant and adjuvant hormone arms.

49. In a subset analysis of pathologically lymph node-positive patients of RTOG 85-31, all of the following are true regarding the addition of androgen deprivation therapy to irradiation except:
   A. The addition of ADT improved disease-specific failure.
   B. The addition of ADT improved metastatic failure.
   C. The addition of ADT improved biochemical control with a PSA level < 1.5 ng/mL.
   D. The addition of ADT did not improve overall survival.

50. All are true regarding immediate versus delayed androgen deprivation therapy in node-positive prostate cancer after prostatectomy as reported by Messing et al. except:
   A. Options for androgen deprivation included goserelin or leuprolide.
   B. Radiotherapy was not allowed.
   C. Immediate androgen deprivation therapy resulted in improved overall survival.
   D. Immediate androgen deprivation therapy resulted in improved prostate cancer-specific survival.

51. All are true regarding the addition of radiotherapy to androgen deprivation therapy in locally advanced prostate cancer as reported in the SPCG-7 study (Widmark et al.) except:
   A. Node-positive patients were allowed.
   B. The overall survival benefit seen with the addition of radiotherapy was limited to men < 65 years.
   C. The number needed to treat to prevent one prostate cancer death was seven in men < 65 years.
   D. While there was a statistically significant increase in toxicity with radiotherapy, quality of life was not worsened.

52. In the SPCG-7 study regarding the addition of radiotherapy to androgen deprivation therapy in locally advanced prostate cancer (Widmark et al.), what was the overall number needed to treat to prevent one prostate cancer death?
    A. 5
    B. 7
    C. 10
    D. 15

53. All of the following are true regarding EORTC 22911 in which patients were randomized to adjuvant radiotherapy or not after prostatectomy except:
    A. Patients had to have either positive surgical margins or pT3 disease.
    B. Total dose to the prostatic fossa was 60 Gy.
    C. Adjuvant radiotherapy did not improve overall survival.
    D. A later subset analysis revealed that only patients with seminal vesicle involvement benefited from adjuvant radiotherapy.

54. All of the following are true regarding the Johns Hopkins retrospective review of salvage radiotherapy after biochemical failure after prostatectomy as reported by Trock et al. except:
    A. Salvage radiotherapy was associated with a threefold improvement in prostate cancer-specific survival.
    B. The addition of hormonal therapy conferred a separate prostate cancer-specific survival benefit, in addition to that seen with salvage radiotherapy.
    C. The benefit of salvage radiotherapy was limited to men with PSA doubling times < 6 months.
    D. There was no benefit for salvage therapy initiated 2 years after recurrence.

55. All of the following are true regarding the SWOG 87-94 trial in which patients were randomized to adjuvant radiotherapy or not after prostatectomy except:
    A. Patients were randomized within 16 weeks of surgery.
    B. The latest update at 15 years still shows no overall survival benefit.
    C. The primary endpoint of the study was metastasis-free survival.
    D. Metastasis-free survival was improved at 15 years with adjuvant radiotherapy.

56. All of the following are true regarding the impact of seminal vesicle invasion (SVI), as reported from data of SWOG 87-94 (Swanson et al.), except:
    A. Those with +SVI had a 10-year biochemical-free survival of 22 %.
    B. Those with −SVI had a 10-year biochemical-free survival of 33 %.
    C. In those with +SVI, all outcomes, including overall survival, improved with RT.
    D. Overall, those with −SVI had improved survival compared to those with +SVI.

57. All of the following are true regarding the duration of androgen deprivation therapy as reported in EORTC 22961 by Bolla et al. except:
    A. Gynecomastia and hot flashes were increased with long-term ADT.
    B. Quality of life was worse in the long-term ADT arm.
    C. Overall survival was improved in the long-term ADT arm.
    D. Almost two-thirds of patients randomized to the long-term ADT arm completed all 3 years.

58. The incidence of testicular cancer is:
    A. Bimodal with germ cell tumors occurring in those aged 25–40 and then again in those 65–70 years
    B. Bimodal with non-germ cell tumors occurring in those aged 25–40 and then again in those 65–70 years
    C. Bimodal with germ cell tumors occurring in those aged 25–40 and then non-germ cell tumors occurring in those 65–70 years
    D. Bimodal with non-germ cell tumors occurring in those age 25–40 and then germ cell tumors occurring in those 65–70 years

59. All of the following are risk factors for the development of testicular cancer except:
    A. History of testicular maldescent
    B. Testicular trauma
    C. Family history of testicular cancer
    D. Gonadal dysgenesis

60. Which is the most common chromosomal change noted in germ cell tumors?
    A. 10p isochromosome
    B. 12p isochromosome
    C. 17q isochromosome
    D. 21q isochromosome

61. Which of the following is not a non-seminomatous germ cell tumor?
    A. Yolk sac tumor
    B. Seminoma
    C. Choriocarcinoma
    D. Mixed germ cell tumors

62. What is the most common testicular tumor in children?
    A. Choriocarcinoma
    B. Yolk sac tumor
    C. Mixed germ cell tumors
    D. Seminoma

63. What immunohistochemical stain is positive in almost all seminomas?
    A. Placental leukocyte alkaline phosphatase
    B. Low-molecular-weight keratins
    C. Blood group antigens
    D. Vimentin

64. Schiller-Duval bodies are seen in which type of testicular tumor?
    A. Choriocarcinoma
    B. Endodermal sinus tumor
    C. Mixed germ cell tumors
    D. Seminoma

65. Which of the following statements about non-seminomatous germ cell tumors
    is false?
    A. Mixed tumors of two or more histologies present at an age intermediate to
       that of seminomatous and non-seminomatous germ cell tumors.
    B. Teratomas are derived from two or more germ cell layers.
    C. Choriocarcinomas manifest with high levels of B-hCG and have a poor
       prognosis.
    D. Yolk sac tumors do not secrete alpha-fetoprotein.

66. All of the following are true regarding lymph node drainage of testicular germ
    cell tumors except:
    A. Right-sided tumors tend to drain to para-caval and intercaval lymph nodes
       due to drainage into the inferior vena cava.
    B. Left-sided tumors drain most commonly to para-aortic lymph nodes.
    C. Supradiaphragmatic spread can occur through the thoracic duct.
    D. Left supraclavicular nodal disease is common both at presentation and at
       time of relapse.

67. What is the most common presenting symptom of a testicular tumor?
    A. Testicular pain
    B. Gynecomastia
    C. Dyspnea
    D. Painless testicular mass

68. Invasion of the spermatic cord constitutes which AJCC T stage?
    A. pT1
    B. pT2
    C. pT3
    D. pT4

69. A healthy, 38-year-old male presents with a painless testicular mass. What is the next step in management?
    A. Antibiotics
    B. Transcrotal biopsy
    C. Radical inguinal orchiectomy
    D. Transcrotal orchiectomy

70. What is the correct AJCC nodal stage for a 2.3 cm inguinal lymph node?
    A. N1
    B. N2
    C. N2b
    D. N3

71. All of the following are acceptable treatment options for stage I seminoma after radical inguinal orchiectomy, except:
    A. Observation
    B. Adjuvant chemotherapy
    C. Adjuvant radiotherapy
    D. Adjuvant chemoradiotherapy

72. What is the 5-year relapse rate of stage I seminoma after observation?
    A. 5 %
    B. 15 %
    C. 25 %
    D. 35 %

73. What is the predominant site of failure for stage I seminoma after observation?
    A. Left supraclavicular nodal region
    B. Inguinal lymph nodes
    C. Para-aortic lymph nodes
    D. Deep pelvic lymph nodes

74. According to the meta-analysis of stage I seminoma managed by surveillance by Warde et al., what two factors predicted for relapse?
    A. Primary tumor size and lymphovascular invasion
    B. Primary tumor size and rete testis invasion
    C. Lymphovascular invasion and rete testis invasion
    D. Lymphovascular invasion and LDH five times normal limit

75. According to the meta-analysis of stage I seminoma managed by surveillance by Warde et al., in those with one of the two defined risk factors, what was the 5-year risk of relapse?
    A. 5 %
    B. 12 %
    C. 16 %
    D. 31 %

76. In a Medical Research Council randomized trial of adjuvant RT versus carboplatin, for stage I seminoma, all of the following are true, except:
    A. Relapse rate was similar in both arms.
    B. There was decreased incidence of second primary testicular germ cell tumors in the carboplatin arm.
    C. The majority of relapses in the carboplatin arm were in the mediastinum.
    D. A single cycle of adjuvant carboplatin was given.

77. Which of the following is not a common site of failure after radiation for stage II seminoma?
    A. Para-aortic lymph nodes
    B. Mediastinal lymph nodes
    C. Supraclavicular lymph nodes
    D. Bone

78. What is the most important prognostic factor for relapse in stage II seminoma?
    A. Rete testis invasion
    B. Primary tumor size
    C. Lymphovascular invasion
    D. Bulk of retroperitoneal disease

79. What is the best next step in management for a residual 2.5 cm retroperitoneal mass after chemotherapy for advanced seminoma?
    A. Observation
    B. Retroperitoneal lymph node dissection
    C. Intraoperative biopsy
    D. Radiation

80. All of the following are true regarding Leydig Cell tumors except:
    A. Initial step in management is radical inguinal orchiectomy.
    B. The majority present in adults as increased virilization.
    C. The most common site of metastasis is to the regional lymph nodes.
    D. There is no role for adjuvant chemotherapy or radiation.

81. All of the following are true regarding mediastinal extragonadal germ cell tumors except:
    A. Local invasion and metastatic disease are common at presentation.
    B. Present with cough, dyspnea, and chest pain.
    C. Seminomatous and non-seminomatous primaries have similar outcomes.
    D. Platinum-based chemotherapy is the backbone of treatment.

82. All are true regarding the MRC Testicular Study Group randomized trial of para-aortic plus pelvic versus para-aortic radiation alone for stage I seminoma except:
    A. Relapse-free survival was not statistically different between the arms.
    B. There was increased diarrhea in the para-aortic alone arm.
    C. Sperm counts were higher in the para-aortic alone arm.
    D. There were four pelvic relapses in the para-aortic alone arm.

83. Regarding the Medical Research Trial TE 18 regarding the optimal dose for stage I seminoma, all of the following are true except:
    A. The radiation field was to the para-aortics alone for all patients.
    B. Acute toxicity was better in the lower-dose arm.
    C. The lower-dose arm was 20 Gy.
    D. Late toxicity was not different between the arms.

84. Human papillomavirus types 16 and 18 are detected in what percentage of penile cancers?
    A. 30–35 %
    B. 40–45 %
    C. 50–55 %
    D. 60–65 %

85. All of the following are risk factors for the development of penile cancer except:
    A. Phimosis
    B. History of genital condylomas
    C. Lichen sclerosis
    D. Neonatal circumcision

86. All of the following regarding HPV and penile cancer are true except:
    A. HPV association is seen more frequently in verrucous than basaloid penile cancers.
    B. HPV-16 and HPV-18 are the most frequently detected subtypes.
    C. HPV presence does not confer a worse prognosis in penile cancer.
    D. Frequency of HPV detection depends on penile cancer subtype.

87. Which of the following is not a common precursor lesion of HPV-associated warty and basaloid penile cancers?
    A. Bowen's disease
    B. Lichen sclerosis
    C. Erythroplasia of Queyrat
    D. Bowenoid papulosis

88. What percentage of those with Erythroplasia of Queyrat will develop squamous cell carcinoma on the prepuce or glans of the penis?
    A. 10–20 %
    B. 40–50 %
    C. 70–80 %
    D. 90–100 %

89. The most common site of penile cancer is the:
    A. Shaft
    B. Glans
    C. Root
    D. Prepuce

90. A cancer found on the skin of the glans will drain to which first and second echelon nodal basins, respectively?
    A. Superficial inguinal, internal iliac
    B. Deep inguinal, internal iliac
    C. Superficial inguinal, external iliac
    D. Deep inguinal, external iliac

91. A poorly differentiated penile cancer is found on the glans and is found to invade into the subepithelial connective tissue. There are two ipsilateral mobile left inguinal lymph nodes. What is the correct AJCC stage?
    A. T1aN2
    B. T1bN2
    C. T1aN1
    D. T1bN1

92. A penile cancer is found to invade into the prostate, and there is a single fixed inguinal mass. What is the correct AJCC stage?
    A. T3N1
    B. T4N1
    C. T3N3
    D. T4N3

93. What percentage of clinically positive lymph nodes are pathologically positive in penile cancers?
    A. 30 %
    B. 40 %
    C. 50 %
    D. 60 %

94. All of the following are reasonable treatment options for a T1 penile cancer of the glans except:
    A. Total penectomy
    B. Partial penectomy
    C. Laser surgery
    D. Interstitial brachytherapy

95. All are true regarding treatment of penile cancer except:
    A. Circumcision is necessary before radiation begins.
    B. Those with >1 cm invasion of the corpus cavernosum cannot be treated with brachytherapy alone.
    C. Those with a primary tumor of larger than 2.5 cm cannot be treated with brachytherapy alone.
    D. When performing inguinal lymph node dissection, the bilateral groins must be dissected.

96. All of the following are true regarding soft tissue necrosis after radiation for penile cancer, except:
   A. It is more common after brachytherapy than external beam radiotherapy.
   B. It is the most common reason for amputation of a tumor-free penis.
   C. The risk of necrosis increases with increasing dose over 45 Gy.
   D. The risk of necrosis increases with a larger number of brachytherapy needles.

Answers and Rationales

1. The correct answer is C. Men have a one in six chance of developing prostate cancer during their lifetime. Michalski J, Pisansky TM, Lawton CA, Potters L, Kuban DA. Prostate cancer. In: Gunderson LL, Tepper JE, editors. Clinical radiation oncology. 3rd ed. Philadelphia: Elsevier Saunders; 2012. p. 1037–97.

2. The correct answer is B. Acinar is the most common adenocarcinoma histology in prostate cancer. Ductal adenocarcinoma is rare, treated with surgery, and does not respond to androgen deprivation therapy. Finamanti M et al. Ductal carcinoma of the prostate: impact on survival and therapeutic controversies of a rare tumor. Urologia. 2011;78(4):283–7.

3. The correct answer is A. Of the listed agents, goserelin is the only LH-releasing analogue. Bicalutamide and flutamide are nonsteroidal antiandrogens, while finasteride is a 5α-reductase inhibitor. Michalski J, Pisansky TM, Lawton CA, Potters L, Kuban DA. Prostate cancer. In: Gunderson LL, Tepper JE, editors. Clinical radiation oncology. 3rd ed. Philadelphia: Elsevier Saunders; 2012. p. 1037–97.

4. The correct answer is C. Finasteride is a 5α-reductase inhibitor, blocking the conversion of testosterone to dihydrotestosterone, without a significant effect on libido, potency, or male musculature. Michalski J, Pisansky TM, Lawton CA, Potters L, Kuban DA. Prostate cancer. In: Gunderson LL, Tepper JE, editors. Clinical radiation oncology. 3rd ed. Philadelphia: Elsevier Saunders; 2012. p. 1037–97.

5. The correct answer is B. The Prostate Cancer Prevention Trial with finasteride reported by Thompson et al. in the 2003 NEJM randomized 18,882 men, aged ≥55, with normal DRE and PSA ≤3.0 ng to receive either 5 mg daily finasteride for 7 years or placebo. There was decreased prostate cancer detected in the finasteride group (18.4 % vs. 24.4 % placebo), for a 24.8 % reduction in prevalence over the 7-year period of the study (95 % CI, 18.6–30.6, $p < 0.001$). However, in those that developed prostate cancer, tumors of a high grade (Gleason 7-10) were more commonly found in the finasteride group (37 % of tumors vs. 22.2 % placebo, $p < 0.001$). Sexual side effects were more common in the finasteride group, while urinary symptoms were more common in the placebo group. Thompson IM et al. The influence of finasteride on the development of prostate cancer. N Engl J Med. 2003;349:215–24.

6. The correct answer is B. In the case–control study by Carter et al. from Johns Hopkins, 16 men without prostate cancer (control group) were compared to 20 men with BPH and 18 men with a histological diagnosis of prostate cancer. All men had multiple PSA and androgen determinations on serum samples obtained

7–25 years prior to diagnosis or exclusion of prostate cancer. At 5 years prior to diagnosis when PSA levels did not differ between subjects with BPH and prostate cancer, the rate of change in PSA level, specifically 0.75 μg/L per year, was found to be significantly greater in those men with prostate cancer. Additional studies have also suggested that a PSA velocity threshold of approximately 0.4 ng/mL per year may be useful for early prostate cancer detection. Carter HB, et al. Longitudinal evaluation of prostate-specific antigen levels in men with or without prostate disease. JAMA. 1992;267(16):2215–20. Carter HB, et al. Detection of life-threatening prostate cancer with prostate-specific antigen velocity during a window of curability. J Natl Cancer Inst. 2006;98(21):1521–7.

7. The correct answer is C. Thiel et al. reported the results of a multicenter clinical performance study of free-to-total PSA ratio, in 1,081 consecutively accrued men presenting with total PSA values between 2.5 and 20 ng/mL. Of the 520 men diagnosed with prostate cancer, only 21 (4 %) had free-to-total PSA ratios >25 %. Of 561 men with benign prostate disease, only 13 (2 %) had free-to-total PSA ratio <7 %, suggesting that a free-to-total PSA of <7 % is highly suspicious for prostate cancer. Additional multicenter data suggests that percent-free PSA <10 % warrants a biopsy. Thiel RP et al. Multicenter comparison of the diagnostic performance of free prostate-specific antigen. Urology. 1996;48(6A Suppl):45–50. Catalona WJ, Partin AW, Slawin KM, et al. Use of percentage of free prostate-specific antigen to enhance differentiation of prostate cancer and benign prostatic disease: a prospective multicenter trial. JAMA. 1998;279:1542–7.

8. The correct answer is C. The half-life of PSA is 2.2 days. Stamey TA et al. Prostate-specific antigen as a serum marker for adenocarcinoma of the prostate. N Engl J Med. 1987;317(15):909–16.

9. The correct answer is D. The Phoenix definition (PSA nadir + 2 ng/mL "at call"/not backdated) is the currently employed definition of PSA failure. Roach M et al. Defining biochemical failure following radiotherapy with or without hormonal therapy in men with clinically localized prostate cancer: recommendations of the RTOG- ASTRO Consensus Conference. Int J Radiat Oncol Biol Phys. 2006;65(4):965–74.

10. The correct answer is D. As the percent-free PSA drops, the risk of cancer increases. The free-to-total ratio is less in prostate cancer versus benign prostatic hypertrophy. Michalski J, Pisansky TM, Lawton CA, Potters L, Kuban DA. Prostate cancer. In: Gunderson LL, Tepper JE, editors. Clinical radiation oncology. 3rd ed. Philadelphia: Elsevier Saunders; 2012. p. 1037–97.

11. The correct answer is B. As the goal of radical prostatectomy is to remove all prostatic and tumor tissue, postoperative PSA level should be undetectable (<0.2 ng/mL), evaluated 30–45 days after surgery. Cookson MS, Aus G, Burnett

AL, et al. Variation in the definition of biochemical recurrence in patients treated for localized prostate cancer: the American Urological Association prostate guidelines for localized prostate cancer update panel report and recommendations for a standard in the reporting of surgical outcomes. J Urol. 2007;177:540–5

12. The correct answer is B. The prostate is composed of three zones: (1) peripheral zone which accounts for 70 % of the prostate volume and is the most common site of carcinoma, (2) transition zone which accounts for 5 % of the prostate volume but enlarges with benign prostatic hypertrophy, and (3) central zone which accounts for 25 % of the prostate volume and contains the ejaculatory ducts. Michalski J, Pisansky TM, Lawton CA, Potters L, Kuban DA. Prostate cancer. In: Gunderson LL, Tepper JE, editors. Clinical radiation oncology. 3rd ed. Philadelphia: Elsevier Saunders; 2012. p. 1037–97.

13. The correct answer is A. The paired neurovascular bundles run along the posterolateral edges of the prostate. Michalski J, Pisansky TM, Lawton CA, Potters L, Kuban DA. Prostate cancer. In: Gunderson LL, Tepper JE, editors. Clinical radiation oncology. 3rd ed. Philadelphia: Elsevier Saunders; 2012. p. 1037–97.

14. The correct answer is C. The internal iliac artery and internal iliac vein, by way of the prostatic venous plexus, provide the arterial supply and venous drainage of the prostate. Michalski J, Pisansky TM, Lawton CA, Potters L, Kuban DA. Prostate cancer. In: Gunderson LL, Tepper JE, editors. Clinical radiation oncology. 3rd ed. Philadelphia: Elsevier Saunders; 2012. p. 1037–97.

15. The correct answer is B. Carcinoma incidentally detected in <5 % of resected tissue is a T stage T1a. T0 implies no evidence of primary tumor. T1b is carcinoma incidentally detected in >5 % of resected tissue, while T1c refers to carcinoma detected on needle biopsy obtained for elevated PSA. Edge SB, Byrd DR, Compton CC, et al., editors. Prostate. AJCC cancer staging handbook. 7th ed. New York: Springer; 2010.

16. The correct answer is D. pT3bN0 is the correct AJCC stage for a prostate adenocarcinoma found to invade into the seminal vesicles, without evidence of lymph node metastasis. The p denotes pathological findings after surgery. T3a refers to extraprostatic extension. Edge SB, Byrd DR, Compton CC, et al., editors. Prostate. AJCC cancer staging handbook. 7th ed. New York: Springer; 2010.

17. The correct answer is C. In prostate cancer, any metastasis to regional lymph nodes is N stage N1 by TNM staging, but AJCC stage IV. Edge SB, Byrd DR, Compton CC, et al., editors. Prostate. AJCC cancer staging handbook. 7th ed. New York: Springer.

18. The correct answer is A. Microscopic invasion into the bladder neck and extra-capsular extension are pT3a. Invasion into the seminal vesicles is pT3b. There is no pT3c. Edge SB, Byrd DR, Compton CC, et al., editors. Prostate. AJCC cancer staging handbook. 7th ed. New York: Springer.

19. The correct answer is C. Roach et al. derived a prediction equation to estimate the risk of lymph node involvement for prostate cancer, incorporating PSA and Gleason score. $\{2/3\ \mathrm{PSA} + [\mathrm{Gleason\ score} - 6] \times 10\}$ Roach, et al. Predicting the risk of lymph node involvement using the pre-treatment prostate specific anti-gen and Gleason score in men with clinically localized prostate cancer. Int J Radiat Oncol Biol Phys. 1994;28:33.

20. The correct answer is A. Roach et al. derived a prediction equation to estimate the risk of extracapsular extension for prostate cancer, incorporating PSA and Gleason score. $\{3/2\ \mathrm{PSA} + [\mathrm{Gleason\ score} - 3] \times 10\}$. Roach et al. Pretreatment prostate-specific antigen and Gleason score predict the risk of extracapsular extension and the risk of failure following radiotherapy in patients with clini-cally localized prostate cancer. Semin Urol Oncol. 2000;18(2):108–14.

21. The correct answer is B. Diaz et al. derived a prediction equation to estimate the risk of seminal involvement for prostate cancer, incorporating PSA and Gleason score. $\{\mathrm{PSA} + [\mathrm{Gleason\ score} - 6] \times 10\}$. Diaz A et al. Indications for and the significance of seminal vesicle irradiation during 3D conformal radiotherapy for localized prostate cancer. Int J Radiat Oncol Biol Phys. 1994;30(2):323–9.

22. The correct answer is A. Six hundred ninety-five men aged ≤ 75 years with early prostate cancer (stage T1b–T2, PSA < 50 ng/mL, moderately to well-differentiated tumor, negative bone scan) and a life expectancy of over 10 years were randomized to undergo either radical prostatectomy or watchful waiting. The majority of tumors (>70 %) were stage T2; only 12 % of patients had T1c disease. At a median of 8.2 years follow-up, the hazard ratio for death from prostate cancer was 0.56 (95 % CI 0.36–0.88) for those that underwent radical prostatectomy. Similarly, radical prostatectomy reduced risks of distant metas-tasis, local progression, and disease-specific mortality. Starting in January 2003, men in either group were allowed to begin hormonal therapy if so advised by their physician. Men in the radical prostatectomy group received less hor-monal therapy, (p<0.01), as well as less palliative radiotherapy (p=0.04). The updated results published in 2011 included three additional years of follow-up to give 15-year estimated results. In the total cohort, the survival benefit of radi-cal prostatectomy persisted. In subgroup analysis by age, the survival benefit seen with radical prostatectomy was confined to men younger than 65 years of age. The number needed to treat to avoid one death was 15 overall and seven for men < 65 years. Notably, among those that underwent radical prostatectomy,

those with extracapsular extension had a 7× risk of death from prostate cancer compared to men without extracapsular extension. Given that men in this study were recruited before widespread PSA screening, the benefit seen with radical prostatectomy in this trial may be reduced in more contemporary populations detected earlier (lead time bias). Bill-Axelson A et al. Radical prostatectomy versus watchful waiting in early prostate cancer. N Engl J Med. 2005;352:1977–84. Bill-Axelson A et al. Radical prostatectomy vs watchful waiting in early prostate cancer. N Engl J Med. 2011;364:1708–17.

23. The correct answer is A. Six hundred ninety-five men aged ≤ 75 years with early prostate cancer (stage T1b–T2, PSA < 50 ng/mL, moderately to well-differentiated tumor, negative bone scan) and a life expectancy of over 10 years were randomized to undergo either radical prostatectomy or watchful waiting. At a median of 8.2 years follow-up, the hazard ratio for death from prostate cancer was 0.56 (95 % CI 0.36–0.88) for those that underwent radical prostatectomy. Similarly, radical prostatectomy reduced risks of distant metastasis, local progression, and disease-specific mortality. The updated results published in 2011 included three additional years of follow-up to give 15-year estimated results. In the total cohort, the survival benefit of radical prostatectomy persisted. In subgroup analysis by age, the survival benefit seen with radical prostatectomy was confined to men younger than 65 years of age. The number needed to treat to avoid one death was 15 overall and seven for men < 65 years. Bill-Axelson A et al. Radical prostatectomy versus watchful waiting in early prostate cancer. N Engl J Med. 2005;352:1977–84. Bill-Axelson A et al. Radical prostatectomy vs. watchful waiting in early prostate cancer. N Engl J Med. 2011;364:1708–17.

24. The correct answer is D. Six hundred ninety-five men aged ≤ 75 years with early prostate cancer (stage T1b-T2, PSA < 50 ng/mL, moderately to well-differentiated tumor, negative bone scan) and a life expectancy of over 10 years were randomized to undergo either radical prostatectomy or watchful waiting. The majority of tumors (>70 %) were stage T2; only 12 % of patients had T1c disease. At a median of 8.2 years follow-up, the hazard ratio for death from prostate cancer was 0.56 (95 % CI 0.36–0.88) for those that underwent radical prostatectomy. Similarly, radical prostatectomy reduced risks of distant metastasis, local progression, and disease-specific mortality. The updated results published in 2011 included three additional years of follow-up to give 15-year estimated results. In the total cohort, the survival benefit of radical prostatectomy persisted. In subgroup analysis by age, the survival benefit seen with radical prostatectomy was confined to men younger than 65 years of age. Notably, among those that underwent radical prostatectomy, those with extracapsular extension had a 7× risk of death from prostate cancer compared to men without extracapsular extension. Bill-Axelson A, et al. Radical prostatectomy versus watchful waiting in early prostate cancer. N Engl J Med. 2005;352:1977–84. Bill-Axelson A et al. Radical prostatectomy vs. watchful waiting in early prostate cancer. N Engl J Med. 2011;364:1708–17.

25. The correct answer is C. Brachytherapy is adequate monotherapy for small (T1–T2a) tumors, low-grade (Gleason 6), low-risk (PSA < 10 ng/mL) prostate cancer. Rosenthal SA, et al. American Society for Radiation Oncology (ASTRO) and American College of Radiology (ACR) practice guideline for the transperineal permanent brachytherapy of prostate cancer. Int J Radiat Oncol Biol Phys. 2011;79(2):335–41.

26. The correct answer is C. Isotopes used for prostate low-dose rate brachytherapy include Pd^{103}, I^{125}, and Au^{89}. Ir^{192} is used for high-dose rate brachytherapy. Michalski J, Pisansky TM, Lawton CA, Potters L, Kuban DA. Prostate cancer. In: Gunderson LL, Tepper JE, editors. Clinical radiation oncology. 3rd ed. Philadelphia: Elsevier Saunders; 2012. p. 1037–97.

27. The correct answer is B. The average energy of I^{125} is 28 keV, while its half-life is 60 days. The half-life of I^{131} is 8 days. The average energy of Pd^{103} is 21 keV. Michalski J, Pisansky TM, Lawton CA, Potters L, Kuban DA. Prostate cancer. In: Gunderson LL, Tepper JE, editors. Clinical radiation oncology. 3rd ed. Philadelphia: Elsevier Saunders; 2012. p. 1037–97.

28. The correct answer is C. The average energy of Pd^{103} is 21 keV, while its half-life is 17 days. The half-life of Ir^{192} is 74 days. The average energy of Pd^{103} is 21 keV. Michalski J, Pisansky TM, Lawton CA, Potters L, Kuban DA. Prostate cancer. In: Gunderson LL, Tepper JE, editors. Clinical radiation oncology. 3rd ed. Philadelphia: Elsevier Saunders; 2012. p. 1037–97.

29. The correct answer is C. The usual prescription dose for prostate brachytherapy using Pd^{103} is 125 Gy. Ninety to one hundred Gy is the usual Pd^{103} brachytherapy boost dose used when treating prostate cancer in conjunction with external beam radiation. Michalski J, Pisansky TM, Lawton CA, Potters L, Kuban DA. Prostate cancer. In: Gunderson LL, Tepper JE, editors. Clinical radiation oncology. 3rd ed. Philadelphia: Elsevier Saunders; 2012. p. 1037–97.

30. The correct answer is D. The usual prescription dose for prostate brachytherapy using I^{125} is 145 Gy. One hundred ten to one hundred twenty Gy is the usual I^{125} brachytherapy boost dose used when treating prostate cancer in conjunction with external beam radiation. Michalski J, Pisansky TM, Lawton CA, Potters L, Kuban DA. Prostate cancer. In: Gunderson LL, Tepper JE, editors. Clinical radiation oncology. 3rd ed. Philadelphia: Elsevier Saunders; 2012. p. 1037–97.

31. The correct answer is D. In this multi-institutional series, 2,693 patients from 11 institutions with T1-2 prostate cancer were treated with either I^{125} (68 %) or Pd^{103} (32 %) brachytherapy as monotherapy for prostate cancer. Among those that underwent I^{125} implant, 8-year PSA relapse-free survival was 93 % in those with a D90 ≥130 Gy, compared to an 8-year PSA relapse-free survival of 76 % in those with a D90 < 130 Gy, $p < 0.001$. Multivariate analysis identified tumor

stage, Gleason score, pretreatment PSA level, treatment year, and isotope used as variables associated with PSA relapse-free survival. Isotope type employed was not significant when only patients with available postimplantation dosimetric information were assessed. The median PSA nadir level was 0.1 ng/mL in those patients free of biochemical relapse at 8 years. Zelefsky MJ, et al. Multiinstitutional analysis of long-term outcome for stages T1-T2 prostate cancer treated with permanent seed implantation. Int J Radiat Oncol Biol Phys. 2007;67(2):327–33.

32. The correct answer is B. Of the listed choices, 30 days is the best choice. Prestidge et al. described their results regarding timing of postimplant computed tomography. In this series, 19 consecutive patients underwent postimplant CT at postoperative days 1, 8, 30, 90, and 180, on which volumes and dose-volume histograms were calculated. They found that the CT scan-determined volume performed on post-op day 1 was an average of 41.4 % greater than the volume on pre-op ultrasound. The average volume also decreased with time, with a corresponding increase in the coverage of the prostate volume by the 80 % isodose volume. They concluded that scans performed on postoperative day 30 adequately describe the time-averaged dose coverage of the prostate. Disadvantages of waiting until day 30 include another visit for the patient, and delay in compensating for underdosing, if present. Prestidge BR, et al. Time of computed tomography-based postimplant assessment following permanent transperineal prostate brachytherapy. Int J Radiat Oncol Biol Phys. 1998;40(5):1111–5.

33. The correct answer is C. In a series of 134 men treated with prostate brachytherapy alone, improved biochemical recurrence-free survival was found to directly increase with the D90. Specifically, those patients with a D90 of >140 Gy had 4-year BRFS of 92 % versus 68 % with a D90 < 140 Gy. This effect was only seen in those with a pretreatment PSA of >10 ng/mL. Stock RG, et al. Dose response study for I-125 prostate implants. Int J Radiat Oncol Biol Phys. 1998;41(1):101–8.

34. The correct answer is D. All of the answer choices are contraindications to brachytherapy except an AUA score of 7, which is favorable. Rosenthal SA, et al. American Society for Radiation Oncology (ASTRO) and American College of Radiology (ACR) practice guideline for the transperineal permanent brachytherapy of prostate cancer. Int J Radiat Oncol Biol Phys. 2011;79(2): 335–41.

35. The correct answer is A. In the dose escalation trial of 70 Gy versus 78 Gy, as initially reported by Pollack et al., the benefit in PSA disease-free survival with higher dose was only seen in those with an initial PSA of >10 ng/mL. This benefit at 6 years was nearly 20 %. No difference in PSA DFS was seen in those with an initial PSA < 10 ng/mL, with both the low- and high-dose arms showing

PSA DFS of approximately 80 %. The 8-year data again showed a statistically significant improvement in freedom from failure with 78 Gy. Looking at PSA, this benefit remained statistically significant only in those with PSA >10 ng/mL (78 % vs. 39 %). Grade 2 and higher gastrointestinal toxicity was statistically significantly doubled in the 78 Gy group (26 % vs. 13 %), genitourinary toxicity was not. Pollack, et al. Prostate cancer radiation dose response: results of the M.D. Anderson phase III randomized trials. Int J Radiat Oncol Biol Phys. 2002;53:1097. Kuban DA et al. Long-term results of the M.D. Anderson randomized dose-escalation for prostate cancer. Int J Radiat Oncol Biol Phys. 70(1):67–74.

36. The correct answer is B. In the PROG 95-09 combination photon and proton dose escalation trial for prostate cancer as reported by Zietman et al., patients were randomized to 70.2GYE versus 79.2GYE. The first 50.4 Gy was delivered with photons. Enrolled patients had early-stage (T1b–T2b) disease with PSA < 15 ng/mL. Five-year PSA disease-free survival was improved almost 20 % in both the low- and intermediate-risk groups. The 10-year update showed a persistent biochemical progression-free survival benefit (83 % vs. 68 %) overall. This benefit is also seen in those with low-risk and intermediate-risk prostate cancer, with no increase in grade 3 toxicities. Zietman AL, et al. A randomized trial comparing conventional dose (70.2GYE) and high dose (79.2GYE) conformal radiation in early stage adenocarcinoma of the prostate: results of an interim analysis of PROG 95-09. JAMA. 2005;294:1233. Zietman AL et al. Randomized trial comparing conventional-dose with high-dose conformal radiation therapy in early-stage adenocarcinoma of the prostate: long-term results from Proton Radiation Oncology Group/American College of Radiology 95-09. J Clin Oncol. 2010;28(7):1106–11.

37. The correct answer is D. In the PROG 95-09 combination photon and proton dose escalation trial for prostate cancer as reported by Zietman et al., patients were randomized to 70.2GYE versus 79.2GYE. The first 50.4 Gy was delivered with photons. Enrolled patients had early-stage (T1b–T2b) disease with PSA < 15 ng/mL. Five-year PSA disease-free survival was improved almost 20 % in both the low- and intermediate-risk groups. The 10-year update showed a persistent biochemical progression-free survival benefit (83 % vs. 68 %) overall. This benefit is also seen in those with low-risk and intermediate-risk prostate cancer, with no increase in grade 3 toxicities. Zietman AL et al. A randomized trial comparing conventional dose (70.2GYE) and high dose (79.2GYE) conformal radiation in early stage adenocarcinoma of the prostate: results of an interim analysis of PROG 95-09. JAMA. 2005;294:1233. Zietman AL et al. Randomized trial comparing conventional-dose with high-dose conformal radiation therapy in early-stage adenocarcinoma of the prostate: long-term results from Proton Radiation Oncology Group/American College of Radiology 95-09. J Clin Oncol. 2010;28(7):1106–11.

38. The correct answer is A. Kupelian et al. reported their experience of treating 770 consecutive patients with hypofractionation (70 Gy/28 fractions) delivered via IMRT. Biochemical failure was calculated by both the ASTRO and nadir +2 ng/mL definitions. With a median follow-up of 45 months, 5-year biochemical relapse-free survival by both definitions was >80 % and 95 %, 85 %, and 68 % in the low-, intermediate-, and high-risk groups, respectively. While there were no acute grade 3 rectal toxicities, there were late grade 3 rectal toxicities in 1.3 % of patients. Late grade 3 urinary toxicity was 0.1 %. Kupelian PA et al. Hypofractionated intensity-modulated radiotherapy (70 Gy at 2.5 Gy per fraction) for localized prostate cancer: Cleveland Clinic experience. Int J Radiat Oncol Biol Phys. 2007;68(5):1424–30.

39. The correct answer is C. Ninety days is the minimum time point needed to define a late radiation complication. LENT, Late Effects Normal Tissue Task Force; RTOG, Radiation Therapy Oncology Group.

40. The correct answer is B. Using the M.D. Anderson prostate dose escalation data of 70 versus 78 Gy, Storey et al. found that keeping the rectal V70 <25 % could reduce grade 2/3 GI toxicity. Keeping the V70 < 25 %, 16 % of patients experienced grade 2/3 GI toxicity, versus 46 % in those with V70 > 25 %. Storey MR et al. Complications from radiotherapy dose escalation in prostate cancer; preliminary results of a randomized trial. Int J Radiat Oncol Biol Phys. 2000;48:635.

41. The correct answer is B. The most frequent secondary malignancies after irradiation for prostate cancer are bladder cancer, rectal cancer, lung cancer, and in-field sarcomas. Brenner DJ et al. Second malignancies in prostate carcinoma patients after radiotherapy compared with surgery. Cancer 2000;54:1063.

42. The correct answer is C. RTOG 86-10 randomized 456 men with bulky ($\geq$25 cm^2) T2-T4 tumors to receive radiation alone (45 Gy to pelvic +/− lower para-aortic LNs, followed by prostatic boost to 65–70 Gy) versus radiation + neoadjuvant and concurrent ADT (monthly 3.6 mg goserelin × 4 months starting 2 months before radiation and 250 mg TID flutamide). While there was a statistically significant benefit for local control, and distant metastasis at both 5 and 8 years of follow-up, there was no overall survival benefit ($p = 0.10$). In a small subset analysis, in centrally reviewed Gleason 2-6 patients, there was a survival benefit at 8 years with the addition of ADT (70 % vs. 52 %, $p = 0.015$). There was no increased treatment toxicity with the addition of ADT. Pilepich MV et al. Phase III Radiation Therapy Oncology Group (RTOG) trial 86-10 of androgen deprivation adjuvant to definitive radiotherapy in locally advanced carcinoma of the prostate. Int J Radiat Oncol Biol Phys. 2001;50:1243.

43. The correct answer is C. To determine the benefit of adjuvant ADT, RTOG 85-31 randomized 945 men with clinical T3, pathological T3, or node-positive prostate cancer to receive either radiation alone (44–46 Gy to the pelvis,

followed by prostatic boost to 65–70 Gy if intact prostate, or 60–65 Gy to prostatic fossa) or radiation with monthly 3.6 mg goserelin beginning the last week of RT and continued indefinitely. The addition of ADT was found to result in statistically significantly decreased local tumor recurrence, distant metastasis, and overall survival. Pilepich MV et al. Androgen suppression adjuvant to definitive radiotherapy in prostate carcinoma: long-term results of phase III RTOG 85-31. Int J Radiat Oncol Biol Phys. 2005;61:1285–90.

44. The correct answer is B. To determine the benefit of androgen deprivation in locally advanced prostate cancer, EORTC 22863 randomized 401 men with either T3-4 or high-grade T1-2 prostate cancer to radiation (50 Gy pelvis + 20 Gy to prostate and SVs) +/– 3 years of monthly 3.6 mg goserelin beginning at the start of radiotherapy. The latest 10-year update in The Lancet shows continued statistically significant improvements in overall survival (58.1 % vs. 39.8 %), disease-free survival (47.7 % vs. 22.7 %), and reduction in prostate cancer mortality (10.3 % vs. 30.4 %). Long-term ADT was not shown to cause increased cardiovascular mortality. Bolla M et al. External irradiation with or without long-term androgen suppression for prostate cancer with high metastatic risk: 10-year results of an EORTC study. Lancet Oncol. 2010;11:1066–73.

45. The correct answer is C. RTOG 92-02 randomized 1,554 men with T2c-4 prostate cancer and a PSA < 150 ng/mL after 4 months of neoadjuvant and concurrent ADT during radiotherapy to observation or long-term androgen deprivation therapy. Neoadjuvant monthly goserelin 3.6 mg and 250 mg flutamide TID began 2 months prior to radiotherapy, radiotherapy was 45–50 Gy to the pelvis, followed by a prostatic boost to 65–70 Gy. After the 4 months of ADT, those randomized to long-term ADT received monthly goserelin for an additional 24 months. Long-term ADT was found to improve local progression, distant metastases, disease-free survival, but not overall survival. In a subset analysis of Gleason 8-10 tumors, there was an overall survival benefit seen with long-term ADT at 10 years (42 % vs. 35 %). Hanks GE et al. Phase III trial of long-term cytoreduction and radiotherapy in locally advanced carcinoma of the prostate: the Radiation Therapy Oncology Group Protocol 92-02. J Clin Oncol. 2003;2:3972. Horwitz EM et al. Ten-year follow-up of Radiation Therapy Oncology Group Protocol 92-02: a phase III trial of the duration of elective androgen deprivation in locally advanced prostate cancer. J Clin Oncol. 2008;26(15):2497–504.

46. The correct answer is D. RTOG 92-02 randomized 1,554 men with T2c-4 prostate cancer and a PSA < 150 ng/mL after 4 months of neoadjuvant and concurrent ADT during radiotherapy to observation or long-term androgen deprivation therapy. Neoadjuvant monthly goserelin 3.6 mg and 250 mg flutamide TID began 2 months prior to radiotherapy, radiotherapy was 45–50 Gy to the pelvis, followed by a prostatic boost to 65–70 Gy. After the 4 months of ADT, those

randomized to long-term ADT received monthly goserelin for an additional 24 months. Long-term ADT was found to improve local progression, distant metastases, disease-free survival, but not overall survival. In a subset analysis of Gleason 8-10 tumors, there was an overall survival benefit seen with long-term ADT at 10 years (42 % vs. 35 %). Hanks GE, et al. Phase III trial of long-term cytoreduction and radiotherapy in locally advanced carcinoma of the prostate: the Radiation Therapy Oncology Group Protocol 92-02. J Clin Oncol. 2003;2:3972. Horwitz EM et al. Ten-year follow-up of Radiation Therapy Oncology Group Protocol 92-02: a phase III trial of the duration of elective androgen deprivation in locally advanced prostate cancer. J Clin Oncol. 2008;26(15):2497–504.

47. The correct answer is B. To determine the benefit of androgen deprivation therapy, 206 men with intermediate-/high-risk prostate cancer (T1b-T2b prostate cancer, PSA $\geq$ 10, Gleason $\geq$ 7, or extracapsular extension/seminal vesicle invasion) were randomized to radiotherapy with or without 6 months of androgen deprivation. Androgen deprivation consisted of leuprolide/goserelin and flutamide, beginning 2 months before the start of radiotherapy. Radiotherapy consisted of 70 Gy to the prostate alone. At 5 years, the addition of ADT was found to improve overall survival (88 % vs. 78 %). This survival benefit persisted at 8 years (74 % vs. 61 %). Post-randomization evaluation of mortality impact via Adult Comorbidity Evalution-27 showed improved overall survival in those with none/minimal comorbidity (90 % vs. 64 %), but not in those with moderate/severe comorbidity. D'Amico AV et al. JAMA. 2008;299(3):289–95.

48. The correct answer is C. To determine the benefit of pelvic node irradiation and the optimal timing of ADT, RTOG 94-13 randomized 1,292 men with an at least 15 % chance of +LN by the Roach formula, or T2c-4 disease, with a PSA <100 ng/mL to one of four arms: (1) whole-pelvis RT + neoadjuvant and concurrent hormones, (2) whole-pelvis RT + adjuvant hormones, (3) prostate-only RT + neoadjuvant and concurrent hormones, and (4) prostate-only RT + adjuvant hormones. ADT consisted of 4 months of a LHRH agonist (3.6 mg goserelin monthly or 7.6 mg leuprolide) and antiandrogen (250 mg TID flutamide). At 4 years, progression-free survival was improved in the whole-pelvis versus prostate-only arms. The 7-year update shows no difference between the whole-pelvis and prostate-only arms and no difference between the neoadjuvant and concurrent versus adjuvant arms. The role of pelvic LN irradiation remains unclear. Lawton CA et al. An update of the phase III trial comparing whole pelvic to prostate only radiotherapy and neoadjuvant to adjuvant total androgen suppression: updated analysis of RTOG 94-13, with emphasis on unexpected hormone/radiation interactions. Int J Radiat Oncol Biol Phys. 2007;69(3):646–55.

49. The correct answer is D. To determine the benefit of adjuvant ADT, RTOG 85-31 randomized 945 men with clinical T3, pathological T3, or node-positive prostate cancer to receive either radiation alone (44–46 Gy to the pelvis,

followed by prostatic boost to 65–70 Gy if intact prostate, or 60–65 Gy to prostatic fossa) or radiation with monthly 3.6 mg goserelin beginning the last week of RT and continued indefinitely. The addition of ADT was found to result in statistically significantly decreased local tumor recurrence, distant metastasis, and overall survival. A subset analysis of the pathologically lymph node-positive patients showed that the addition of ADT to radiation improved all endpoints: disease-specific failure, metastatic failure, biochemical failure with PSA < 1.5 ng/mL, and overall survival. Absolute survival at 9 years was 38 % for patients receiving ADT only at the time of relapse versus 62 % for those who received immediate hormonal manipulation with irradiation, $p < 0.03$. Pilepich MV et al. Androgen suppression adjuvant to definitive radiotherapy in prostate carcinoma: long-term results of phase III RTOG 85-31. Int J Radiat Oncol Biol Phys. 2005;61:1285–90. Lawton CA et al. Androgen suppression plus radiation vs. radiation alone for patients with D1 (pN+) adenocarcinoma of the prostate: updated results based on a national prospective randomized trial, RTOG 85-31. J Clin Oncol. 2005;23:800.

50. The correct answer is A. The ECOG EST-3886 Trial as reported by Messing et al. randomized men with positive LNs after prostatectomy to either immediate or delayed androgen deprivation therapy (at progression). Androgen deprivation therapy consisted of either bilateral orchiectomy or goserelin. Radiotherapy was not allowed. The latest update at 12 years shows a persistent progression-free survival, prostate cancer-specific survival, and overall survival benefit with immediate androgen deprivation. Messing EM et al. Immediate versus deferred androgen deprivation treatment in patients with node-positive prostate cancer after radical prostatectomy and pelvic lymphadenectomy. Lancet Oncol. 2006;7(6):472–9.

51. The correct answer is A. To determine the benefit of adding radiotherapy to androgen deprivation therapy in locally advanced prostate cancer (T1b-T2b G2-3, or T3), the Scandinavian Prostate Cancer Group Study-7 randomized 875 men with node-negative prostate cancer and a PSA < 70 ng/mL to either androgen deprivation therapy alone or androgen deprivation therapy + 50 Gy to pelvis followed by boost to total of 70 Gy to the prostate and seminal vesicles. Androgen deprivation therapy consisted of 3 months of total androgen blockade with leuprolide, followed by continuous 250 mg TID flutamide. The latest update at 15 years shows an overall survival benefit in those men < 65 years who received radiation in addition to ADT. The NNT is 15 overall and 7 in men < 65 years. Fransson et al. reported the quality of life findings from the SPCG-7 study in which 99 % of participants contributed QOL information. While radiotherapy did statistically significantly worsen 4-year urinary moderate/severe bother scores (18 % vs. 12 %), dysuria (4 % vs. 2 %), bowel bother scores (11 % vs. 7 %), and erectile dysfunction (85 % vs. 72 %), quality of life was reported as similar between those who did and did not receive radiation. As such, given the overall survival benefit, adjuvant radiotherapy in addition to

ADT is recommended for locally advanced prostate cancer. Widmark A et al. Endocrine treatment, with or without radiotherapy, in locally advanced prostate cancer (SPCG-7/SFUO-3): an open randomised phase III trial. Lancet. 2009;373(9660):301–8. Fransson P et al. Quality of life in patients with locally advanced prostate cancer given endocrine treatment with or without radiotherapy: 4-year follow-up of SPCG-7/SFUO-3, an open-label, randomised, phase III trial. Lancet Oncol. 2009;4:370–80.

52. The correct answer is D. To determine the benefit of adding radiotherapy to androgen deprivation therapy in locally advanced prostate cancer (T1b-T2b G2-3, or T3), the Scandinavian Prostate Cancer Group Study-7 randomized 875 men with node-negative prostate cancer and a PSA < 70 ng/mL to either androgen deprivation therapy alone or androgen deprivation therapy + 50 Gy to pelvis followed by boost to total of 70 Gy to the prostate and seminal vesicles. Androgen deprivation therapy consisted of 3 months of total androgen blockade with leuprolide, followed by continuous 250 mg TID flutamide. The latest update at 15 years shows an overall survival benefit in those men < 65 years who received radiation in addition to ADT. The NNT is 15 overall and seven in men < 65 years. Fransson et al. reported the quality of life findings from the SPCG-7 study in which 99 % of participants contributed QOL information. While radiotherapy did statistically significantly worsen 4-year urinary moderate/severe bother scores (18 % vs. 12 %), dysuria (4 % vs. 2 %), bowel bother scores (11 % vs. 7 %), and erectile dysfunction (85 % vs. 72 %), quality of life was reported as similar between those who did and did not receive radiation. As such, given the overall survival benefit, adjuvant radiotherapy in addition to ADT is recommended for locally advanced prostate cancer. Widmark A et al. Endocrine treatment, with or without radiotherapy, in locally advanced prostate cancer (SPCG-7/SFUO-3): an open randomised phase III trial. Lancet. 2009;373(9660):301–8. Fransson P et al. Quality of life in patients with locally advanced prostate cancer given endocrine treatment with or without radiotherapy: 4-year follow-up of SPCG-7/SFUO-3, an open-label, randomised, phase III trial. Lancet Oncol. 2009;4:370–80.

53. The correct answer is D. To determine the benefit of adjuvant radiotherapy after prostatectomy, EORTC 22911 randomized 1,005 men with extracapsular extension, + SM, or seminal vesicle invasion after surgery to observation versus radiation (60 Gy). With a median follow-up of 5 years, biochemical progression-free survival was improved with radiotherapy, 72.2 % versus 51.8 %, ($p < 0.001$), as was clinical progression-free survival. There was no overall survival benefit. A subsequent subset analysis found that only patients with positive margins benefited from adjuvant RT. Bolla M et al. Post-operative radiotherapy (P-XRT) after radical prostatectomy (PX) improves progression-free survival (PFS) in pT3N0 prostate cancer (PC) (EORTC 22911). Int J Radiat Oncol Biol Phys.

2004;60(Suppl):S186. Van der Kwast TH et al. J Clin Oncol. 2007;25(27): 4178–86.

54. The correct answer is B. Trock et al. reported the Johns Hopkins experience of salvage radiotherapy after radical prostatectomy. In this retrospective review of 635 men, 397 had no adjuvant therapy, 160 had salvage radiotherapy alone, and 78 had salvage radiotherapy plus hormonal therapy. With a median of 6 years after recurrence, salvage radiation was found to confer a threefold increase in prostate cancer-specific survival (HR = 0.32) and overall survival. There was no additional benefit of hormonal therapy to salvage radiotherapy. The survival benefit of radiation was limited to men with PSA doubling times of <6 months. There was no prostate cancer-specific survival benefit for salvage radiotherapy initiated 2 years after recurrence. In men whose PSA did not become undetect-able after salvage radiotherapy, there was no prostate cancer-specific survival benefit from salvage radiotherapy. A separate analysis at Duke suggests that the survival benefit of salvage radiotherapy may extend to patients with PSA dou-bling time >6 months. Trock BJ et al. Prostate cancer-specific survival follow-ing salvage radiotherapy vs. observation in men with biochemical recurrence after radical prostatectomy. JAMA. 2008;299(23):2760–9. Cotter SE et al. Salvage radiation in men after prostate-specific antigen failure and the risk of death. Cancer. 2011;117(17):3925–32.

55. The correct answer is B. To determine the benefit of adjuvant radiotherapy after prostatectomy, SWOG 87-94 randomized 473 men within 16 weeks of radical prostatectomy and with one of three adverse pathological features (extracapsu-lar extension, positive margins, or seminal vesicle invasion) to observation or adjuvant radiotherapy to the prostatic fossa (60–64 Gy). The primary endpoint was metastasis-free survival. At 10 years, the use of prostatic fossa radiotherapy was found to improve both biochemical progression-free survival (64 % vs. 35 %) and clinical progression-free survival (61 % vs. 47 %), though there was no overall survival benefit. The most recent update at 15 years now shows an improvement in metastasis-free survival and overall survival, 59 % versus 48 %, (p = 0.023). Notably, 70 of 211 of the patients on the observation arm ultimately received RT. Thompson et al. Adjuvant radiotherapy for pathological T3N0M0 prostate cancer significantly reduces risk of metastases and improves survival: long-term follow-up of a randomized clinical trial. J Urol. 2009;181(3): 956–62.

56. The correct answer is C. SWOG 87-94 performed a subset analysis of 139 patients with seminal vesicle involvement versus 286 patients without. Overall, those with +SVI had poorer 10-year biochemical-free survival (22 % vs. 33 % in those with −SVI, p = 0.04). Those with +SVI also had worse metastasis-free and overall survival, (p = 0.005 and p = 0.02), respectively. With the addition of

adjuvant radiation, those with +SVI experienced improved 10-year biochemical failure-free survival (12–36 %, $p = 0.001$), but not overall or metastasis-free survival. Swanson GP et al. J Urol. 2008;180(6):2453–7.

57. The correct answer is B. To determine the optimal duration of ADT, EORTC 22961 randomized 970 men with locally advanced prostate cancer (T1c-T2b pN1-2 or cT2c-T4 N0-N2) to receive radiotherapy (50 Gy to pelvis followed by boost to 70 Gy) with either short-term (6 months) or long-term (3 years) androgen deprivation therapy, starting on day 1 of radiation. Seventy-two percent of those randomized to the long-term ADT arm completed all 3 years. Five-year overall survival was improved in those that received long-term ADT. While hot flashes and gynecomastia were increased in the long-term ADT arm, quality of life was comparable between the two arms. Bolla M et al. Duration of androgen suppression in the treatment of prostate cancer. N Engl J Med. 2009;360(24):2516–7.

58. The correct answer is C. The incidence of testicular cancer is bimodal with the first peak occurring in young adults aged 25–40 years, with germ cell histology. The second peak occurs later, in those aged 65–75 years, with non-germ cell histology (most commonly lymphoma). Warde PR, Hogg D, Gospodarowicz MK. Testicular cancer. In: Gunderson LL, Tepper JE, editors. Clinical radiation oncology. 3rd ed. Philadelphia: Elsevier Saunders; 2012. p. 903–33.

59. The correct answer is B. Well-established risk factors for the development of testicular cancer include a history of testicular maldescent, a family history of testicular cancer, presence of a contralateral testicular tumor, and gonadal dysgenesis. Cryptorchidism increases the risk of developing testicular cancer five times. There is no evidence that testicular trauma leads to the development of testicular cancer. Dieckmann KP et al. Clinical epidemiology of testicular germ cell tumors. World J Urol. 2004;22:2–14.

60. The correct answer is B. The 12p isochromosome (two chromosome 12 short arms) is the most common chromosomal change found in germ cell tumors, occurring in over 80 % of cases. It is also found in testicular carcinoma in situ. Oosterhuis JW et al. Current views on the pathogenesis of testicular germ cell tumors and perspectives for futures research: highlights of the 5h Copenhagen Workshop on Carcinoma in situ and Cancer of the Testis. APMIS. 2003;111:280–9. Atkin N et al. High chromosome numbers of testicular germ cell tumors. Cancer Genet Cytogenet. 1995;88:90.

61. The correct answer is B. Of the listed histologies, all are non-seminomatous germ cell tumors except the seminoma. Overall, 60 % of germ cell tumors are of seminomatous histology, 30 % are non-seminomatous, and 10 % are mixed tumors. McGlynn KA et al. Trends in the incidence of testicular germ cell tumors in the United States. Cancer. 2003;97:63–70.

62. The correct answer is B. Yolk sac (endodermal sinus) tumors are the most common testicular tumor in children. Warde PR, Hogg D, Gospodarowicz MK. Testicular cancer. In: Gunderson LL, Tepper JE, editors. Clinical radiation oncology. 3rd ed. Philadelphia: Elsevier Saunders; 2012. p. 903–33.

63. The correct answer is A. Placental leukocyte alkaline phosphatase is expressed by almost all seminomas on immunohistochemistry. Warde PR, Hogg D, Gospodarowicz MK. Testicular cancer. In: Gunderson LL, Tepper JE, editors. Clinical radiation oncology. 3rd ed. Philadelphia: Elsevier Saunders; 2012. p. 903–33.

64. The correct answer is B. Schiller-Duval bodies are a cellular feature seen in endodermal sinus tumors. It consists of a central vessel surrounded by tumor cells, with the whole structure often contained in a cystic space. Warde PR, Hogg D, Gospodarowicz MK. Testicular cancer. In: Gunderson LL, Tepper JE, editors. Clinical radiation oncology. 3rd ed. Philadelphia: Elsevier Saunders; 2012. p. 903–33.

65. The correct answer is D. Non-seminomatous germ cell tumors present at a median age of 27 years, seminomatous germ cell tumors present at a median age of 16 years, and mixed germ cell tumors present intermediately at a median age of 33 years. Teratomas are derived from two or more of germ cell layers (endoderm, ectoderm, mesoderm). Choriocarcinomas are relatively rare, present with high levels of B-hCG, metastases, and a poor prognosis. Yolk sac tumors, also known as endodermal sinus tumors, produce alpha-fetoprotein and are the most common variant of childhood germ cell tumor. Thomas R et al. An analysis of surveillance for state I combined teratoma-seminoma of the testis. Br J Cancer. 1996;74:59–62.

66. The correct answer is D. Lymph node drainage accounts for the distribution of lymph node metastases in testicular germ cell tumors. Due to drainage of the right testicular vein into the inferior vena cava, right-sided tumors metastasize most commonly to para-caval and intercaval lymph nodes. The left testicular vein drains into the left renal vein, and lymph node metastases are most commonly para-aortic. Supradiaphragmatic spread can occur through the thoracic duct, and while rare at presentation, left supraclavicular nodal disease is frequent at the time of relapse. Donohue J et al. Distribution of nodal metastases in nonseminomatous testicular cancer. Br J Cancer. 1996;128:315–20.

67. The correct answer is D. The most common presenting symptom of a testicular tumor is a painless mass. The next most common symptom is testicular pain. Gynecomastia from B-hCG-producing malignancies and symptoms from metastases (back pain, dyspnea) are less common presenting symptoms. Warde PR, Hogg D, Gospodarowicz MK. Testicular cancer. In: Gunderson LL, Tepper

JE, editors. Clinical radiation oncology. 3rd ed. Philadelphia: Elsevier Saunders; 2012. p. 903–33.

68. The correct answer is C. Invasion of the spermatic cord constitutes AJCC T stage pT3. Edge SB, Byrd DR, Compton CC, et al., editors. Testis. AJCC cancer staging handbook. 7th ed. New York: Springer; 2010.

69. The correct answer is C. In a healthy male with a painless testicular mass in his late thirties, the most likely diagnosis is a testicular tumor. Initial management is radical inguinal orchiectomy, which is both diagnostic and therapeutic. Transcrotal orchiectomy is not recommended and does not allow high division of the spermatic cord. Transcrotal biopsy to establish a diagnosis would be an acceptable next step in management for a patient with life-threatening metastatic disease, with likely germ cell malignancy, who needs to start systemic therapy. Fleshner N et al. Controversies in the management of testicular seminoma. Semin Urol Oncol. 2002;20:227–230. Sharir S et al. Progression detection of stage I nonseminomatous testicular cancer on surveillance: implication for the follow-up protocol. J Urol. 1999;161:474–6. Schmoll HJ et al. European consensus on diagnosis and treatment of germ cell cancer: a report of the European Germ Cell Cancer Consensus Group (EGCCCG). Ann Oncol. 2004;15:1377–99.

70. The correct answer is B. A 2.3 cm inguinal lymph node is AJCC nodal stage N2. Lymph nodes <2 cm are N1; those >5 cm are N3. There is no N2b. Edge SB, Byrd DR, Compton CC, et al., editors. Testis. AJCC cancer staging handbook. 7th ed. New York: Springer; 2010.

71. The correct answer is D. Viable treatment options after radical orchiectomy for a stage I seminoma include observation, adjuvant chemotherapy, and adjuvant radiation. Close observation prevents treatment-related morbidity, while maintaining cure rates at 100 %. Low-dose radiotherapy is an option, though there can be adverse effects of spermatogenesis, gastrointestinal symptoms, and cardiac disease. Horwich A. Surveillance for stage I seminoma of the testis. In: Horwich A, editor. Testicular cancer. Investigation and management. London: Chapman and Hall Medical; 1991, p. 109–16. Warde P et al. Results of adjuvant radiation therapy and surveillance in stage I seminoma. Br J Urol. 1997;80(A1144):291. Zagars GK et al. Mortality after cure of testicular seminoma. J Clin Oncol. 2004;22:640–7. Hamilton CR et al. Gastrointestinal morbidity of adjuvant radiotherapy in stage I malignant teratoma of the testis. Radiother Oncol. 1987;10:85–90. Huddart RA et al. Cardiovascular disease as a long-term complication of treatment for testicular cancer. J Clin Oncol. 2003;21:1513–23.

72. The correct answer is B. A meta-analysis of four surveillance series of stage I seminoma included 638 patients and found an overall 5-year relapse-free rate

of 82.3 %. Warde P et al. Prognostic factors for relapse in stage I seminoma managed by surveillance: a pooled analysis. J Clin Oncol. 2002;15(22):4448–52.

73. The correct answer is C. In both the Princess Margaret surveillance study (Warde et al.) and the Danish Testicular Cancer Study Group DATECA study, the most common site of relapse was the para-aortic lymph nodes, 85 % and 82 %, respectively. Warde P et al. Results of adjuvant radiation therapy and surveillance in stage I seminoma. Br J Urol. 1997;80:A1144-291. Von der Maase H et al. Surveillance following orchidectomy for stage I seminoma of the testis. Eur J Cancer. 1993;14:1931–4.

74. The correct answer is B. A meta-analysis of four surveillance series of stage I seminoma included 638 patients and found on multivariate analysis that the factors that significantly predicted for relapse were primary tumor size and rete testis invasion. Hazard ratio for tumor size >4 cm alone was 2.0 (95 % CI, 1.2–3.2), hazard ratio for rete testis involvement was 1.7 (95 % CI, 1.1–2.6), and hazard ratio with both factors was 3.4 (95 % CI, 2.0–6.1). Warde P et al. Prognostic factors for relapse in stage I seminoma managed by surveillance: a pooled analysis. J Clin Oncol. 2002;15(22):4448–52.

75. The correct answer is C. A meta-analysis of four surveillance series of stage I seminoma included 638 patients and found on multivariate analysis that the factors that significantly predicted for relapse were primary tumor size and rete testis invasion. Hazard ratio for tumor size >4 cm alone was 2.0 (95 % CI, 1.2–3.2), hazard ratio for rete testis involvement was 1.7 (95 % CI, 1.1–2.6), and hazard ratio with both factors was 3.4 (95 % CI, 2.0–6.1). With no risk factors, the 5-year risk of relapse was 12.2 %. With one and two risk factors, the risks of 5-year relapse were 15.9 % and 31.5 %, respectively. Warde P et al. Prognostic factors for relapse in stage I seminoma managed by surveillance: a pooled analysis. J Clin Oncol. 2002;15(22):4448–52.

76. The correct answer is C. A Medical Research Council study in the United Kingdom randomized 1,447 patients s/p orchiectomy for stage I seminoma to undergo either adjuvant radiation (20–30 Gy) or a single course of carboplatin (AUC=7). Relapse rate was similar in both arms, with the majority of the carboplatin relapses occurring in the retroperitoneal nodes. There were fewer second primary testicular germ cell tumors in the chemotherapy arm as well. Oliver RT et al. Randomized trial of carboplatin versus radiotherapy for stage I seminoma: mature results on relapse and contralateral testicular cancer rates in MRC TE19/EORTC 30982 study (ISRCTN27163214). J Clin Oncol. 2001;29(6):957–62.

77. The correct answer is A. Following radiotherapy for stage II seminoma, the most common sites of relapse are the mediastinal and supraclavicular lymph nodes, the lung, and bone. Crook J, Mazeron J-J. Penile cancer. In: Gunderson

LL, Tepper JE, editors. Clinical radiation oncology. 3rd ed. Philadelphia: Elsevier Saunders; 2012. p. 903–33.

78. The correct answer is D. While primary tumor size and rete testis involvement are the most important prognostic factors for relapse in stage I seminoma, bulk of retroperitoneal disease is the most important factor in stage II seminoma. A Princess Margaret series of 95 stage II seminoma patients treated with radiotherapy showed that bulk of retroperitoneal disease was the only prognostic factor for relapse. Those with nodal disease < 5 cm (stage IIA/B) had a 5-year relapse-free survival of 91 % compared to 44 % in those with stage IIC disease. Chung PW et al. Stage II testicular seminoma: patterns of recurrence and outcome of treatment. Eur Urol. 2004;45:754–9. Discussion 759–760.

79. The correct answer is A. It is not uncommon to find a residual mass after treatment of a stage II seminoma. Memorial Sloan Kettering Cancer Center reported their experience of managing residual retroperitoneal masses in 1997. Fifty-five of 104 patients with a residual mass underwent either formal retroperitoneal lymph node dissection ($n = 32$) or multiple intraoperative biopsy ($n = 23$). In those with a residual mass of <3 cm, no residual tumor was found pathologically, whereas 30 % of those with a tumor >3 cm had residual tumor. As such, patients with residual masses <3 cm can be safely observed with serial imaging. Herr HW et al. Surgery for a post-chemotherapy residual mass in seminoma. J Urol. 1997;157:860–2.

80. The correct answer is B. Leydig cell tumors can present in either children (25 %), with signs of prepubertal virilization, or more commonly in adults (75 %), with a painless testicular mass. The initial step in management is radical inguinal orchiectomy, though there is no role for adjuvant chemotherapy or radiation. The most common site of metastasis is to the regional lymph nodes. Thrasher J, et al. Non-germ cell testicular tumors. Probl Urol. 1994;8:167. Kim I et al. Leydig cell tumors of the testis: a clinicopathological analysis of 40 cases and review of the literature. Am J Surg Pathol. 1985;9:177–92.

81. The correct answer is C. Mediastinal extragonadal germ cell tumors (EGCTs) frequently present with local invasion and/or metastases. Symptoms of cough, dyspnea, and chest pain are common. The mainstay of therapy is cisplatin-based chemotherapy; there is no role for routine radiotherapy. An international analysis of 635 patients with EGCTs showed improved outcomes in patients with pure seminoma versus non-seminomatous histology. Long-term cure rates of seminoma were 89 % regardless of primary site, whereas non-seminomatous EGCTs in the mediastinum had a worse outcome (5y survival 45 %), compared to those with a retroperitoneal primary site (5y survival 63 %). Bokemeyer C et al. Extragonadal germ cell tumors of the mediastinum and retroperitoneum: results from an international analysis. J Clin Oncol. 2002;20:1864–73.

82. The correct answer is B. The MRC Trial TE 10 sought to determine the optimal field size for treatment of stage I seminoma with radiation. Four hundred seventy-eight men were randomized to receive 30 Gy radiation to para-aortic + pelvic LNs versus para-aortic LNs alone. There was no statistical difference in relapses between the arms, though there were four pelvic relapses in the para-aortic alone arm, compared to none in the para-aortic + pelvic arm. Acute toxicity was decreased in the para-aortic alone arm, and sperm counts were significantly higher. This trial established para-aortic fields as standard for stage I seminoma treatment. Fossa SD et al. Optimal planning target volume for stage I testicular seminoma: a Medical Research Council randomized trial. Medical Research Council Testicular Tumor Working Group. J Clin Oncol. 1999;17(4):1146.

83. The correct answer is A. The MRC Trial TE 18 sought to determine the optimal dose for treatment of stage I seminoma with radiation. Six hundred twenty-five men were randomized to receive 30 Gy versus 20 Gy radiation to para-aortic LNs (para-aortic + pelvic in those with prior inguinal surgery). There was no statistical difference in relapses between the arms. Acute toxicity at 4 weeks was significantly better in the 20 Gy arm, though there was no difference between the arms at 12 weeks. This trial established 20 Gy as an acceptable dose for treatment of stage I seminoma. Jones WG et al. Randomized trial of 30 versus 20 Gy in the adjuvant treatment of stage I Testicular Seminoma: a report on Medical Research Council Trial TE18, European Organisation for the Research and Treatment of Cancer Trial 30942 (ISRCTN18525328). J Clin Oncol. 2005;23(6):1200–8.

84. The correct answer is B. Human papillomavirus types 16 and 18 are detected in 40–45 % of penile cancers. Rubin MA et al. Detection and typing of human papillomavirus DNA in penile carcinoma: evidence for multiple independent pathways of penile carcinogenesis. Am J Pathol. 2001;159:1211–8. McCance DJ et al., Human papillomavirus types 16 and 18 in carcinomas of the penis from Brazil. Int J Cancer. 1986;37:55–9.

85. The correct answer is D. All are risk factors for the development of penile cancer except neonatal circumcision, which is associated with a threefold decrease in the risk of penile carcinoma. Dillner J et al. Etiology of squamous cell carcinoma of the penis. Scand J Urol Nephrl Suppl. 2000;Suppl 205:189–93.

86. The correct answer is A. The frequency of HPV detection does depend on the histologic subtype of penile cancer. Verrucous subtypes are less commonly associated with HPV (35 %), whereas basaloid and warty subtypes are commonly associated (80–100 %). HPV 16 and HPV 18 are the most frequently detected subtypes. HPV presence does not confer a worse prognosis. Rubin MA et al. Detection and typing of human papillomavirus DNA in penile carcinoma: evidence for multiple independent pathways of penile carcinogenesis. Am J Pathol.

2001;159:1211–8. Bezerra AL et al. Human papillomavirus as a prognostic factor in carcinoma of the penis: analysis of 82 patients treated with amputation and bilateral lymphadenectomy. Cancer. 2001;91:2315–21.

87. The correct answer is B. All are known precursor lesions for warty and basaloid penile cancers except lichen sclerosis, which tends to be associated with non-HPV variants of penile carcinoma. Gross G et al. Role of human papillomavirus in penile cancer, penile intraepithelial squamous cell neoplasias and in genital warts. Med Microbiol Immunol (Berl). 2004;193:35–44. Perceau G et al. Lichen sclerosus is frequently present in penile squamous cell carcinomas but is not always associated with oncogenic human papillomavirus. Br J Dermatol. 2003;148:924–38. Velazquez EF et al. Lichen sclerosus in 68 patients with squamous cell carcinoma of the penis: frequent atypias and correlation with special carcinoma variants suggests a precancerous role. Am J Surg Pathol. 2003;27:1448–53.

88. The correct answer is A. Approximately 10–20 % of those with Erythroplasia of Queyrat will develop squamous cell carcinoma on the prepuce or glans of the penis. Crook J, Mazeron J-J. Penile cancer. In: Gunderson LL, Tepper JE, editors. Clinical radiation oncology. 3rd ed. Philadelphia: Elsevier Saunders; 2012. p. 903–33.

89. The correct answer is B. The glans is the most common site of primary tumors (48 %), with the prepuce as the second most common site (25 %). The shaft is the least commonly involved site (2 %). Stancik I et al. Penile cancer: review of the recent literature. Curr Opin Urol. 2003;13:467–72.

90. The correct answer is C. A penile cancer of the glans will drain first to the superficial inguinal LNs and then to the external iliac lymph nodes. A lesion involving the corpus cavernosum or posterior urethra may drain to the internal iliac LNs. Crook J, Mazeron J-J. Penile cancer. In: Gunderson LL, Tepper JE, editors. Clinical radiation oncology. 3rd ed. Philadelphia: Elsevier Saunders; 2012. p. 903–33.

91. The correct answer is B. A poorly differentiated penile cancer with invasion into the subepithelial connective tissue is T1b. Lymphovascular space invasion in a lesion that invades into the subepithelial connective tissue is also T1b. Multiple ipsilateral mobile inguinal lymph nodes are N2. A single mobile inguinal lymph node is N1. Bilateral inguinal lymph nodes are N2. The presence of pelvic lymph nodes is N3, as is a fixed inguinal mass. Edge SB, Byrd DR, Compton CC, et al., editors. Penis. AJCC cancer staging handbook. 7th ed. New York: Springer; 2010.

92. The correct answer is D. Invasion of the prostate is now classified as T4, a change in the new AJCC staging system. It was previously T3, now only urethral invasion is T3. A single fixed inguinal mass is N3. Edge SB, Byrd DR,

Compton CC, et al., editors. Penis. AJCC cancer staging handbook. 7th ed. New York: Springer; 2010.

93. The correct answer is C. Approximately half of clinically suspicious lymph nodes are pathologically positive in penile cancers. Narayana AS et al. Carcinoma of the penis: analysis of 219 cases. Cancer. 1982;49:2185–91.

94. The correct answer is A. A T1 penile carcinoma of the glans could be most reasonably treated by laser surgery, which has been reported to yield a superior functional and cosmetic results compared to standard surgical techniques. Partial penectomy given the distal location is a reasonable surgical option. Total penectomy is an option but may be extreme for the size and location of the tumor. Interstitial brachytherapy is an excellent treatment option for a T1 tumor of the glans, offering 5y local control rates of over 70 % and penile preservation rates of 72–83 %. Malek RS. Laser treatment of premalignant and malignant squamous cell lesions of the penis. Lasers Surg Med. 1992;12:246–53. Windahl T et al. Combined laser treatment for penile carcinoma: results after long-term follow-up. J Urol. 2003;169:2118–21. Mazeron JJ et al. Interstitial radiation therapy for carcinoma of the penis using iridium 192 wires: the Henri Mondor experience (1970–1979). Int J Radiat Oncol Biol Phys. 1984;10:1891–5. Crook JM et al. Penile brachytherapy results for 49 patients. Int J Radiat Oncol Biol Phys. 2005;62:460.

95. The correct answer is C. Due to the high incidence of pathologically positive lymph nodes and contralateral lymph nodes, when performing groin dissection, it is important to dissect bilaterally. If Cloquet's node is positive, a pelvic lymph node dissection should then be performed. For early lesions, brachytherapy alone is contraindicated for lesions with >1 cm invasion of corpus cavernosa or for a primary of size >4 cm. Before beginning RT, it is important to perform circumcision to minimize RT-induced toxicity (edema and/or phimosis). Crook J, Mazeron J-J. Penile cancer. In: Gunderson LL, Tepper JE, editors. Clinical radiation oncology. 3rd ed. Philadelphia: Elsevier Saunders; 2012. p. 903–33.

96. The correct answer is C. Soft tissue necrosis is one of the most common late complications of radiotherapy for penile cancer and is more common after brachytherapy than external beam radiotherapy. The risk of necrosis increases with increasing dose over 60 Gy, as well as with an increasing number of brachytherapy needles. There is also an increasing risk of necrosis with T3 tumors. Necrosis is the most common reason for amputation of a tumor-free penis. Jackson S. The treatment of carcinoma of the penis. Br J Surg. 1966;53:33–5. Mazeron JJ et al. Interstitial radiation therapy for carcinoma of the penis using iridium 192 wires: the Henri Mondor experience (1970–1979). Int J Radiat Oncol Biol Phys. 1984;10:1891–95. Crook JM et al. Penile brachytherapy results for 49 patients. Int J Radiat Oncol Biol Phys. 2005;62:460.

Chapter 11
Gynecologic Malignancies

Joseph G. Waller, Celine Bicquart Ord, and Subhakar Mutyala

Questions

1. What is the appropriate AJCC 7th edition/FIGO 2008 staging for a 36-year-old female diagnosed with an HPV-positive 4.5 cm clinically visible squamous cell carcinoma of the cervix with a horizontal spread of 9 mm, with lymphovascular space invasion, but without evidence of invasion of the vagina, parametrium, bladder, or evidence of hydronephrosis?
   A. T1b2/IB2
   B. T1b1/IB1
   C. T2a2/IIA2
   D. T3a/IIIA

2. All of the following have been identified as risk factors for the development of cervical cancer EXCEPT:
   A. DES exposure in utero
   B. Immunosuppression
   C. Smoking
   D. HPV 6 and 11

J.G. Waller, MD, MPH (✉)
Department of Radiation Medicine, Oregon Health & Science University,
3181 SW Sam Jackson Park Rd, KPV4, Portland, OR 97239-3098, USA
e-mail: wallerj@ohsu.edu

C.B. Ord, MD
Department of Radiation Oncology, Scott & White Memorial Hospital,
2401 S. 31st Street, 76508 Temple, TX, USA

S. Mutyala, MD
Department of Radiation Oncology, Scott & White Healthcare System
and Texas A&M College of Medicine, 2401 S. 31st Street, 76508 Temple, TX, USA

C.B. Ord et al. (eds.), *Radiation Oncology Study Guide*,   289
DOI 10.1007/978-1-4614-6400-6_11, © Springer Science+Business Media New York 2013

3. Which of the following recommendations regarding cervical cancer screening is recommended by the United States Preventative Services Task Force (USPSTF)?
   A. Annual screening within 1 year of the onset of vaginal intercourse.
   B. Annual screening starting no later than 18 years of age.
   C. Women >65 years old with prior negative screening and no risk factors do not need further screening.
   D. Women >30 years old with three consecutive negative Pap smears do not need further screening if no new sexual partners.

4. The risks of pelvic lymph node involvement for stage IB, IIB, and IIIB cervical cancer are best estimated as (respectively):
   A. 15 %, 30 %, 50 %
   B. 5 %, 20 %, 35 %
   C. 5 %, 40 %, 60 %
   D. 10 %, 15 %, 30 %

5. The most common site of distant metastases in cervical cancer following irradiation alone is:
   A. Liver
   B. Para-aortic nodes
   C. Lung
   D. Bone

6. Which of the following risk factors is least prognostic in cervical cancer?
   A. Tumor size
   B. Anemia
   C. Angiolymphatic space involvement
   D. Depth of invasion

7. According to the GOG 120 trial, chemoradiation with EBRT + cisplatin alone had superior overall survival and progression-free compared to which other treatment?
   A. Radiation + hydroxyurea
   B. Radiation + hydroxyurea/cisplatin/5-FU
   C. Hydroxyurea alone
   D. Hydroxyurea/cisplatin/5-FU alone

8. The RTOG 79-20 trial (Rotman et al.), which randomized high-risk cervical cancer to standard pelvic versus extended-field radiation, reported what outcomes for extended-field radiation?
   A. Improved OS and DFS
   B. Improved OS but not DFS
   C. Improved DFS but not OS
   D. No improvement in either OS or DFS

9. Which chemoradiation trial showed a survival benefit for definitive chemora-
   diation compared to extended-field radiation alone for cervical cancer?
   A. GOG 120
   B. GOG 123
   C. RTOG 90-01
   D. NCIC

10. Regarding the GOG 123 trial (Keys et al.) comparing neoadjuvant radiation
    alone versus chemoradiation followed by LDR brachytherapy and hysterec-
    tomy in patients with bulky stage IB2 cervical cancer, all of the following are
    true EXCEPT:
    A. There was a statistically significant increase in pathologic complete
       response rate in the chemoradiation arm.
    B. The 3-year overall survival rates for the radiation alone and chemoradiation
       arms were 74 % and 83 %, respectively.
    C. Total radiation dose was 75 Gy to point A and 55 Gy to point B.
    D. Node-positive patients had a statistically significant increase in the rate of
       distant failures for the radiation-alone arm.

11. Which of the following is true regarding the Intergroup 0107 trial reported by
    Peters et al., comparing adjuvant radiation alone versus adjuvant concurrent
    chemoradiation for high-risk cervical cancer?
    A. The radiation-alone arm consisted of EBRT to 45 Gy in 25 fractions fol-
       lowed by an LDR boost to 75 Gy to point A.
    B. Chemotherapy consisted of cisplatin alone (70 mg/m^2; weekly ×6).
    C. The difference in relapse pattern was statistically significant between the
       two groups.
    D. Inclusion criteria included patients who were found to have positive pelvic
       nodes, positive margins, and/or positive parametrial involvement.

12. Which of the following is not an indication for postoperative chemoradiation
    after surgery for cervical cancer?
    A. Tumor size >4 cm
    B. Positive margins
    C. Parametrial involvement
    D. Lymph node positivity

13. Which of the following is NOT a valid criticism of the NCIC trial comparing
    bulky IB/IIA or stage IIB–IVA cervical cancer treated with either definitive
    radiation alone or chemoradiation?
    A. Poor quality control of radiation
    B. Small sample size
    C. Lack of surgical staging
    D. Use of cisplatin alone

14. A class II extended or modified radical hysterectomy includes all of the following EXCEPT:
    A. Unroofing of the ureters
    B. Mobilization of the ureters, bladder, and rectum to remove parametrial tissue to pelvic sidewall
    C. Removal of 1–2 cm of the vaginal cuff
    D. Removal of the cardinal and uterosacral ligaments

15. A Canadian study by Grogan et al. studied the prognostic significance of hemoglobin levels during definitive RT. Their study concluded all of the following EXCEPT:
    A. Patients who were transfused to the goal hemoglobin 12 g/dL had worse outcomes to pts who maintained hemoglobin levels naturally.
    B. Maintaining hemoglobin levels at 12 g/dL resulted in statistically significantly improved local control.
    C. Maintaining hemoglobin levels at 12 g/dL results in statistically significantly improved rates of distant metastasis.
    D. Average weekly nadir of hemoglobin was statistically significant on both univariate and multivariate analysis.

16. Which of the following is correct regarding outcomes of Landoni et al. comparing radiation alone versus surgery for stage IB/IIA cervical cancer?
    A. 5-year overall survival was better in the RT arm.
    B. 5-year overall survival was better in the surgical arm.
    C. Severe morbidity rates were similar in both arms.
    D. Severe morbidity rates were increased in the surgery arm.

17. Conization is NOT appropriate in which of the following patients?
    A. A 40-year-old woman with preinvasive disease where the entire transformational zone is has not been well visualized.
    B. A 32-year-old woman with FIGO stage IA disease, who wishes to maintain fertility.
    C. A 74-year-old woman with FIGO stage IB disease with multiple medical comorbidities.
    D. A 54-year-old woman with preinvasive disease but marked discrepancy between Pap smear results and colposcopy.

18. The GOG 92 trial randomized patients following radical hysterectomy and PLND to adjuvant RT versus observation based on what inclusion criteria?
    A. Negative lymph nodes and ≥2 of the following risk factors: >1/3 stromal invasion, +ALI, size >4 cm
    B. Positive lymph nodes or ≥2 of the following risk factors: >1/3 stromal invasion, +ALI, size >4 cm
    C. Negative lymph nodes and ≥1 of the following risk factors: >1/3 stromal invasion, +ALI, size >4 cm
    D. Positive lymph nodes or ≥1 of the following risk factors: >1/3 stromal invasion, +ALI, size >4 cm

19. Which of the following is a finding of the GOG 71 phase III trial by Keys et al. evaluating adjuvant hysterectomy for bulky stage IB cervical cancers?
    A. Adjuvant hysterectomy does improve OS.
    B. Adjuvant hysterectomy increases G3/G4 adverse effects.
    C. Adjuvant hysterectomy does not improve LC.
    D. There are tumors that will benefit from adjuvant hysterectomy.

20. What dose and fractionation did Spanos et al. use for palliation of pelvic malignancies in the RTOG 85-02 phase I/II trial?
    A. 800 cGy × 1 fraction
    B. 300 cGy × 10 fractions
    C. 500 cGy × 3 fractions
    D. 370 cGy × 4 fractions delivered BID

21. Which of the following correctly identifies a measurement of point A based on the Manchester system?
    A. 2 cm superior and 5 cm lateral to the cervical os along the axis of the tandem
    B. 2 cm superior and 5 cm lateral to the cervical os along the midline of the patient
    C. 2 cm superior and 3 cm lateral to the cervical os along the midline of the patient
    D. 2 cm superior and 2 cm lateral to the cervical os along the axis of the tandem

22. Recommended dose rate to point A using LDR brachytherapy is:
    A. 10 cGy/h
    B. 50 cGy/h
    C. 100 cGy/h
    D. 200 cGy/h

23. The GOG currently recommends a total radiation dose to point A for intact cervix of:
    A. 45 Gy
    B. 85 Gy
    C. 100 Gy
    D. 120 Gy

24. All of the following are advantages or potential advantages of HDR brachytherapy to LDR except:
    A. Reduced radiation exposure to healthcare personnel
    B. Reduced cost
    C. Increased therapeutic ratio
    D. Reduced need for hospitalization

25. All of the following situations favor the use of interstitial brachytherapy over intracavitary brachytherapy boost except:
    A. Persistent, palpable disease on the pelvic sidewall
    B. Necrotic tumor still visible on the posterior cervical lip
    C. Inability to see or feel the cervical os
    D. Vaginal disease thicker than 5 mm

26. In HDR, target rectal point dose limits are _____% of the daily fraction dose to point A.
    A. 10 %
    B. 30 %
    C. 50 %
    D. 70 %

27. Prolonging a course of radiotherapy beyond approximately 7 weeks is associated with a _____% decrease in pelvic control per extra day.
    A. 0.1 %
    B. 1 %
    C. 5 %
    D. 10 %

28. In the United States, endometrial cancer is the _____ most common gynecologic malignancy and the _____ most common malignancy in women overall:
    A. 1st, 4th
    B. 2nd, 4th
    C. 1st, 10th
    D. 2nd, 10th

29. All of the following are risk factors for endometrial cancer EXCEPT:
    A. Obesity
    B. Multiparity
    C. Late menopause
    D. Prior use of tamoxifen

30. Women diagnosed with any of the following are at increased risk of developing endometrial cancer except:
    A. HNPCC (Lynch syndrome)
    B. Polycystic ovarian syndrome (PCOS)
    C. Von Hippel-Lindau disease (VHL)
    D. Peutz-Jeghers

31. The majority of patients with endometrial cancer present at which stage?
    A. Stage I
    B. Stage II
    C. Stage III
    D. Stage IV

32. Regarding endometrial hyperplasia, which of the following is true?
    A. Prophylactic hysterectomy is not recommended for women with known hyperplasia with atypia.
    B. Progression from simple hyperplasia with atypia to carcinoma occurs in <2 % of patients.
    C. Endometrial adenocarcinoma frequently arises from atypical hyperplasia.
    D. Atypical nuclear changes can be associated with both simple and complex hyperplasia.

33. Which of the following has the worst prognosis?
    A. Villoglandular adenocarcinoma
    B. Secretory adenocarcinoma
    C. Endometrioid adenocarcinoma with squamous differentiation
    D. Uterine papillary serous adenocarcinoma (UPSC)

34. All of the following are characteristic of type II endometrial cancer EXCEPT:
    A. Estrogen dependent
    B. Precursor lesion is intraepithelial carcinoma
    C. Usually diagnosed in older, postmenopausal patients
    D. Poorer prognosis than type I

35. HER2 mutations have been identified in up to 80 % of serous adenocarcinoma (UPSC), making which of the following a promising therapeutic strategy?
    A. Tamoxifen
    B. Herceptin
    C. Erlotinib
    D. Cetuximab

36. A woman presents with a 5 cm grade 3, endometrial adenocarcinoma, invading 7 mm of 15 mm thick myometrium, extending into the glandular epithelium of the endocervix, without involvement of the serosa, adnexa, vagina, bladder, or bowel and with no evidence of nodal involvement. What is the correct AJCC 7th ed./FIGO 2008 stage?
    A. T1a/IA
    B. T1b/IB
    C. T1c/IC
    D. T2/II

37. What is the correct AJCC 7th edition/FIGO 2008 stage for a woman with a 2 cm G3 endometrioid adenocarcinoma with 8 mm invasion of a 16 mm myometrium, no cervical stromal, serosa, adnexa, vagina, bowel, or bladder involvement and with no pelvic nodes but a single positive para-aortic node?
    A. T3cN1/IIIC1
    B. T3cN2/IIIC2
    C. T1bN1/IIIC1
    D. T1bN2/IIIC2

38. According to GOG 33, what is the approximate risk of pelvic lymph node involvement for a woman with stage IC, grade 2 endometrial adenocarcinoma?
   A. 6 %
   B. 12 %
   C. 18 %
   D. 27 %

39. Regarding the MRC ASTEC randomized control trial comparing surgery +/− lymphadenectomy, which of the following is true?
   A. Lymphadenectomy provided an OS benefit only.
   B. Lymphadenectomy provided a PFS benefit only.
   C. Lymphadenectomy provided both an OS and PFS benefit.
   D. Lymphadenectomy did not provide either an OS or PFS benefit.

40. In the Norwegian trial (Aalders et al. 1980) comparing surgery + brachytherapy +/− whole pelvis RT (WPRT), radiation was delivered in what dose and fractionation?
   A. VC LDR 60 Gy to surface +/− 40 Gy/20 fxs
   B. VC LDR 45 Gy to surface +/− 45 Gy/25 fxs
   C. VC HDR 30 Gy/5 fxs to surface +/− 45 Gy/25 fxs
   D. VC HDR 21 Gy/3 fxs to surface +/− 50 Gy/25 fxs

41. According to the Aalders trial, LRR for the surgery + adjuvant brachytherapy-alone arm versus the adjuvant brachytherapy + EBRT arm was:
   A. 7 % versus 2 %
   B. 15 % versus 4 %
   C. 15 % versus 14 %
   D. 22 % versus 11 %

42. All of the following stage/grade combinations met inclusion criteria for the PORTEC-1 trial EXCEPT:
   A. IC, G2
   B. IB, G2
   C. IB, G3
   D. IC, G3

43. In the PORTEC-1 trial, what percent of failures occurred in the vaginal vault?
   A. 35 %
   B. 55 %
   C. 75 %
   D. 95 %

44. Women in the PORTEC-1 trial were randomized after TAH-BSO to:
   A. VC brachytherapy +/− EBRT
   B. VC brachytherapy versus EBRT
   C. Observation versus EBRT
   D. Observation versus VC brachytherapy

45. In the GOG 99 trial, the high-intermediate risk (HIR) was defined by all of the following EXCEPT:
    A. Age ≥70 with only one other risk factor
    B. Any age but surgically inoperable
    C. Age ≥50 with two other risk factors
    D. Any age with three risk factors

46. Which of the following was not a risk factor for characterization of "high-intermediate" risk in the GOG 99 trial?
    A. Intermediate grade
    B. High grade
    C. 50 % MMI invasion
    D. +LVSI

47. Regarding the GOG 99 trial, what were the rates of local recurrence at 2 years for the high-intermediate-risk (HIR) cohorts in the observation arm and adjuvant RT arm, respectively?
    A. 12 % versus 3 %
    B. 26 % versus 6 %
    C. 6 % versus 2 %
    D. 22 % versus 19 %

48. The PORTEC-2 trial made what conclusions regarding the use of vaginal brachytherapy (VBT) compared to whole pelvis radiation therapy (WPRT) in the adjuvant setting?
    A. VBT significantly improved vaginal cuff recurrence.
    B. Patient reported quality of life was better in the VBT arm.
    C. There was no difference in the rates of pelvic recurrence between the two arms.
    D. Both progression-free survival and overall survival were significantly improved in the WPRT arm.

49. All of the following are true regarding the GOG 122 trial comparing whole abdominal radiation therapy (WART) versus combination chemotherapy in advanced stage endometrial cancer except:
    A. WART improved 5-year OS (42 % versus 55 %) and DFS (38 % versus 50 %).
    B. WART included para-aortic boost if pelvic LN+ or no LN sampling.
    C. Chemotherapy consisted of combination doxorubicin and cisplatin.
    D. Chemotherapy increased the grade 3–4 hematological, gastrointestinal, and cardiac toxicity.

50. What was the rate of pelvic relapse at 2 years in the Ontario Canada group phase II trial of sandwich chemoRT?
    A. 55 %
    B. 33 %
    C. 15 %
    D. 3 %

51. The most common histology in uterine sarcomas is:
    A. Carcinosarcoma (malignant mixed mullerian tumor)
    B. Leiomyosarcoma
    C. Adenosarcoma
    D. Endometrial stromal sarcoma

52. What is the most appropriate therapy for a 50-year-old woman s/p TAH/BSO but
    no lymph node sampling, who is found to have a grade 3 endometrioid adenocar-
    cinoma with invasion of the outer one third of the myometrium, no lymphovas-
    cular space invasion, negative margins, but cervical stromal involvement?
    A. Pelvic RT alone
    B. Pelvic and para-aortic lymph node dissection
    C. Pelvic RT + vaginal brachytherapy
    D. Chemotherapy with doxorubicin + cisplatin alone

53. The dose limit for the upper vaginal mucosa, in equivalent dose in 2 Gy fractions
    (EQD2), is:
    A. 60–70 Gy
    B. 80–90 Gy
    C. 110 Gy
    D. 140 Gy

54. All of the following are true regarding uterine sarcomas except:
    A. Postoperative radiation improves locoregional control but not overall survival.
    B. Carcinosarcoma tends to fail in the lymph nodes.
    C. Leiomyosarcoma tends to fail in the lung.
    D. Leiomyosarcoma tends to present at more advanced stages.

55. Which of the following pairings is incorrect regarding the drainage of the uterus?
    A. Upper uterus can drain via the ovarian artery to the para-aortic lymph nodes.
    B. Middle uterus drains to internal iliac lymph nodes.
    C. Lower uterus drains to the internal iliac lymph nodes.
    D. Lower uterus drains to the inguinofemoral lymph nodes.

56. What is the 5-year survival for FIGO stage II vulvar cancer?
    A. 90 %
    B. 75 %
    C. 50 %
    D. 20 %

57. What percentage of vulvar intraepithelial neoplasia 3 (VIN 3) lesions
    progresses to invasive carcinoma?
    A. <5 %
    B. 10 %
    C. 15 %
    D. 20 %

58. All of the following are true about subtypes of vulvar cancer except:
    A. Melanoma is the second most common tumor of the vulva.
    B. Vulvar cancer with a trabecular growth pattern often spreads to regional lymph nodes.
    C. Verrucous cancers require postoperative radiation due to the propensity for lymph node involvement.
    D. Vulvar cancers arising from Bartholin's glands are not usually squamous cell carcinomas.

59. In the pathological surgical margin study of resection for vulvar cancers, Heaps et al. found no recurrences in patients in whom margins were equal to or greater than _____mm.
    A. 5 mm
    B. 6 mm
    C. 7 mm
    D. 8 mm

60. According to Heaps et al., what was the approximate local recurrence rate of a vulvar cancer resected with a 5 mm clear margin?
    A. 20 %
    B. 30 %
    C. 40 %
    D. 50 %

61. What are the first echelon lymph nodes for vulvar cancer?
    A. Inguinal
    B. Deep femoral
    C. External iliac
    D. Para-aortic

62. What is the risk of developing a secondary lung malignancy in those with either a vaginal or vulvar cancer?
    A. 2×
    B. 4×
    C. 6×
    D. 10×

63. Which of the following vulvar lesions is associated with a "cake-icing" appearance?
    A. Verrucous
    B. Paget's
    C. HPV-associated squamous cell carcinoma
    D. Melanoma

64. What is the risk of positive contralateral inguinal nodes with negative ipsilateral lymph nodes in vulvar cancer?
    A. <1 %
    B. 3 %
    C. 5 %
    D. 7 %

65. What is the risk of lymph node positivity with >5 mm depth of invasion of a primary vulvar lesion?
    A. 5 %
    B. 10 %
    C. 25 %
    D. 35 %

66. What is an absolute indication for postoperative radiation for vulvar cancer that has undergone groin dissection?
    A. One positive lymph node on groin dissection
    B. One positive lymph node of 2 cm on groin dissection
    C. Two positive lymph nodes on groin dissection
    D. Primary tumor size of 2.5 cm

67. In GOG 88, as reported by Stehman et al., what was the groin recurrence rate with radiation alone to the groin?
    A. 0 %
    B. 8 %
    C. 12 %
    D. 18 %

68. In GOG 88, as reported by Stehman et al., to what depth in the groin was the radiation prescribed?
    A. 2 cm
    B. 3 cm
    C. 4 cm
    D. 5 cm

69. All are true regarding methods and outcomes of GOG 88 as reported by Stehman et al. except:
    A. Overall survival was improved with the addition of bilateral inguinofemoral lymph node dissection.
    B. Groin recurrences were not improved with the addition of bilateral inguino-femoral lymph node dissection.
    C. Progression-free survival was worse in those that did not undergo bilateral inguinofemoral lymph node dissection.
    D. Those with positive lymph nodes on bilateral inguinofemoral lymph node dissection received postoperative radiotherapy to the groin.

70. In GOG 37, as reported by Homesley et al., all are true regarding the methods except:
    A. All patients underwent groin dissection.
    B. Patients were randomized to observation versus postoperative radiotherapy.
    C. Postoperative radiotherapy was delivered to the groin and to the primary site.
    D. Only patients with positive lymph nodes were eligible for randomization of postoperative radiotherapy.

71. What was the rate of groin relapse with and without groin irradiation, respectively, as reported in GOG 37?
    A. 5 % and 24 %
    B. 24 % and 5 %
    C. 0 % and 15 %
    D. 15 % and 0 %

72. In the 6-year update of GOG 37 published in 2009 (Kunos et al.), what ipsilateral lymph node burden positivity was found to significantly benefit from pelvic and inguinal radiotherapy?
    A. 10 %
    B. 20 %
    C. 30 %
    D. 40 %

73. What is the most common site of distant metastasis in vulvar cancer?
    A. Bone
    B. Liver
    C. Brain
    D. Lung

74. A 60-year-old woman presents with a 2.5 cm primary vulvar lesion and two ipsilateral inguinal lymph nodes, each 4 mm. What is the correct FIGO stage?
    A. IB
    B. II
    C. IIIA
    D. IIIB

75. What is the correct FIGO stage for a vulvar cancer that has extracapsular extension of an inguinal lymph node?
    A. IIIA
    B. IIIB
    C. IIIC
    D. IVA

76. What is the correct FIGO stage for a vulvar cancer that has fixed, ulcerated inguinal adenopathy?
    A. IIIB
    B. IIIC
    C. IVA
    D. IVB

77. What is the correct FIGO stage for a vulvar cancer that has positive common iliac adenopathy?
    A. IIIB
    B. IIIC
    C. IVA
    D. IVB

78. All of the following are correct regarding vaginal cancers related to DES exposure except:
    A. The median age of presentation is younger than non-DES-related vaginal cancers.
    B. Most present with an advanced stage at diagnosis.
    C. There is a greater risk for vaginal than cervical cancers.
    D. Clear cell adenocarcinoma has been linked to in utero exposure of DES.

79. Which is the most common site for vaginal intraepithelial neoplasia (VAIN)?
    A. Upper one third of vagina.
    B. Middle one third of vagina.
    C. Lower one third of vagina.
    D. VAIN is evenly seen in all thirds of the vagina.

80. What is the second most common histology of cancers found in the vagina?
    A. Adenocarcinoma
    B. Melanoma
    C. Sarcoma
    D. Metastases

81. Which of the pathways of spread or lymph node drainage pairings is incorrect?
    A. Proximal third of vagina by inguinal-femoral nodes to external iliac nodes.
    B. Lower third of vagina to inguinal-femoral nodes then pelvic nodes.
    C. Rectovaginal lesions to pararectal and presacral nodes.
    D. Upper two-thirds of vagina can spread to bladder.

82. What is the 5-year pelvic control rate of a FIGO stage I vaginal cancer treated with radical radiotherapy as reported by Frank et al.?
    A. 92 %
    B. 86 %
    C. 84 %
    D. 80 %

83. Which of the following statements regarding relapse site after primary treatment of vaginal cancers is incorrect?
    A. Most squamous cell cancers of the vagina fail locoregionally.
    B. Most melanomas of the vagina fail distantly.
    C. Clear cell adenocarcinomas of the vagina have a higher rate of distant relapse than squamous cell carcinomas of the vagina.
    D. Clear cell adenocarcinomas of the vagina most commonly fail locoregionally.

84. A 65-year-old woman presents with a 1.0 cm lesion on the vagina that extends onto the lower lip of the external cervical os. What is the correct FIGO stage?
    A. I
    B. IIA
    C. IIB
    D. III

85. Pelvic sidewall involvement in a vaginal cancer is what FIGO stage?
    A. IIA
    B. IIB
    C. III
    D. IVA

86. Which is the most common pathologic type of ovarian cancer?
    A. Germ cell tumors
    B. Serous cystadenocarcinoma
    C. Mucinous adenocarcinoma
    D. Endometrioid adenocarcinoma

87. All of the following are true regarding ovarian papillary serous carcinoma, except:
    A. These are associated with early lymphatic and myometrial invasion.
    B. Mixed tumors with <25 % papillary serous carcinoma behave like adenocarcinoma.
    C. Most failures are distant.
    D. Half have positive lymph nodes.

88. All of the following are true regarding borderline tumors of low malignant potential, except:
    A. Serous and mucinous are histological subtypes.
    B. Fertility drug use is a risk factor.
    C. These typically present with early-stage disease.
    D. Oral contraceptive use is a risk factor.

89. Which is the only type of ovarian tumor to always require postoperative radiotherapy?
    A. Dysgerminoma
    B. Serous cystadenocarcinoma
    C. Serous borderline tumor of low malignant potential
    D. Mucinous borderline tumor of low malignant potential

Answers and Rationales

1. The correct answer is B. T1a disease is limited to microscopically identified disease limited to <5 mm depth and >7 mm in horizontal spread. T1b disease is clinically visible and further classified based on size ≤ or >4 cm. T2 and T3 disease can be thought of in a similar fashion with T2a and T3a involving the upper two third and lower one third of the vagina, respectively, and T2b and T3b involving the parametria and pelvic sidewall, respectively. Hydronephrosis is classified as T3b even without sidewall involvement. AJCC 7th edition staging remained relatively unchanged to the AJCC 6th edition staging with the exception of further clarifying T2a into T2a1 and T2a2 based on size ≤ or > 4 cm. Age, histology, HPV status, and LVSI are not accounted for in cervical cancer staging. Edge SB, Byrd DR, Compton CC, et al., editors. Cervix uteri. AJCC cancer staging handbook. 7th ed. New York, NY: Springer; 2010.

2. The correct answer is D. HPV 16 and 18 are identified as the cause of 70 % of cervical cancer diagnoses. HPV 16 and 18 have been strongly associated with cervical malignancies, whereas types 6 and 11 are associated with benign condylomata and low- grade abnormalities. Risk factors for HPV infection and subsequent cervical cancer include early age at first coitus, multiple sex partners, multiparity, and previous STDs. Diethylstilbestrol (DES) exposure in utero is associated with clear cell carcinoma of the cervix. Hariri S. Dunne E. Human papillomavirus: Chapter 5-1. In. Roush SW, McIntire L, editors. Centers for disease control and prevention. Manual for the surveillance of vaccine-preventable diseases. Atlanta, GA: Centers for disease control and prevention; 2011.

3. The correct answer is C. In June 2012, updated recommendations were released from both the United States Preventive Services Task Force (USPSTF) and from the partnership of the American Cancer Society/American Society for Colposcopy and Cervical Pathology/American Society for Clinical Pathology (ACS/ASCCP/ASCP). These new recommendations mark a change from previous recommendations for annual cancer screening. Importantly, those women less than 21 years of age (regardless of age of sexual initiation or other risk factors), as well as women over 65 years of age with adequate prior screening and not at high risk for cervical cancer, should not be screened. Screening was also not recommended for women "who have had a hysterectomy with removal of the cervix and who do not have a history of high-grade precancerous lesion (cervical intraepithelial neoplasia 2 or 3) or cervical cancer (D recommendation)." In women younger than 30, screening for cervical cancer with HPV testing, alone or in combination with cytology, is not recommended. Moyer V. On behalf of the U.S. preventive services task force. Screening for cervical cancer: U.S. Preventive services task force recommendation statement. Ann Intern Med. 2012;156(12):880–91.

4. The correct answer is A. The risk of both pelvic and para-aortic lymph node involvement has been shown to correlate with depth of invasion, parametrial involvement, angiolymphatic space invasion, and even age. Pelvic nodal involvement for stages IB, IIB, and IIIB is estimated at 15 %, 30 %, and 50 %, respectively. Generally speaking, the para-aortic risk is one-half that of pelvic nodal involvement. Lagasse LD et al. Results and complications of operative staging in cervical cancer: experience of the Gynecologic Oncology Group. Gynecol Oncol. 1980;9(1):90–8. Delgado G et al. A prospective surgical pathological study of stage I squamous carcinoma of the cervix: a Gynecologic Oncology Group Study. Gynecol Oncol. 1989;35(3):314–20.

5. The correct answer is C. Fagundes et al. published retrospective data for over 1,200 pts and found 10-year rates of distant metastases of 16 %, 31 %, 26 %, and 39 % for stages IB, IIA, IIB, and III, respectively. The most common site was lung, with the second most common being the para-aortics (22 %) and third being the bone (16 %). The most common bony site was the lumbothoracic spine. Other organic sites of disease included the liver, abdominal cavity, and GI tract. Fagundes H et al. Distant metastases after irradiation alone in carcinoma of the cervix. Int J Radiat Oncol Biol Phys. 1992;24(2):197–204.

6. The correct answer is B. Two large studies through the GOG found that the single most important prognostic variable was nodal involvement. One of these studies, by Stehman et al. (Cancer 1991), prospectively analyzed 626 pts and found para-aortic lymph node involvement overwhelmingly predicted relapse and survival. Other risk factors included tumor size, depth of invasion into the cervical stroma, and angiolymphatic invasion. Cell type, grade, and pretreatment hematocrit were not significant when accounting for these other factors. Many other studies as far back as 1983 however have established anemia as a significant prognostic factor. Stehman FB et al. Carcinoma of the cervix treated with radiation therapy. A multi-variate analysis of prognostic variables in the Gynecologic Oncology Group. Cancer. 1991;67(11):2776–85.

7. The correct answer is A. GOG 120 is a phase III trial which randomized 526 patients with advanced stage cervical cancer (FIGO IIB–IVA) without para-aortic involvement to radiation and one of three chemotherapy arms: (1) hydroxyurea alone (control arm), (2) hydroxyurea/cisplatin/5-FU, (3) cisplatin alone (40 mg/m^2 weekly during EBRT). Both cisplatin-based arms showed significantly improved 10-year PFS (46 % vs. 26 %) and 10-year OS (53 % vs. 34 %) compared to hydroxyurea alone. There was no added benefit to combined therapy compared to cisplatin alone, and the cisplatin-alone arm had significantly less acute toxicity compared to the three-drug regimen. There were no radiation-alone or chemotherapy-alone arms in this trial. Rose PG et al. Concurrent cisplatin-based radiotherapy and chemotherapy for locally advanced cervical cancer. N Engl J Med. 1999;340(15):1144–53.

8. The correct answer is B. RTOG 79-20 found improved OS but not DFS for extended-field RT. The authors suggest that this is a result of lower rates of first distant failure in the extended-field arm and improved outcomes in survival following first failure. Rotman et al. Prophylactic extended-field irradiation of para-aortic lymph nodes in stages IIB and bulky IB and IIA cervical carcinomas. Ten-year treatment results of RTOG 79-20. JAMA. 1995;274(5):387–93.

9. The correct answer is C. RTOG 90-01 randomized patients to either extended-field radiation alone (to include para-aortic nodes) or pelvic radiation with concurrent chemotherapy (cisplatin/5-FU). The addition of chemotherapy statistically significantly improved 5-year OS for the CRT arm (73 % vs. 58 %, $p=0.004$). GOG 120 compared chemoradiation with either hydroxyurea or a cisplatin-based regimen. GOG 123 compared neoadjuvant radiation (standard field) versus neoadjuvant chemoradiation. The NCIC trial compared definitive chemoradiation versus radiation alone, but the radiation was a standard pelvic field. The NCIC trial was the only trial of these four that did not show a survival advantage for chemoradiation. This trial has been criticized for its lack of surgical staging. Morris M et al. Pelvic radiation with concurrent chemotherapy compared with pelvic and para-aortic radiation for high-risk cervical cancer. N Engl J Med. 1999;340(15):1137–43. Rose PG et al. Concurrent cisplatin-based radiotherapy and chemotherapy for locally advanced cervical cancer. N Engl J Med. 1999;340(15):1144–53. Keys HM et al. Cisplatin, radiation, and adjuvant hysterectomy compared with radiation and adjuvant hysterectomy for bulky stage IB cervical carcinoma. N Engl J Med. 1999;340(15):1154–61. Pearcey R et al. Phase III trial comparing radical radiotherapy with and without cisplatin chemotherapy in patients with advanced squamous cell cancer of the cervix. J Clin Oncol. 2002;20(4):966–72.

10. The correct answer is D. GOG 123 examined pts with bulky early-stage disease (≥ 4 cm; stage IB2). Patients received EBRT to 45 Gy in 25 fractions followed by an LDR boost to cumulative dose of 75 Gy to point A and 55 Gy to point B. Chemotherapy was concurrent weekly cisplatin 40 mg/m^2×6. All patients subsequently went on to extrafascial hysterectomy (class I). There was a SS increase in pathologic CR for the chemoradiation arm (52 % vs. 41 %), 3-year OS (83 % vs. 74 %), LC, and PFS. Node-positive patients were excluded from this study. Keys HM et al. Cisplatin, radiation, and adjuvant hysterectomy compared with radiation and adjuvant hysterectomy for bulky stage IB cervical carcinoma. N Engl J Med. 1999;340(15):1154–61.

11. The correct answer is D. The Intergroup 0107 trial evaluated the benefit of adjuvant therapy after class III radical hysterectomy in 243 patients found to have high-risk pathologic features including positive pelvic nodes, positive margins, and/or positive parametrial involvement. Radiation alone consisted of 49.3 Gy in 29 fractions without a brachytherapy boost. Chemotherapy included both cisplatin and 5-FU delivered during days 1 and 22 of radiation, followed by an additional two cycles after the completion of radiation. There was a statistically significant

improvement in 4-year OS (81 % vs. 71 %, $p=0.007$) for chemoradiation versus RT alone. There was no difference in relapse patterns between the two groups. Peters WA et al. Concurrent chemotherapy and pelvic radiation therapy compared with pelvic radiation therapy alone as adjuvant therapy after radical surgery in high-risk early-stage cancer of the cervix. J Clin Oncol. 2000;18(8):1606–13.

12. The correct answer is A. Per Sedlis et al., tumor size >4 cm is an indication for postoperative radiation, not chemoradiation. Postoperative chemoradiation is indicated for positive lymph nodes, positive margins, or parametrial involvement (Peters et al.). Sedlis A et al. A randomized trial of pelvic radiation therapy versus no further therapy in selected patients with stage IB carcinoma of the cervix after radical hysterectomy and pelvic lymphadenectomy: a Gynecologic Oncology Group Study. Gynecol Oncol. 1999;73(2):177–83. Peters WA et al. Concurrent chemotherapy and pelvic radiation therapy compared with pelvic radiation therapy alone as adjuvant therapy after radical surgery in high-risk early-stage cancer of the cervix. J Clin Oncol. 2000;18(8):1606–13.

13. The correct answer is A. The NCIC trial was the only chemoradiation trial that did not find a PFS or OS benefit for the addition of chemotherapy to radiation. Multiple reasons have been formulated for this and include a lack of surgical staging, small sample size ($n = 259$), reduced hemoglobin in the chemoradiation arm (a known prognostic factor), and the omission of 5-FU to the chemotherapy regimen (synergistic). One suggestion for the lack of benefit was that cisplatin chemotherapy exerted its largest benefit in patients who receive suboptimal/prolonged radiation courses, but this is controversial. There was careful quality control of the radiation with requirements to complete radiation within 7 weeks. Pearcey R et al. Phase III trial comparing radical radiotherapy with and without cisplatin chemotherapy in patients with advanced squamous cell cancer of the cervix. J Clin Oncol. 2002;20(4):966–72.

14. The correct answer is B. Details of the classes of hysterectomies are as follows:

Class I (total abdominal hysterectomy; extrafascial): removal of cervix, small rim of vaginal cuff, and outside of the pubocervical fascia
Class II (modified radical hysterectomy; extended): unroofing of ureters to resect parametrial and paracervical tissue medial to ureters (cardinal and uterosacral ligaments) and vaginal cuff (1–2 cm)
Class III (radical abdominal hysterectomy; Wertheim-Meigs): mobilization of ureters, bladder, and rectum to remove parametrial tissue to pelvic sidewall and vaginal cuff (upper 1/3–1/2), and lymphadenectomy
Class IV (extended radical hysterectomy): removal of superior vesicular artery, part of ureter and bladder, and more vaginal cuff

Bermudez RS, Huang K, Hsu I-C. Cervical cancer. In: Hansen EW, Roach M, editors. Handbook of evidence-based radiation oncology. 2nd ed. New York: Springer; 2010.

15. The correct answer is A. A multicenter retrospective analysis of 605 patients sought to determine the importance of hemoglobin (Hgb) level. A cutoff level of 12 g/dL was used as the reference point. Both presenting and average weekly nadir Hgb correlated with LC, OS, and PFS on univariate analysis; only the weekly nadir was positive on multivariate analysis. Patients who were transfused to keep Hgb ≥12 g/dL had similar outcomes to untransfused patients with Hgb levels ≥12 g/dL (univariate analysis only). Patients with Hgb >12.0 g/dL had statistically significantly improved LC, OS, and DM. Five-year OS was 74 % for pts with Hgb >12.0 g/dL, 52 % for Hgb 11.0–11.9 g/dL, and 45 % for Hgb <11.0 g/dL ($p < 0.0001$). An attempted GOG phase III trial using transfusions and erythropoietin to maintain Hgb > 12.0–13.0 g/dL was closed prematurely due to an increased incidence of thromboembolic events. Grogan M et al. The important of hemoglobin levels during radiotherapy for carcinoma of the cervix. Cancer. 1999;86(8):1528–36.

16. The correct answer is D. The Landoni trial established radiation as a reasonable alternative to surgery for definitive treatment of early-stage cervical cancer. In this trial, 343 patients with stage IB/IIA disease were randomized to either surgery with radical hysterectomy + pelvic LND or definitive radiation with 47 Gy EBRT followed by a brachytherapy boost to 76 Gy to point A. Adjuvant radiotherapy to 50.4 Gy was allowed for high-risk pathologic factors (stage > IIA, <3 mm uninvolved stroma, +margins, or +LN). In total, 63 % of patients in the surgery arm received adjuvant RT. There was no difference in 5-year OS (83 %), DFS (74 %), or recurrence (25 %) between the two arms. Severe morbidity however was worse in the surgery +/− RT arm (28 % vs. 12 %). Landoni F et al. Randomised study of radical surgery versus radiotherapy for stage Ib-IIa cervical cancer. Lancet. 1997;350(9077):535–40.

17. The correct answer is C. Conization may be a reasonable option for women with preinvasive disease when ablative treatment is contraindicated, as is the case if the entire transformation zone has not been well visualized, if there is marked discrepancy between Pap smear results and colposcopy or if colposcopy evaluation with biopsies leaves unresolved the presence of invasive disease. It may also be reasonable for a select group of women with FIGO stage IA microinvasive disease who wish to maintain fertility and who agree to close follow-up. Conization is NOT appropriate for IB disease. Brachytherapy is recommended for surgically inoperable patients with reported 10-year progression-free survival of 98–100 %. Age by itself is not a factor when considering the appropriateness of conization. Koh W, Moore DH. Cervical cancer. In Gunderson LL, Tepper JE, editors. Clinical radiation oncology. 3rd ed. Philadelphia: Elsevier Saunders; 2012. p. 1183–213.

18. The correct answer is A. GOG 92 is a phase III RCT which randomized patients s/p radical hysterectomy + PLND with negative lymph nodes to adjuvant RT if they had two or more of the following risk factors: >1/3 stromal invasion, +ALI,

or size >4 cm versus observation. RT was to 46–50.4 Gy EBRT delivered over 23–28 fractions. The most recent update in 2006 shows a reduction in local recurrence with the addition of postoperative radiation (20.7 vs.13.9 %), though adjuvant RT did not improve OS (RT 97 %, observation 91 %; $p = 0.074$). Sedlis A et al. A randomized trial of pelvic radiation therapy versus no further therapy in selected patients with stage IB carcinoma of the cervix after radical hysterectomy and pelvic lymphadenectomy: a Gynecologic Oncology Group Study. Gynecol Oncol. 1999;73(2):177–83. Rotman M et al. A phase III randomized trial of postoperative pelvic irradiation in Stage IB cervical carcinoma with poor prognostic features: follow-up of a gynecologic oncology group study. Int J Radiat Oncol Biol Phys. 2006;65(1):169–76.

19. The correct answer is D. GOG 71 was a phase III trial evaluating the benefit of adjuvant extrafascial hysterectomy (type I) following radiation for bulky stage IB tumors. This study found a trend for improved 5-year LC for the hysterectomy arm (27 % vs. 14 %) but did not find an OS benefit. Subset analysis did suggest an OS benefit for adjuvant hysterectomy in women with tumors <7 cm (RR 0.60; $p = 0.007$) with worse outcomes for tumors >7 cm (RR 2.03). The authors recognize that the study was not powered to evaluate survival as a function of tumor size. G3/G4 toxicity was similar (10 %) between treatment groups. Keys HM et al. Radiation therapy with and without extrafascial hysterectomy for bulky stage IB cervical carcinoma: a randomized trial of Gynecologic Oncology Group. Gynecol Oncol. 2003;89(3):343–453.

20. Spanos et al. initially published a trial of 1,000 cGy × 1 delivered three times with 4-week intervals and found unacceptably high late GI toxicity (35–40 %; RTOG 79-05). They therefore attempted a second trial using 370 cGy × 4 fractions delivered BID × 3 courses to a total of 4,400 cGy based on a linear-quadratic model of acute and late toxicities. With this dose and fractionation, they found a significant reduction in toxicity without a reduction in tumor control. Spanos WJ et al. Radiation palliation of cervical cancer. J Natl Cancer Inst Monogr. 1996;(21):127–30.

21. The correct answer is D. Point A is defined as 2 cm superior and 2 cm lateral to the cervical os along the axis of the tandem or midline and approximates where the uterine vessels cross the ureter. Point B is defined as 2 cm superior and 5 cm lateral to the cervical os along the midline of the patient and approximates the pelvic sidewall. Tod M, Meredith W. Treatment of cancer of the cervix uteri- a revised "Manchester method". Br J Radiol. 1953;(26): 252–57.

22. The correct answer is B. The recommended dose rate to point A using LDR brachytherapy is 50 cGy/h. ICRU 38 (1985) Dose and Volume Specification for Reporting Intracavitary Therapy in Gynecology.

23. The correct answer is B. The GOG recommends a total of 85 Gy, which is accounted for by the combination of 45 Gy delivered by EBRT plus either 40 Gy LDR or 30 Gy HDR (6 Gy×5 which using the LQ model equates to a biological equivalent dose of 40 Gy LDR).

24. The correct answer is C. There is no evidence that the larger HDR fractions improve the therapeutic ratio. With larger fractions, there is the possibility of a reduction in the therapeutic ratio between tumor control and normal tissue toxicity. LDR allows for sublethal repair thus potentially improving toxicity to normal tissue. HDR does offer increased control in terms of optimization of dwell positions and perhaps dose optimization. Clear benefits of HDR include reduced radiation exposure to personnel and reduced hospitalization. Eifel PJ. High-dose-rate brachytherapy for carcinoma of the cervix: high tech or high risk? Int J Radiat Oncol Biol Phys. 1992;24 (2):383–86; discussion 387–388. Lertsanguansinchai P et al. Phase III randomized trial comparing LDR and HDR brachytherapy in treatment of cervical carcinoma. Int J Radiat Oncol Biol Phys. 2004;59(5):1424–31.

25. The correct answer is B. Inability to see or feel the cervical os, vaginal disease thicker than 5 mm, and persistent, palpable disease on the pelvic sidewall are all situations in which interstitial brachytherapy is preferred over intracavitary brachytherapy boost. Bulky lesions, a narrow vagina, and lower vaginal extension are also indications for interstitial brachytherapy. Nag S et al. The American brachytherapy society recommendations for high-dose-rate brachytherapy for carcinoma of the cervix. Int J Radiat Oncol Biol Phys. 2000;48:201–11.

26. The correct answer is D. In HDR, target rectal point dose limits are 70 % of the daily fraction dose to point A, based on biological equivalency dosing to late reacting tissues ($\alpha/\beta=3$). Viani GA et al. Brachytherapy for cervix cancer: low-dose rate or high-dose rate brachytherapy—a meta-analysis of clinical trials. J Exp Clin Cancer Res. 2009;28(1):47.

27. The correct answer is B. Prolonging a course of radiotherapy beyond approximately 7 weeks is associated with a 1 % decrease in pelvic control per extra day. Lanciano RM et al. The influence of treatment time on outcome for squamous cell cancer of the uterine cervix treated with radiation: a patterns-of-care study. Int J Radiat Oncol Biol Phys. 1993;25(3):391–97.

28. The correct answer is A. In the United States, endometrial cancer is the most common gynecologic malignancy and the fourth most common malignancy in women overall. Incidence rates in the USA are 25 per 100,000 and this represents the highest rate in the world. In 2012, there will be 47,130 estimated new cases of endometrial cancer, with 8,010 estimated deaths. The incidence in European countries is 20 per 100,000 and is lower in the rest of the world. Jemal A et al. Cancer statistics, 2006. CA Cancer J Clin. 2006;56:106–30. American Cancer Society. Cancer Facts and Figures 2012.

29. The correct answer is B. Risk factors for endometrial cancer are most commonly related to unopposed estrogen. Sources of unopposed estrogen include nulliparity, early menarche, late menopause, obesity, and oral contraceptive use. Tamoxifen is an estrogen receptor antagonist in the breast but is a weak agonist in the endometrium. Gambrell RD Jr. et al. Role of estrogens and progesterone in the etiology and prevention of endometrial cancer: review. Am J Obstet Gyneol. 1983;146:696–707. Purdie DM, Green AC. Epidemiology of endometrial cancer. Best Pract Res Clin Obstet Gynaecol. 2001;15:341–54. Shapiro S et al. Risk of localized and widespread endometrial cancer in relation to recent and discontinued use of conjugated estrogens. New Engl J Med. 1985;313:969–72. Fisher B et al. Endometrial cancer in tamoxifen-treated breast cancer patients: findings from the National Surgical Adjuvant Breast and Bowel Project (NSABP) B-14. J Natl Cancer Inst. 1994;86:527–37.

30. The correct answer is C. Women with Lynch II syndrome are at a significantly increased risk of developing endometrial cancer with as much as a 60 % risk by age 60. Polycystic ovarian syndrome (PCOS) is thought to increase risk through the unopposed estrogen in anovulation. The most common extra-gastrointestinal malignancies in Peutz-Jeghers syndrome are gynecologic. Cowden syndrome is a rare autosomal dominant syndrome with mutation in the *PTEN* tumor suppressor gene; women with this syndrome have an approximate 20–25 % lifetime risk of endometrial cancer. Those with Von Hippel-Lindau disease have an increased risk of renal cell carcinoma, hemangioblastomas, pheochromocytomas, and neuroendocrine tumors of the pancreas but are not associated with increased risk of endometrial cancer. Aarnio M et al. Cancer risk in mutation carriers of DNA-mismatch- repair genes. Int J Cancer. 1999;81:214–18. Wijnen J et al. Familial endometrial cancer in female carriers of MSH6 germline mutations. Nat Genet. 1999;23:142–44. Lynch HT et al. Genetics, natural history, tumor spectrum, and pathology of hereditary nonpolyposis colorectal cancer: an updated review. Gastroenterology. 1993;104:1535–49.

31. The correct answer is A. The majority (almost three-quarters) of patients with endometrial cancer present with early, uterine-confined stage I disease. Creutzberg CL, Fleming GF. Endometrial cancer. In Gunderson LL, Tepper JE, editors. Clinical radiation oncology. 3rd ed. Philadelphia: Elsevier Saunders;2012. 1215–39.

32. The correct answer is C. Endometrial hyperplasia often, but not always, precedes endometrial carcinoma. Hyperplasia is designated as simple and complex based on cellular architecture. Both can be associated with atypia. Prophylactic hysterectomy is recommended for any woman with hyperplasia with atypia because of the cancer risk. Progression from simple hyperplasia to carcinoma is rare (<2 %), but any hyperplasia with atypia carries a 30–40 % risk of progression to carcinoma. Kurman RJ et al. The behavior of endometrial hyperplasia. A long-term study of "untreated" hyperplasia in 170 patients. Cancer. 1985;56:403–12. Lindahl B, Willen R. Spontaneous endometrial hyperplasia; a

prospective, 5 year follow-up of 246 patients after abrasio only, including 380 patients followed up for 2 years. Anticancer Res. 1994;14: 2141–46. Baloglu H et al. Atypical endometrial hyperplasia shares genomic abnormalities with endometrioid carcinoma by comparative genomic hybridization. Hum Pathol. 2001;32: 615–22.

33. The correct answer is D. Endometrioid adenocarcinomas include answer choices A–C and compromise 75 % of all endometrial cancers. Non-endometrioid adenocarcinomas include serous, mucinous, and clear cell carcinomas. They have a poorer prognosis, similar to a grade III endometrioid carcinoma, and are often diagnosed at a more advanced stage with a higher risk of intra-abdominal dissemination. Serous adenocarcinoma is also referred to as uterine papillary serous carcinoma (UPSC). Kurman RF, editor. Blaustein's pathology of the female genital tract: endometrial carcinoma. 4th ed. New York: Springer-Verlag; 1994. p. 439–86. Christopherson WM et al. Carcinoma of the endometrium. V. An analysis of prognosticators in patients with favorable subtypes and stage I disease. Cancer. 1983;51:1705–09. Hendrickson M et al. Uterine papillary serous carcinoma: a highly malignant form of endometrial adenocarcinoma. Am J Surg Pathol. 1982;6:93–108. Eifel PJ et al. Adenocarcinoma of the endometrium. Analysis of 256 cases with disease limited to the uterine corpus: treatment comparisons. Cancer. 1983;52:1026–31.

34. The correct answer is A. Type I endometrial cancers are typically low-grade, estrogen-dependent endometrioid-type cancers with a good prognosis. They tend to be preceded by hyperplasia. Type II tumors are estrogen independent, high grade, and are often found in atrophic endometrium. They are preceded by intraepithelial carcinoma and often serous and clear cell carcinomas. They are frequently seen in older, postmenopausal women and have a poor prognosis. Ambros RA et al. Endometrial intraepithelial carcinoma: a distinctive lesion specifically associated with tumors displaying serous differentiation. Hum Pathol. 1995;26:1260–67.

35. The correct answer is B. HER2 mutations have been identified in up to 80 % of serous adenocarcinomas (UPSC) making Herceptin (trastuzumab), a monoclonal antibody to HER2, a promising therapy. Erlotinib and cetuximab are EGFR tyrosine kinase inhibitors, which may also have some activity against type II endometrial cancers but are not related to HER2. Tamoxifen has weak estrogen receptor agonist activity and is a risk factor for type I endometrial adenocarcinomas. It has no clinical benefit in endometrial cancer. Khalifa MA et al. Expression of EGFR, HER-2/neu, P53, and PCNA in endometrioid, serous papillary, and clear cell endometrial adenocarcinoma. Gynecol Oncol. 1994;53:84–92. Jasas KV et al. Phase II study of erlotinib (OSI 774) in women with recurrent or metastatic endometrial cancer: NCIC CTG IND-148. 2004 ASCO annual meetings proceedings. J Clin Oncol. 2005; 5019.

36. The correct answer is A. Staging for endometrial cancer is surgical, as opposed to the clinical staging of cervical cancer. IA is <50 % myometrial invasion, IB ≥50 % myometrial invasion. This changed from the AJCC 6th edition. IC is no longer a category. Stage II includes cervical stromal involvement without extension beyond the uterus; endocervical involvement is no longer stage IIA and is now still considered stage I disease. IIIA involves serosa/adnexa; IIIB is vaginal involvement. Pelvic and para-aortic nodal involvement is staged IIIC1 and IIIC2, respectively. This subdivision is new compared to prior staging. Stage IVA includes bladder and bowel involvement. IVB is for M1 disease. Uterine sarcomas are now staged uniquely. Grade is not taken into consideration for staging. Edge SB, Byrd DR, Compton CC, et al., editors. Corpus uteri. AJCC cancer staging handbook. 7th ed. New York: Springer; 2010.

37. The correct answer is D. The AJCC 7th edition T stage for this pt with ≥50 % depth invasion without invasion of other structures remains T1b regardless of nodal positivity. Presence of para-aortic nodes, regardless of pelvic nodal status, is N2. T1bN2 disease is consistent with FIGO stage IIIC2. Edge SB, Byrd DR, Compton CC, et al., editors. Corpus uteri. AJCC cancer staging handbook. 7th ed. New York: Springer; 2010.

38. The correct answer is C. GOG 33 (Creasman et al.) was a landmark prospective surgical trial of 1,180 patients that examined pelvic and para-aortic node positivity based on grade and depth of invasion (clinical stage). Nodal risk for stage I disease can be estimated by multiplying the grade (1, 2, or 3) with the stage (IA=1, IB=2, IC=3) times three (rule of 3s). In this question, the pelvic nodal risk would be $2 \times 3 \times 3 = 18$. In GOG 33, the reported IC, grade 2 pelvic lymph node positivity was reported as 19 %. Para-aortic risk is approximately two third that of the estimated pelvic nodal risk. Creasman WT et al. Surgical pathologic spread patterns of endometrial cancer. A Gynecologic Oncology Group Study. Cancer. 1987;60 (Suppl 8):2035–41.

39. The correct answer is D. The MRC ASTEC trial randomized 1,408 women with clinically suspected uterine-confined disease to TAH/BSO/pelvic washings/ PALN palpation +/− lymphadenectomy to assess for therapeutic advantage of additional lymph node sampling. With adjustment for baseline characteristics and pathology, there was no overall or progression-free survival benefit for the addition of lymphadenectomy. The avoidance of lymphadenectomy and use of adjuvant RT was also supported by similar outcomes of the PORTEC-1 and GOG 99 trials. The PORTEC-1 trial did not include lymphadenectomy and had similar LRR and OS and lower toxicity compared to pts in the GOG 99 trial. Patients at intermediate/high risk (high grade, IC/IIA) were subsequently randomized to the ASTEC adjuvant radiation trial. Kitchener H et al. Efficacy of systematic pelvic lymphadenectomy in endometrial cancer (MRC ASTEC trial): a randomized study. Lancet. 2009;373(9658):125–36.

40. The correct answer is A. The Norwegian Aalders trial randomized 540 women with stage I adenocarcinoma after hysterectomy + vaginal cuff brachytherapy with LDR to 60 Gy prescribed to the surface to +/− whole pelvis RT to 40 Gy in 20 fractions with a midline block after 20 Gy. This trial did not include HDR brachytherapy. Aalders J et al. Postoperative external irradiation and prognostic parameters in stage I endometrial carcinoma: clinical and histopathologic study of 540 patients. Obstet Gynecol. 1980;56(4):419–27.

41. The correct answer is A. The addition of WPRT to surgery + VC LDR brachytherapy resulted in a statistically significant decrease in LRR from 7 % to 2 % with the addition of whole pelvis RT (WPRT). There was no OS benefit for the groups overall (90 % for both groups) which was explained by an increase in DM rate for the WPRT arm (5 % vs. 10 %). However, a subset analysis revealed that in the IC, grade 3 group, overall survival was improved with the addition of WPRT (82 % vs. 72 %), due to the large LR benefit (20 % vs. 5 % with WPRT). Aalders J et al. Postoperative external irradiation and prognostic parameters in stage I endometrial carcinoma: clinical and histopathologic study of 540 patients. Obstet Gynecol. 1980;56(4):419–27.

42. The correct answer is D. The PORTEC-1 trial included all patients with grade 1 and ≥50 myometrial invasion, grade 2 with any invasion, and grade 3 with ≤50 % myometrial invasion. IC, grade 3 patients were excluded. Stage II disease was included in PORTEC-2, not PORTEC-1. Creutzberg CL et al. Surgery and postoperative radiotherapy versus surgery alone for patients with stage-1 endometrial carcinoma: multicentre randomized trial. PORTEC Study Group. Post Operative Radiation Therapy in Endometrial Carcinoma. Lancet. 2000;355(9213):1401–11.

43. The correct answer is C. Almost three-quarters (73 %) of failures were in the vaginal vault. Creutzberg CL et al. Surgery and postoperative radiotherapy versus surgery alone for patients with stage-1 endometrial carcinoma: multicentre randomized trial. PORTEC Study Group. Post Operative Radiation Therapy in Endometrial Carcinoma. Lancet. 2000;355(9213):1401–11.

44. The correct answer is C. The PORTEC-1 trial randomized women post TAH-BSO to either observation or EBRT to 46 Gy in 23 fractions. The EBRT arm had improved 5-year LC (14 % → 5 %) without an improvement in 10-year overall survival. Women with stage IB, G2 tumors were found to have extremely low LRR (5 %). Risk factors for relapse were high grade, >50 % myometrial invasion, and age >60 year. The latest update at 15 years still shows a local control benefit for the addition of radiation, though these patients had significant increases in urinary incontinence, diarrhea, fecal leakage, and limitation in daily activity. Foil A was the randomization for the Aalders trial. Foil B was the randomization for PORTEC-2. Creutzberg CL et al. Surgery and postoperative radiotherapy versus surgery alone for patients with stage-1 endometrial

carcinoma: multicentre randomized trial. PORTEC Study Group. Post Operative Radiation Therapy in Endometrial Carcinoma. Lancet. 2000;355(9213):1401–11. Nout RA et al. Long-term outcome and quality of life of patients with endometrial carcinoma treated with or without pelvic radiotherapy in the Post Operative Radiation Therapy in Endometrial Carcinoma 1 (PORTEC-1) Trial. J Clin Oncol. 2011;29(13):1692–1700.

45. The correct answer is B. GOG 99 defined a high-intermediate-risk group (HIR) based on age and three risk factors: grade 2 or 3, outer one third myometrial invasion (MMI), and the presence of lymphovascular space invasion (LVSI). The HIR group was defined by answer choices A, C, and D. The low-intermediate-risk (LIR) group included anyone who did not fit the definition of HIR. All patients in this trial were surgical candidates and all underwent TAH-BSO prior to randomization to either observation or EBRT. This definition differed from the high-risk group in the PORTEC trials which defined high risk as having any two of the following: age >60, grade 3, or >50 % MMI for PORTEC-1 and age >60 and stage IC G1-2 or stage IB G3, or any age and stage IIA grade 1–2 or stage IIA grade 3 with <50 % MMI for PORTEC-2. Keys HM et al. A phase III trial of surgery with or without adjunctive external pelvic radiation therapy in intermediate-risk endometrial adenocarcinoma: a Gynecologic Oncology Group study. Gynecol Oncol. 2004;92(3):744–51.

46. The correct answer choice is C. Both intermediate and high-grade tumors were considered as risk factors. Remember that tumors had to have >2/3 myometrial invasion reaching the outer one third of the myometrium to be considered HIR. Lymphovascular space invasion was also considered a risk factor in the HIR category. Keys HM et al. A phase III trial of surgery with or without adjunctive external pelvic radiation therapy in intermediate-risk endometrial adenocarcinoma: a Gynecologic Oncology Group study. Gynecol Oncol. 2004;92(3):744–51.

47. The correct answer is B. The GOG 99 trial showed improved recurrence rates with adjuvant RT compared to observation following TAH-BSO + lymphadenectomy for stage IB, IC, or IIA disease. Overall recurrence rate improved from 12 % to 3 % (foil A). The HIR subgroup showed the largest benefit from 26 % to 6 %. The LIR subgroup showed the smallest benefit (6 % vs. 2 %; foil C). These results are very similar to the PORTEC-1 trial, which did not include lymphadenectomy, an important difference between the two trials. Keys HM et al. A phase III trial of surgery with or without adjunctive external pelvic radiation therapy in intermediate-risk endometrial adenocarcinoma: a Gynecologic Oncology Group study. Gynecol Oncol. 2004;92(3):744–51.

48. The correct answer is B. The PORTEC-2 trial randomized 427 women with HIR disease (age ≥60 and stage IC, G1-2 or stage IB, G3, or any age and stage IIA grade 1–2 or stage IIA grade 3 with <50 % MMI) to receive either adjuvant vaginal brachytherapy (VBT – 21Gy HDR in three fractions or 30 Gy LDR) or

whole pelvis radiation therapy (WPRT – 46 Gy/23 fractions). With a median follow-up of 45 months, disease-free survival and overall survival were not different (84.8 % vs. 79.6 %, $p = 0.57$). WPRT reduced isolated pelvic recurrence from 1.5 % to 0.5 %, but the 5-year rates of vaginal cuff recurrence were not different—1.8 % VBT (95 % CI 0.6–5.9) versus 1.6 % WPRT (95 % CI 0.5–4.9), $p = 0.74$. The prospectively obtained patient reported quality of life scores were higher in the VBT arm. At the completion of radiotherapy, reported acute grade 1–2 GI toxicity was 15 % versus 54 % favoring the brachytherapy arm. Nout RA et al. Vaginal brachytherapy versus pelvic external beam radiotherapy for patients with endometrial cancer of high- intermediate risk (PORTEC-2): an open-label, non-inferiority, randomised trial. Lancet. 2010;375(9717):816–23.

49. The correct answer is A. The GOG 122 trial randomized women with advanced stage endometrial cancer to either whole abdomen radiation therapy (WART) (30 Gy/20 fractions + 15 Gy pelvic boost) or chemotherapy with doxorubicin and cisplatin q3 week×7 cycles followed by a single cycle of cisplatin alone. The radiation arm did include a 15 Gy para-aortic boost for pelvic LN+ or the lack of lymph node sampling during surgery. The chemotherapy arm had improved 5-year overall survival and disease-free survival compared to WART, but did have increased grade 3/4 gastrointestinal, hematologic, and cardiac toxicity. Treatment-related deaths were 4 % for chemo and 2 % for WART. Randall ME et al. Randomized phase III trial of whole-abdominal irradiation versus doxorubicin and cisplatin chemotherapy in advanced endometrial carcinoma: a Gynecologic Oncology Group Study. J Clin Oncol. 2006;24(1):36–44.

50. The correct answer is D. The GOG 122 trial showed superior DFS and OS for chemotherapy alone compared to WART alone, but pelvic relapse rates were very high (55 %). The Ontario Canada group trial examined carboplatin/paclitaxel q3 week×4 cycles followed by pelvic radiotherapy to 45 Gy followed by two additional cycles of carbo/taxol. Two-year disease-free survival and overall survival were 55 % (similar to GOG 122), but pelvic relapse rates were extremely low (3 %). Randall ME et al. Randomized phase III trial of whole-abdominal irradiation versus doxorubicin and cisplatin chemotherapy in advanced endometrial carcinoma: a Gynecologic Oncology Group Study. J Clin Oncol. 2006;24(1):36–44. Lupe K et al. Adjuvant paclitaxel and carboplatin chemotherapy with involved field radiation in advanced endometrial cancer: a sequential approach. Int J Radiat Oncol Biol Phys. 2007;67:110–6.

51. The correct answer is A. Carcinosarcoma, or malignant mixed mullerian tumor (MMMT), is the most common type of uterine sarcoma (45 %). Leiomyosarcomas are second most common (40 %) and endometrial stromal sarcomas are third most common (10–15 %). All other forms are rare. Kurman RF, editor. Blaustein's pathology of the female genital tract: endometrial carcinoma. 4th ed. New York: Springer-Verlag; 1994. p. 439–86. Brooks SE et al. Surveillance, epidemiology, and end results analysis of 2,677 cases of uterine sarcoma 1989–1999. Gynecol Oncol. 2004;93(1):204.

52. The correct answer is C. There is no benefit of lymphadenectomy (per MRC ASTEC) and pelvic RT is generally recommended when surgical staging has not been performed. Chemotherapy alone has similar outcomes to RT alone in advanced stage endometrial cancer, but LRR remains unacceptably high. Involvement of the cervix necessitates the addition of VC brachytherapy to WPRT. Creutzberg CL et al. PORTEC Study Group. Fifteen-year radiotherapy outcomes of the randomized PORTEC-1 trial for endometrial carcinoma. Int J Radiat Oncol Biol Phys. 2001;81(4):631–38. Barton DP et al. Efficacy of systematic pelvic lymphadenectomy in endometrial cancer (MRC ASTEC Trial): a randomized study. Int J Gynecol Cancer. 2009;19(8):1465.

53. The correct answer is D. The upper vaginal mucosa can tolerate doses up to 140 Gy. The lower two-thirds of the vaginal mucosa should be limited to 80–85 Gy. Remember that typical point A doses reach 85–95 Gy with vaginal wall doses reaching nearly 150 % of the prescription dose. Fletcher GH. Textbook of radiotherapy. Philadelphia: Lea & Febiger; 1992. Eifel PJ et al. Radiation therapy for cervical carcinoma. In Dilts PV Jr, Sciarra JJ, editors. Gynecology and obstetrics. Philadelphia: JB Lippincott; 1993. p. 1–25.

54. The correct answer is D. Leiomyosarcoma is the second most common uterine sarcoma, tends to present at earlier stages, and tends to fail in the lung. Carcinosarcoma, also known as mixed mullerian tumor, is the most common uterine sarcoma and tends to fail in the lymph nodes. The addition of postoperative radiotherapy improves locoregional control, but does not improve overall survival. Brooks SE et al. Surveillance, epidemiology, and end results analysis of 2,677 cases of uterine sarcoma 1989–1999. Gynecol Oncol. 2004;93(1):204. Gertszten K et al. The impact of adjuvant radiotherapy on carcinoma of the uterus. Gynecol Oncol. 1998;68:8–13. Salazar OM et al. Uterine sarcoma: analysis of failures with special emphasis on the use of adjuvant radiation therapy. Cancer. 1978;42:1161–70.

55. The correct answer is C. The other pairings are correct. Creutzberg CL, Fleming GF. Endometrial cancer. In Gunderson LL, Tepper JE, editors. Clinical radiation oncology. 3rd ed. Philadelphia: Elsevier Saunders; 2012. p. 1215–39.

56. The correct answer is B. The 5-year survival for FIGO stage II vulvar cancer is 77 %. The 5-year survival for FIGO stages I–IV is 90 %, 77 %, 51 %, and 18 %, respectively. Benedet JL et al. Squamous carcinoma of the vulva: results of treatment 1938–1976. Am J Obstet Gynecol. 1979;134:201–7. Boutselis JG. Radical vulvectomy for invasive squamous cell carcinoma of the vulva. Obstet Gynecol. 1972;39:827–36. Cavanaugh D, Shepherd JH. The place of pelvic exenteration in the primary management of advanced carcinoma of the vulva. Gynecol Oncol. 1982;13:318–22. Hacker NF et al. Management of regional lymph nodes and their prognostic influence in vulvar cancer. Obstet Gynecol. 1983;61:408–12. Morley GW: Infiltrative carcinoma of the vulva: results of surgical treatment. Am J Obstet Gynecol. 1976;874–88. Rutledge F et al. Carcinoma of the vulva. Am J Obstet Gynecol. 1970;106:1117–30.

57. The correct answer is A. Of all VIN-3 lesions, only 2–5 % progress to invasive carcinoma. Buscema J et al. Carcinoma in situ of the vulva. Obstet Gynecol. 1980;55:225–30.

58. The correct answer is C. Vulvar cancer is predominantly squamous cell in histology (80–90 %), though tumors of Bartholin's glands are more frequently adenocarcinoma. Melanoma is the second most common malignancy in the vulva. Poorly differentiated tumors with a trabecular, infiltrative pattern frequently metastasize to regional lymph nodes and should be considered for postoperative radiation after surgery. Verrucous cancers, though warty and exophytic, rarely metastasize to regional nodes and are treated with radical local excision. Foye G et al. Verrucous carcinoma of the vulva. Obstet Gynecol. 1969;34:484–8. Gallousis S. Verrucous carcinoma. Report of three vulvar cases and review of the literature. Obstet Gynecol. 1972;40:502–7. Russell AH. Cancer of the vulva. In Leibel SA, Phillips TL, editors. Textbook of radiation oncology. Philadelphia: WB Saunders; 2004. p. 1674. Gualco M et al. Morphologic and biologic studies on ten cases of verrucous carcinoma of the vulva supporting the theory of a discrete clinico-pathologic entity. In J Gynecol Cancer. 2003;13:317–24.

59. The correct answer is D. Heaps et al. reported their findings regarding surgical margin status and local recurrence. Of 115 patients that underwent resection for vulvar cancer, in those with surgical margins ≥8 mm, there were no local recurrences in 91 patients. In 44 patients with surgical margins <8 mm, 21 (48 %) recurred. Heaps JM et al. Surgical-pathologic variables predictive of local recurrence in squamous cell carcinoma of the vulva. Gynecol Oncol. 1990;38:309–14.

60. The correct answer is D. Heaps et al. reported their findings regarding surgical margin status and local recurrence. Of 115 patients that underwent resection for vulvar cancer, in those with surgical margins ≥8 mm, there were no local recurrences in 91 patients. In 44 patients with surgical margins <8 mm, 21 (48 %) recurred. Heaps JM et al. Surgical-pathologic variables predictive of local recurrence in squamous cell carcinoma of the vulva. Gynecol Oncol. 1990;38:309–14.

61. The correct answer is A. The first echelon lymph nodes for vulvar cancer are the inguinal lymph nodes. Russell AH, Van der Zee GJ. Vulvar and vaginal carcinoma. In Gunderson, LL, Tepper JE, editors. Clinical radiation oncology. 3rd ed. Philadelphia: Elsevier Saunders; 2012. p. 1241–76.

62. The correct answer is B. Women with either a vulvar or vaginal cancer have a fourfold risk of developing a secondary lung malignancy. Frisch M, Melbye M. Risk of lung cancer in pre- and post- menopausal women with anogenital malignancies. Int J Cancer. 1995;62:508–11.

63. The correct answer is B. Extramammary Paget's disease of the vulva is associated with a "cake-icing" appearance. Dubeuilh W. Paget's disease of the vulva. Brit J Dermatol. 1901;13:407.

64. The correct answer is B. In a vulvar cancer with negative ipsilateral lymphadenopathy, there is an approximately 3 % chance of positive contralateral lymphadenopathy. Stehman FB et al. Early stage I carcinoma of the vulva treated with ipsilateral superficial inguinal lymphadenectomy and modified radical hemivulvectomy: a prospective study of the Gynecologic Oncology Group. Obstet Gynecol. 1992;79:490–7. Hoffman JS et al. Microinvasive squamous carcinoma of the vulva: search for a definition. Obstet Gynecol. 1983;61:615–8. Burke TW et al. Radical wide excision and selective inguinal node dissection for squamous cell carcinoma of the vulva. Gynecol Oncol. 1990;38:328–32. Lin JY et al. Morbidity and recurrence with modifications of radical vulvectomy and groin dissection. Gynecol Oncol. 1992;47:80–6. Andrews SJ et al. Therapeutic implication of lymph nodal spread in lateral T1 and T2 squamous cell carcinoma of the vulva. Gynecol Oncol. 1994;55:41–6. Tham KF et al. Early vulval cancer: the place of conservative management. Eur J Surg Oncol. 1993;19:361–7. Farias- Eisner R et al. Conservative and individualized surgery for early squamous carcinoma of the vulva: the treatment of choice for Stage I and II (T1-2N0-1M0) disease. Gynecol Oncol. 1994;53:55–8.

65. The correct answer is D. With >5 mm depth of invasion in a vulvar primary, the risk of positive inguinal lymph node positivity is >35 %. Wilkinson EJ et al. Microinvasive carcinoma of the vulva. Int J Gynecol Pathol. 1982;1:29–39. Kneale BLG et al. Microinvasive carcinoma of the vulva: clinical features and management. In Coppleson M, editor. Gynecologic oncology. Edinburgh: Churchill Livingstone; 1981. p. 320. Hacker NF et al. Individualization of treatment of stage I squamous cell vulvar carcinoma. Obstet Gynecol. 1984;63:155–62. Magrina JF et al. Stage I squamous cell cancer of the vulva. Am J Obstet Gynecol. 1979;134:453–9. Parker RT et al. Operative management of early invasive epidermoid carcinoma of the vulva. Am J Obstet Gynecol. 1975;123:349–55. Hoffman JS et al. Microinvasive squamous carcinoma of the vulva: search for a definition. Obstet Gynecol. 1983;61:615–8.

66. The correct answer is C. The presence of two positive lymph nodes on groin dissection is an absolute indication for postoperative radiotherapy; as with ≥ 2 positive groin nodes, the risk of positive pelvic lymph nodes increases to 15–25 %. Benedet JL et al. Squamous carcinoma of the vulva: results of treatment 1938–1976. Am J Obstet Gynecol. 1979;134:201–7. Morley GW. Infiltrative carcinoma of the vulva: results of surgical treatment. Am J Obstet Gynecol. 1976;124:874–88. Rutledge F et al. Carcinoma of the vulva. Am J Obstet Gynecol. 1970;106:1117–30. Krupp PJ, Bohm JW. Lymph gland metastases in invasive squamous cell cancer of the vulva. Am J Obstet Gynecol. 1978;130:943–52.

67. The correct answer is D. GOG 88 (Stehman et al.) sought to determine if groin irradiation was superior to and less morbid than groin dissection in those with non-suspicious (N0-1) inguinal lymph nodes. Fifty-eight patients with T2-3 or T1 with +ALI, SCCA of the vulva, and non-suspicious groin nodes were randomized after radical vulvectomy to undergo either bilateral inguinofemoral groin dissection or radiotherapy to the groin (50 Gy/25 fractions, prescribed to 3 cm depth). Those with positive lymph nodes on groin dissection ($n = 5$) received 50 Gy to the groin and hemi-pelvis. After interim analysis showed excessive groin relapses in the radiation-alone arm, 18 % versus 0 % after groin dissection, the study was prematurely closed. Progression-free survival and overall survival were significantly better with groin dissection, ($p = 0.03$ and $p = 0.04$), respectively. A major criticism of this study was the poor radiation technique, as the groin radiation was prescribed to 3 cm depth from the surface, while the deep inguinal/femoral lymph nodes are located at 5–8 cm depth. Stehman et al. Groin dissection versus groin radiation in carcinoma of the vulva: a Gynecologic Oncology Group Study. Int J Radiat Oncol Biol Phys. 1992;24(2):389–96.

68. The correct answer is B. GOG 88 (Stehman et al.) sought to determine if groin irradiation was superior to and less morbid than groin dissection in those with non-suspicious (N0-1) inguinal lymph nodes. Fifty-eight patients with T2-3 or T1 with +ALI, SCCA of the vulva, and non-suspicious groin nodes were randomized after radical vulvectomy to undergo either bilateral inguinofemoral groin dissection or radiotherapy to the groin (50 Gy/25 fractions, prescribed to 3 cm depth). Those with positive lymph nodes on groin dissection ($n = 5$) received 50 Gy to the groin and hemi-pelvis. After interim analysis showed excessive groin relapses in the radiation-alone arm, 18 % versus 0 % after groin dissection, the study was prematurely closed. Progression-free survival and overall survival were significantly better with groin dissection, ($p = 0.03$ and $p = 0.04$), respectively. A major criticism of this study was the poor radiation technique, as the groin radiation was prescribed to 3 cm depth from the surface, while the deep inguinal/femoral lymph nodes are located at 5–8 cm depth. Stehman et al. Groin dissection versus groin radiation in carcinoma of the vulva: a Gynecologic Oncology Group Study. Int J Radiat Oncol Biol Phys. 1992;24(2):389–96.

69. The correct answer is B. GOG 88 (Stehman et al.) sought to determine if groin irradiation was superior to and less morbid than groin dissection in those with non-suspicious (N0-1) inguinal lymph nodes. Fifty-eight patients with T2-3 or T1 with +ALI, SCCA of the vulva, and non-suspicious groin nodes were randomized after radical vulvectomy to undergo either bilateral inguinofemoral groin dissection or radiotherapy to the groin (50 Gy/25 fractions, prescribed to 3 cm depth). Those with positive lymph nodes on groin dissection ($n = 5$) received 50 Gy to the groin and hemi-pelvis. After interim analysis showed

excessive groin relapses in the radiation-alone arm, 18 % versus 0 % after groin dissection, the study was prematurely closed. Progression-free survival and overall survival were significantly better with groin dissection, ($p = 0.03$ and $p = 0.04$), respectively. A major criticism of this study was the poor radiation technique, as the groin radiation was prescribed to 3 cm depth from the surface, while the deep inguinal/femoral lymph nodes are located at 5–8 cm depth. Stehman et al. Groin dissection versus groin radiation in carcinoma of the vulva: a Gynecologic Oncology Group Study. Int J Radiat Oncol Biol Phys. 1992;24(2):389–96.

70. The correct answer is C. GOG 37 (Homesley et al.) randomized 114 patients s/p radical vulvectomy and bilateral inguinal lymph node dissection with POSITIVE lymph nodes to undergo either bilateral pelvic lymph node dissection or bilateral inguinal and pelvic radiation (45–50 Gy). No radiation was given to the primary site. After interim analysis showed decreased groin recurrences in the radiation arm, 5 % versus 24 % with surgery alone, the study was prematurely closed. Disease-free survival and overall survival were improved with radiotherapy, especially in those with ≥2 + LNs, with the benefit due to the significant decrease in groin recurrences. The 6-year update in 2009 shows the persistent disease-free survival benefit and the overall survival benefit in those with cN2-3 disease and 2+ groin lymph nodes. Additionally, a significant benefit for radiotherapy was seen in those with ≥20 % ipsilateral + LN burden. Homesley HD et al. Radiation therapy versus pelvic node resection for carcinoma of the vulva with positive groin nodes. Obstet Gynecol. 1986;68(6):733–40. Kunos C et al. Radiation therapy compared with pelvic node resection for node-positive vulvar cancer: a randomized controlled trial. Obstet Gynecol. 2009;114(3):537–46.

71. The correct answer is A. GOG 37 (Homesley et al.) randomized 114 patients s/p radical vulvectomy and bilateral inguinal lymph node dissection with POSITIVE lymph nodes to undergo either bilateral pelvic lymph node dissection or bilateral inguinal and pelvic radiation (45–50 Gy). No radiation was given to the primary site. After interim analysis showed decreased groin recurrences in the radiation arm, 5 % versus 24 % with surgery alone, the study was prematurely closed. Disease-free survival and overall survival were improved with radiotherapy, especially in those with ≥2 + LNs, with the benefit due to the significant decrease in groin recurrences. The 6-year update in 2009 shows the persistent disease-free survival benefit and the overall survival benefit in those with cN2-3 disease and 2+ groin lymph nodes. Additionally, a significant benefit for radiotherapy was seen in those with ≥20 % ipsilateral + LN burden. Homesley HD et al. Radiation therapy versus pelvic node resection for carcinoma of the vulva with positive groin nodes. Obstet Gynecol. 1986;68(6):733–40. Kunos C et al. Radiation therapy compared with pelvic node resection for node-positive vulvar cancer: a randomized controlled trial. Obstet Gynecol. 2009;114(3):537–46.

72. The correct answer is B. GOG 37 (Homesley et al.) randomized 114 patients s/p radical vulvectomy and bilateral inguinal lymph node dissection with POSITIVE lymph nodes to undergo either bilateral pelvic lymph node dissection or bilateral inguinal and pelvic radiation (45–50 Gy). No radiation was given to the primary site. After interim analysis showed decreased groin recurrences in the radiation arm, 5 % versus 24 % with surgery alone, the study was prematurely closed. Disease-free survival and overall survival were improved with radiotherapy, especially in those with ≥2 + LNs, with the benefit due to the significant decrease in groin recurrences. The 6-year update in 2009 shows the persistent disease-free survival benefit and the overall survival benefit in those with cN2-3 disease and 2+ groin lymph nodes. Additionally, a significant benefit for radiotherapy was seen in those with ≥20 % ipsilateral + LN burden. Homesley HD et al. Radiation therapy versus pelvic node resection for carcinoma of the vulva with positive groin nodes. Obstet Gynecol. 1986;68(6):733–40. Kunos C et al. Radiation therapy compared with pelvic node resection for node-positive vulvar cancer: a randomized controlled trial. Obstet Gynecol. 2009;114(3):537–46.

73. The correct answer is D. The most common site of distant metastasis for vulvar cancer is the lung. Russell AH, Van der Zee GJ. Vulvar and vaginal carcinoma. In Gunderson LL, Tepper JE, editors. Clinical radiation oncology. 3rd ed. Philadelphia: Elsevier Saunders; 2012. p. 1241–76.

74. The correct answer is C. A single 2.5 cm vulvar lesion without lymphadenopathy would be stage IB. However, with 2 LNs measuring 4 mm, the correct FIGO stage is IIIA. Edge SB, Byrd DR, Compton CC, et al., editors. Vulva. AJCC cancer staging handbook. 7th ed. New York: Springer; 2010.

75. The correct answer is C. The presence of extracapsular extension in a mobile inguinal lymph node is FIGO stage IIIC. Edge SB, Byrd DR, Compton CC, et al., editors. Vulva. AJCC cancer staging handbook. 7th ed. New York: Springer; 2010.

76. The correct answer is C. Any fixed or ulcerated inguinal lymph node is FIGO stage IVA. Edge SB, Byrd DR, Compton CC, et al., editors. Vulva. AJCC cancer staging handbook. 7th ed. New York: Springer: 2010.

77. The correct answer is D. Para-aortic or pelvic adenopathy is FIGO stage IVB. Edge SB, Byrd DR, Compton CC, et al., editors. Vulva. AJCC cancer staging handbook. 7th ed. New York: Springer; 2010.

78. The correct answer is B. The clear cell variant of vaginal adenocarcinoma has been linked to in utero exposure of diethylstilbestrol (DES), with a peak age of presentation of 26 years. Most cases (90 %) are stage I/II at presentation. DES has been linked to both cervical and vaginal cancers, with the latter being more frequent. Herbst AL, Scully RE. Adenocarcinoma of the vaginal in

adolescence: analysis of 325 cases. Cancer. 1984;53:1978–84. Herbst AL. Diethylstilbestrol and adenocarcinoma of the vagina. Am J Obstet Gynecol. 1999;181:1576–8, discussion 1579.

79. The correct answer is A. Vaginal intraepithelial neoplasia is most commonly seen in the upper one third of the vagina. Russell AH, Van der Zee GJ. Vulvar and vaginal carcinoma. In Gunderson LL, Tepper JE, editors. Clinical radiation oncology. 3rd ed. Philadelphia: Elsevier Saunders; 2012. p. 1241–76.

80. The correct answer is B. Melanoma is the second most common histologic type of cancer seen in the vagina. Squamous cell carcinoma accounts for 80 % of vaginal lesions. Most adenocarcinomas found in the vagina are metastases from other primary sites, excluding primary clear cell adenocarcinomas. Russell AH, Van der Zee GJ. Vulvar and vaginal carcinoma. In Gunderson LL, Tepper JE, editors. Clinical radiation oncology. 3rd ed. Philadelphia: Elsevier Saunders: 2012. p. 1241–76.

81. The correct answer is A. The proximal third of vagina drains by obturator nodes to external iliac, hypogastric, and common iliac nodes. The lower third of the vagina drains first to the inguinal-femoral nodes, then pelvic nodes, necessitating treatment of the groins in lower one third vaginal cancers. Rectovaginal lesions can spread to pararectal and presacral nodes. Lesions in the upper two-thirds of the vagina can primarily spread to involve the bladder, rectum, or parametrium. Russell AH, Van der Zee GJ. Vulvar and vaginal carcinoma. In Gunderson LL, Tepper JE, editors. Clinical radiation oncology. 3rd ed. Philadelphia: Elsevier Saunders; 2012. p. 1241–76.

82. The correct answer is B. Frank et al. reported the results of primary irradiation in 193 previously untreated patients with vaginal cancer. The 5-year pelvic control rate of FIGO stage I cancers was 86 %, 84 % in FIGO stage II, and 69 % in FIGO stage III. Frank et al. Definitive radiation therapy for squamous cell carcinoma of the vagina. Int J Radiat Oncol Biol Phys. 2005;62:138–47.

83. The correct answer is B. Squamous cell carcinomas of the vagina, melanoma of the vagina, and clear cell adenocarcinoma of the vagina all tend to relapse locoregionally, rather than distantly. Clear cell adenocarcinoma does have a higher rate of distant metastasis compared to squamous cell carcinoma of the vagina. Frank et al. Definitive radiation therapy for squamous cell carcinoma of the vagina. Int J Radiat Oncol Biol Phys. 2005;62:138–47. Waggoner SE et al. Influence of in utero diethylstilbestrol exposure on the prognosis and biologic behavior of vaginal clear-cell adenocarcinoma. Gynecol Oncol. 1994;55:238–44.

84. The correct answer is B. Any cancer that involves the cervix is staged as a cervical cancer. Involvement of the upper two third of the vagina is FIGO stage IIA. Edge SB, Byrd DR, Compton CC, et al., editors. Vagina. AJCC cancer staging handbook. 7th ed. New York: Springer: 2010.

85. The correct answer is C. Pelvic sidewall involvement in vaginal cancer is FIGO stage III. Edge SB, Byrd DR, Compton CC, et al., editors. Vagina. AJCC cancer staging handbook. 7th ed. New York: Springer; 2010.

86. The correct answer is B. Serous cystadenocarcinoma is the most common pathological type of ovarian cancer, with 30 % of these occurring bilaterally. Elevation of CA-125 is commonly seen. Mucinous and endometrioid types each have an approximately 15 % incidence and tend to have better outcomes. Vicus D, Small Jr W, Covens A. Ovarian cancer. In Gunderson LL, Tepper JE, editors. Clinical radiation oncology. 3rd ed. Philadelphia: Elsevier Saunders; 2012. p. 1277–97.

87. The correct answer is C. Ovarian papillary serous carcinoma is frequently associated with early lymphatic and myometrial invasion, and 50 % have positive lymph nodes. Ovarian papillary serous carcinoma tends to spread intraperitoneally, and most failures occur in the abdomen, either alone or concurrently with other sites. Mixed tumors comprised of <25 % PSC behave more like adenocarcinoma, whereas those with >25 % PSC behave like the more aggressive PSC. Vicus D, Small Jr W, Covens A. Ovarian cancer. In Gunderson LL, Tepper JE, editors. Clinical radiation oncology. 3rd ed. Philadelphia: Elsevier Saunders; 2012. p. 1277–97.

88. The correct answer is D. Borderline ovarian tumors of low malignant potential comprise 15 % of overall ovarian tumors. There are two histological subtypes: serous and mucinous subtypes. While the use of fertility drugs is a risk factor for the development of borderline ovarian tumors of low malignant potential, oral contraceptive use and breastfeeding decrease the risk. These tumors tend to present with early-stage disease and large tumors. Serous type tumors are bilateral 35–75 % of the time. Vicus D, Small Jr W, Covens A. Ovarian cancer. In Gunderson LL, Tepper JE, editors. Clinical radiation oncology. 3rd ed. Philadelphia: Elsevier Saunders; 2012. p. 1277–97.

89. The correct answer is A. Dysgerminoma is the most common type of germ cell tumor and is bilateral 10 % of the time. These tumors occur most frequently in Asians and Blacks, and tend to present in the early 20s. This is the only ovarian tumor to always receive postoperative radiotherapy after bilateral salpingo-oophorectomy. Vicus D, Small Jr W, Covens A. Ovarian cancer. In Gunderson LL, Tepper JE, editors. Clinical radiation oncology. 3rd ed. Philadelphia: Elsevier Saunders; 2012. p. 1277–97.

Chapter 12
Hematologic Malignancies

Patrick J. Gagnon, Celine Bicquart Ord, and Carol Marquez

1. The International Prognostic Score (IPS) for advanced Hodgkin lymphoma includes all of the following except:
   A. Age ≥45
   B. Albumin < 3.5 g/dL
   C. Hemoglobin < 10.5 g/dL
   D. Leukocytosis defined as WBC > 15,000/mm^3

2. Lymphocyte-predominant Hodgkin lymphoma is most frequently characterized by the following typical immunophenotype:
   A. CD20+, CD45+, CD3−, CD15−, CD30−
   B. CD20+, CD45−, CD3−, CD15+, CD30+
   C. CD20−, CD45+, CD3+, CD15−, CD30+
   D. CD20−, CD45−, CD3+, CD15+, CD30−

P.J. Gagnon, MD, MS (✉)
Department of Radiation Oncology, Southcoast Centers for Cancer Care,
206 Mill Road, 02719 Fairhaven, MA, USA
e-mail: bceagles@gmail.com

C.B. Ord, MD
Department of Radiation Oncology, Scott & White Memorial Hospital,
2401 S. 31st Street, 76508 Temple, TX, USA
e-mail: cord@sw.org

C. Marquez, MD
Department of Radiation Medicine, Oregon Health and Science University,
3181 SW Sam Jackson Park Rd, KPV4, 97239 Portland, OR, USA
e-mail: marquezc@ohsu.edu

C.B. Ord et al. (eds.), *Radiation Oncology Study Guide*,
DOI 10.1007/978-1-4614-6400-6_12, © Springer Science+Business Media New York 2013

3. Classical Hodgkin lymphoma is most frequently characterized by the following typical immunophenotype:
   A. CD20+, CD45+, CD3–, CD15–, CD30–
   B. CD20+, CD45–, CD3–, CD15+, CD30+
   C. CD20–, CD45+, CD3+, CD15–, CD30+
   D. CD20–, CD45–, CD3+, CD15+, CD30–

4. Which is the most common subtype of Hodgkin lymphoma?
   A. Lymphocyte predominant
   B. Lymphocyte depleted
   C. Nodular sclerosing
   D. Mixed cell type

5. Which one of the following subtypes of Hodgkin lymphoma is most likely to be treated with radiation alone?
   A. Lymphocyte predominant
   B. Lymphocyte depleted
   C. Nodular sclerosing
   D. Mixed cell type

6. Which one of the following subtypes of Hodgkin lymphoma is most likely to present with abdominal disease or in the bone marrow with little adenopathy?
   A. Lymphocyte predominant
   B. Lymphocyte depleted
   C. Nodular sclerosing
   D. Mixed cell type

7. What is the most common location of Hodgkin lymphoma at presentation?
   A. Abdominal mass
   B. Cervical adenopathy
   C. Mediastinal mass
   D. Inguinal adenopathy

8. What is the most commonly involved extranodal site in Hodgkin lymphoma?
   A. Liver
   B. Pancreas
   C. Spleen
   D. Small bowel

9. What percentage of patients has bone marrow involvement at presentation with Hodgkin lymphoma?
   A. 90 %
   B. 50 %
   C. 20 %
   D. <5 %

10. Which subtype of Hodgkin lymphoma can be seen more frequently in children <10 years old?
    A. Mixed cellularity
    B. Lymphocyte depleted
    C. Lymphocyte predominant
    D. Lymphocyte equivalent

11. Which of the following was not an arm of the NCIC HD6 trial for early-stage, favorable Hodgkin lymphoma?
    A. Subtotal lymphoid irradiation alone
    B. ABVD × 2 cycles →PR →ABVD × 4 cycles
    C. ABVD × 2 cycles → CR → ABVD × 2 cycles
    D. ABVD × 2 cycles → PR →BEACOPPesc × 2 cycles

12. Based on the German Hodgkin Study Group HD10 trial, ABVD × 2 followed by IFRT to 20 Gy would be appropriate for all of the following patients except:
    A. Age 40; nodular sclerosing histology; bilateral hilar, mediastinal, and unilateral supraclavicular disease (non-bulky by GHSG definition); ESR of 45; no B symptoms
    B. Age 26; nodular sclerosing histology; mediastinal, bilateral supraclavicular, and left axillary disease (non-bulky by GHSG definition); ESR of 38; no B symptoms
    C. Age 34; nodular sclerosing histology; bilateral cervical disease (non-bulky by GHSG definition); ESR of 25; 15 % weight loss over 2 months prior to presentation, drenching night sweats, no fevers
    D. Age 52, lymphocyte-depleted histology, unilateral axillary and supraclavicular disease (non-bulky by GHSG definition), ESR of 42, no B symptoms

13. All of the following are true regarding the methods of the 4-arm German HD 10 trial for early-stage, non-bulky Hodgkin lymphoma except:
    A. Patients were randomized to either 2 or 4 cycles of ABVD.
    B. Patients were randomized to either 20 Gy or 30 Gy radiation.
    C. Radiation volume was subtotal nodal irradiation.
    D. Patients were stratified by age, systemic symptoms, albumin level, and supradiaphragmatic versus infradiaphragmatic disease.

14. Which of the following is a conclusion from the German HD 10 trial for early-stage, non-bulky Hodgkin lymphoma?
    A. Decreased radiation dose leads to decreased secondary malignancies.
    B. Decreased chemotherapy leads to decreased secondary malignancies.
    C. Decreased radiation dose does not decrease toxicity.
    D. Decreased chemotherapy does decrease toxicity.

15. All of the following are true regarding the German HD8 trial of extended- versus involved-field RT except:
    A. Regardless of field size, 30 Gy was delivered, with no subsequent boost.
    B. All patients received COPP/ABVD × 2 cycles prior to radiation.
    C. There was no difference in overall or progression-free survival between the arms.
    D. Subset analysis of elderly patients >60 years showed worse survival in the extended-field arm.

16. Involved nodal radiation therapy (INRT) has been utilized in which randomized clinical trials?
    A. GHSG HD10
    B. ECOG 2496
    C. EORTC H10U
    D. None of the above

17. Escalated BEACOPP would be appropriate first-line therapy for which of the following patients based on the NCCN guidelines?
    A. 22-year-old male with stage IV mixed cellularity Hodgkin lymphoma with an IPS of 3
    B. 63-year-old female with stage II non-bulky nodular sclerosing Hodgkin lymphoma with ESR of 125 and an IPS of 4
    C. 50-year-old male with stage III non-bulky lymphocyte-predominant Hodgkin lymphoma with an IPS of 3
    D. 48-year-old male with stage III nodular sclerosing Hodgkin lymphoma with ESR of 25 and an IPS of 4

18. The 8-week Stanford V regimen would be appropriate for all of the following patients except:
    A. 24-year-old female with non-bulky IIA nodular sclerosing Hodgkin lymphoma with ESR of 80 and mediastinal, left axillary, and left supraclavicular disease
    B. 24-year-old male with IIA nodular sclerosing Hodgkin lymphoma with ESR of 30 and left hilar and mediastinal disease measuring 11 cm
    C. 50-year-old female with IIA nodular sclerosing Hodgkin lymphoma with ESR of 90, bilateral supraclavicular, bilateral hilar, mediastinal disease measuring 5 cm, and bilateral axillary disease
    D. 50-year-old male with non-bulky stage I nodular sclerosing Hodgkin lymphoma with ESR of 70, unilateral cervical disease, 5 % weight loss over the past 6 months

19. Waldeyer's ring includes all of the following except:
    A. Base of tongue
    B. Palatine tonsil
    C. Nasopharynx
    D. Soft palate

20. Twelve weeks of Stanford V chemotherapy for stage III/IV Hodgkin lymphoma is followed by 36 Gy of IFRT within 3 weeks to the following sites:
    A. All initially involved sites
    B. Sites with any residual disease as measured by CT
    C. Initial sites > 5 cm
    D. Initial sites > 10 cm and/or mediastinal disease with an MMR > 0.33

21. A 22-year-old female with stage IIB Hodgkin lymphoma previously treated with ABVD×4 and IFRT to 30 Gy at age 20, now presents with pathologically confirmed isolated relapse in a cervical lymph node within her original radiation therapy fields. Which of the following is the most appropriate salvage regimen?
    A. ICE chemotherapy followed by autologous stem cell transplant
    B. Re-induction with ABVD×2 followed by ESHAP×2 followed by allogeneic stem cell transplant
    C. ICE chemotherapy followed by re-irradiation to 20 Gy then autologous stem cell transplant
    D. ESHAP chemotherapy followed by total lymphoid irradiation to 30 Gy

22. Which of the following chemotherapy regimens correctly matches the listed abbreviation?
    A. ABVD = doxorubicin, bleomycin, vincristine, dacarbazine
    B. BEACOPP = bleomycin, etoposide, doxorubicin, carboplatin, vincristine, prednisone, dacarbazine
    C. Stanford V = mechlorethamine, vincristine, prednisone, doxorubicin, bleomycin, vinblastine, etoposide
    D. MOPP = mechlorethamine, vinblastine, procarbazine, prednisone

23. Using involved-field instead of subtotal nodal irradiation substantially reduces the risk of which second malignancy?
    A. Breast cancer
    B. Lung cancer
    C. Leukemias
    D. Colorectal

24. Which of the following subtypes of Hodgkin lymphoma would be expected to respond to single-agent rituximab?
    A. Lymphocyte depleted
    B. Mixed cellularity
    C. Lymphocyte predominant
    D. None of the above

25. Which is the most common subtype of non-Hodgkin lymphoma?
    A. Follicular lymphoma
    B. Diffuse large B-cell lymphoma
    C. Peripheral T-cell lymphoma
    D. Mycosis fungoides

26. Follicular lymphoma is most frequently characterized by the following typical immunophenotype:
    A. CD5+, CD10+, CD43+
    B. CD5-, CD10+, CD43+
    C. CD5+, CD10+, CD43-
    D. CD5-, CD10+, CD43-

27. Mantle-cell lymphoma is most frequently characterized by the following typical immunophenotype:
    A. CD5+, CD 10+, CD23+
    B. CD5+, CD10-, CD23-
    C. CD5-, CD10+, CD23+
    D. CD5-, CD10-, CD23-

28. MALT lymphoma is most frequently characterized by the following typical immunophenotype:
    A. CD5+, CD10+, CD23+
    B. CD5+, CD10-, CD23+
    C. CD5-, CD10+,CD23-
    D. CD5-, CD10-, CD23-

29. The following translocations and diseases are correctly matched except:
    A. t(14;18) – Follicular lymphoma
    B. t(11;14) – Mantle-cell lymphoma
    C. t(11;18) – Diffuse large B-cell lymphoma
    D. t(8;14) – Burkitt's lymphoma

30. Which of the following best represents the percentage of patients with bone marrow involvement in newly diagnosed follicular lymphoma?
    A. 10 %
    B. 30 %
    C. 40 %
    D. >50 %

31. The most appropriate primary treatment for stage I/II non-bulky grade 1 follicular lymphoma in a young patient with a good performance status is:
    A. Close observation and treatment at progression
    B. IFRT to 4 Gy in 2 fractions
    C. IFRT to 30–36 Gy
    D. 3 cycles of R-CHOP followed by IFRT to 30–36 Gy

32. The Follicular Lymphoma International Prognostic Index (FLIPI) predicts progression-free survival based on all of the following except:
    A. Age ≥ 60
    B. Hemoglobin < 12 g/dL
    C. Number of nodal sites ≥ 5
    D. Ann Arbor Stage ≥ II

33. The highest rate of malignant transformation to diffuse large B-cell lymphoma occurs with which of the following?
    A. Mixed cellularity Hodgkin lymphoma
    B. Gastric MALT lymphoma
    C. NK/T-cell lymphoma
    D. Follicular lymphoma

34. EBV DNA viral load may be used as a prognostic and monitoring tool for which of the following diseases?
    A. Non-Hodgkin lymphoma involving Waldeyer's ring
    B. NK/T-cell lymphoma, nasal type
    C. Extranodal diffuse large B-cell lymphoma
    D. Burkitt's lymphoma

35. A patient with early-stage, non-bulky diffuse large B-cell lymphoma should be treated with the following regimen:
    A. R-CHOP × 3 followed by 36 Gy IFRT
    B. R-CHOP × 6 followed by 20 Gy IFRT
    C. Dose dense R-CHOP × 3 followed by 36 Gy IFRT
    D. R-EPOCH × 6 followed by 45 Gy IFRT

36. The ECOG E1482 (Horning et al.) trial randomized patients with stage I/II non-Hodgkin lymphoma to CHOP × 8 +/− IFRT. What was the radiotherapy dose given to those sustaining a complete response after chemotherapy?
    A. 20 Gy
    B. 30 Gy
    C. 40 Gy
    D. 50 Gy

37. The ECOG E1482 (Horning et al.) trial randomized patients with stage I/II non-Hodgkin lymphoma to CHOP × 8 +/− IFRT. What was the radiotherapy dose given to those sustaining a partial response to chemotherapy?
    A. 20 Gy
    B. 30 Gy
    C. 40 Gy
    D. 50 Gy

38. The SWOG 8736 trial (Miller et al.) randomized patients with stage I/II non-bulky non-Hodgkin lymphoma to chemotherapy alone versus chemotherapy followed by IFRT. Which of the following was not a treatment regimen of this trial?
    A. CHOP × 8
    B. CHOP × 3 + IFRT (50 Gy for partial responders)
    C. CHOP × 3 + IFRT (40 Gy for partial responders)
    D. CHOP × 3 + IFRT (40 Gy for complete responders)

39. Following all initial therapy for early-stage diffuse large B-cell lymphoma, restaging with PET/CT should be done at which interval to minimize the risks of false positives based on NCCN guidelines?
    A. 2 weeks
    B. 4 weeks
    C. 8 weeks
    D. 12 weeks

40. The international prognostic index (IPI) for non-Hodgkin lymphoma stratifies patients into risk groups based on all of the following factors except:
    A. Age > 60 years
    B. >2 sites of extranodal involvement
    C. Serum LDH elevated above the normal range
    D. Stage III or IV disease

41. The FIT trial randomized patients with advanced-stage follicular lymphoma in first remission after standard chemotherapy to observation versus consolidation radioimmunotherapy with Y-90 ibritumomab (Zevalin). Which of the following is false?
    A. Consolidation with yttrium-90 ibritumomab prolonged median progression-free survival.
    B. Consolidation with yttrium-90 ibritumomab prolonged median progression-free survival in all Follicular Lymphoma International Prognostic Index risk subgroups.
    C. Of those patients with a partial response after induction, less than one-half were converted to a complete response.
    D. Final complete response rate is approximately 85 %.

42. Quadruple therapy for gastric MALT lymphoma includes all of the following except:
    A. Metronidazole
    B. Tetracycline
    C. Omeprazole
    D. Doxycycline

43. Local skin-directed therapies for stage IA (< 10 % of skin surface area involvement) cutaneous T-cell lymphoma (mycosis fungoides) appropriately include which of the following as first-line therapy?
    A. PUVA therapy
    B. UVB therapy
    C. Local RT
    D. Total skin electron beam therapy

44. Sezary syndrome is defined as:
    A. Skin involvement of >80 % and circulating Sezary cells in the peripheral blood
    B. Skin involvement of >50 % and biopsy positive lymph node for Sezary cells
    C. Skin involvement of >80 % and bone marrow positive for Sezary cells
    D. Skin involvement of >50 % and circulating Sezary cells in the peripheral blood

45. Which subtype of primary cutaneous B-cell lymphoma carries the worst prognosis?
    A. Primary cutaneous diffuse large B-cell lymphoma, leg type.
    B. Primary cutaneous follicle center lymphoma.
    C. Primary cutaneous marginal zone lymphoma.
    D. They all carry equivalent excellent prognosis.

46. What percentage of primary CNS lymphoma also has concurrent ocular involvement?
    A. 5 %
    B. 15 %
    C. 30 %
    D. 45 %

47. Of those with isolated ocular lymphoma, what percentage will subsequently develop primary CNS lymphoma?
    A. 15 %
    B. 30 %
    C. 50 %
    D. 90 %

48. What is the most important prognostic factor in primary CNS lymphoma?
    A. Age
    B. Increased cerebrospinal fluid protein level
    C. LDH serum level
    D. Response to initial therapy

49. Primary first-line therapy for elderly (age > 60), good performance status patients with biopsy proven CNS diffuse large B-cell lymphoma should include:
    A. Steroids + whole brain radiation therapy to 30 Gy
    B. Steroids + systemic high-dose methotrexate + intrathecal methotrexate followed by whole brain radiation therapy to 30 Gy
    C. Steroids + systemic high-dose methotrexate + systemic cytarabine
    D. Steroids + intrathecal methotrexate + systemic cytarabine + whole brain radiation to 24 Gy with a boost to gross residual disease to 45 Gy

50. Which of the following regimens is appropriate for palliation in an advanced-stage follicular lymphoma?
    A. 8 Gy in 1 fraction
    B. 30 Gy in 20 fractions
    C. 4 Gy in 2 fractions
    D. 40 Gy in 20 fractions

51. Accepted first-line treatment options for localized early-stage mantle-cell lymphoma include which of the following?
    A. IFRT alone to 36 Gy.
    B. HyperCVAD + rituximab alone.
    C. HyperCVAD + rituximab followed by IFRT to 30 Gy.
    D. All of the above are accepted regimens for first-line therapy.

52. Which of the following lymphomas has been associated with breast implants?
    A. Diffuse large B-cell lymphoma
    B. Anaplastic large-cell lymphoma
    C. Burkitt's lymphoma
    D. Hairy cell leukemia

53. Primary mediastinal B-cell lymphoma often has an indistinguishable histology with which of the following lymphomas?
    A. Nodular sclerosing Hodgkin lymphoma
    B. Diffuse large B-cell lymphoma
    C. Follicular lymphoma
    D. Non-gastric marginal zone lymphoma

54. What percentage of orbital lymphomas are bilateral?
    A. 40–45 %
    B. 30–35 %
    C. 20–25 %
    D. 10–15 %

55. What is the most common histology of orbital lymphoma?
    A. Marginal zone
    B. Mantle cell
    C. Follicular lymphoma
    D. T-cell lymphoma

56. What radiotherapy dose is typically employed for orbital lymphomas and has been shown to yield local control >95 %?
    A. 15 Gy
    B. 20 Gy
    C. 30 Gy
    D. 36 Gy

57. Diagnosis of solitary plasmacytoma requires which of the following?
    A. Bone marrow biopsy demonstrating < 10 % plasma cells
    B. M protein in serum < 30 g/L
    C. No hypercalcemia > 11.5 mg/dL
    D. All of the above

58. Plasma cells are most frequently characterized by the following typical immunophenotype:
    A. CD5+, CD20+, CD38+
    B. CD5+, CD20+, CD38−
    C. CD5−, CD20−, CD38+
    D. CD5−, CD20−, CD38−

59. Despite a negative serum protein electrophoresis, Bence Jones proteins will be seen on urine protein electrophoresis in what percentage of patients with multiple myeloma?
    A. 10 %
    B. 20 %
    C. 30 %
    D. 40 %

60. What percentage of monoclonal gammopathy of undetermined significance (MGUS) will proceed to a B-cell neoplasm within 1 year?
    A. 10 %
    B. 6 %
    C. 4 %
    D. 2 %

61. Which of the following would exclude a diagnosis of POEMS syndrome?
    A. Polyneuropathy
    B. Serum M protein level of 4 g/dL
    C. Solitary osteosclerotic lesion
    D. Bone marrow with 5 % plasma cells

62. True or false: The risk of transformation to multiple myeloma is higher in solitary extraosseous plasmacytoma than in solitary osseous plasmacytoma.
    A. True
    B. False

63. Which is the most common site of extramedullary plasmacytoma?
    A. Head and neck
    B. Skin
    C. Lung
    D. Breast

64. Solitary osseous plasmacytoma should be treated with which of the following doses?
    A. 8 Gy
    B. 30 Gy
    C. 40 Gy
    D. 50 Gy

65. Which therapy used in multiple myeloma is incorrectly associated with a treatment-related adverse event?
    A. Bisphosphonates – Osteonecrosis of the jaw
    B. Thalidomide – Deep venous thrombosis
    C. Bortezomib – Hepatitis B reactivation
    D. Dexamethasone – Pneumocystis pneumonia

Answers and Rationales

1. The correct answer is B. The International Prognostic Score (IPS) is useful to determine prognosis of advanced-stage (stages III–IV) Hodgkin lymphoma. The score includes the following factors: hemoglobin < 10.5 g/dL, age ≥ 45, lymphocytopenia (lymphocyte count < 8 % of the WBC and/or lymphocyte count < 600/mm^3), stage IV, leukocytosis (WBC > 15,000/mm^3), albumin < 4 g/dL, and male gender. A useful mnemonic to recall this is HAL SWAM. In this question, B is the correct answer as the albumin level should be < 4 g/dL, not 3.5 g/dL. Hasenclever et al. A prognostic score for advanced Hodgkin's disease. International Prognostic Factors Project on Advanced Hodgkin's Disease. N Eng J Med 1998;339:1506–14.

2. The correct answer is A. Lymphocyte-predominant Hodgkin lymphoma is characterized by A: CD20+, CD45+, CD3−, CD15−, CD30−. Classical Hodgkin lymphoma is characterized by B: CD20+ (<40% of cases), CD45−, CD3−, CD15+, CD30+. Note that the reliable expression of CD20 in LPHL has led to use of rituximab, an anti-CD20 antibody. The German Hodgkin Study Group showed an overall response rate of 100 % and a 36-month PFS benefit of 81 % in 28 patients. This may inspire investigations including anti-CD20 antibody-based therapy. NCCN Guidelines. Hodgkin Lymphoma. Version 2.2012. Eichenauer et al. Phase 2 study of rituximab in newly diagnosed stage IA nodular lymphocyte-predominant Hodgkin lymphoma: a report from the German Hodgkin Study Group. Blood 2011;118:4363–5.

3. The correct answer is B. Classical Hodgkin lymphoma is characterized by B: CD20+ (<40 % of cases), CD45−, CD3−, CD15+, CD30+. Ng AK, Weiss L, LaCasce AS. Hodgkins lymphoma. In: Gunderson LL, Tepper JE, editors. Clinical radiation oncology. 3rd ed. Philadelphia: Elsevier Saunders; 2012. p. 1527–43.

4. The correct answer is C. Approximately 2/3 of Hodgkin lymphoma is nodular sclerosing type. It commonly presents in neck and mediastinal sites in young adults. Ng AK, Weiss L, LaCasce AS. Hodgkins lymphoma. In: Gunderson LL, Tepper JE, editors. Clinical radiation oncology. 3rd ed. Philadelphia: Elsevier Saunders; 2012. p. 1527–43.

5. The correct answer is A. Lymphocyte-predominant Hodgkin lymphoma, which presents frequently in peripheral nodal sites, can be treated with radiation alone to 36Gy. Bodis S et al. Clinical presentation, course, and prognostic factors in lymphocyte-predominant Hodgkin's disease. J Clin Oncol. 1997;15:3060–6.

6. The correct answer is B. Lymphocyte-depleted Hodgkin lymphoma is more common in the elderly and presents with abdominal disease and bone marrow involvement, with little adenopathy. Ng AK, Weiss L, LaCasce AS. Hodgkins lymphoma. In: Gunderson LL, Tepper JE, editors. Clinical radiation oncology. 3rd ed. Philadelphia: Elsevier Saunders; 2012. p. 1527–43.

7. The correct answer is B. Cervical adenopathy is by far the most common location of Hodgkin disease at presentation (>70 %). Mediastinal disease is the second most common mode of presentation. Ng AK, Weiss L, LaCasce AS. Hodgkins lymphoma. In: Gunderson LL, Tepper JE, editors. Clinical radiation oncology. 3rd ed. Philadelphia: Elsevier Saunders; 2012. p. 1527–43.

8. The correct answer is C. The spleen is the most commonly involved extranodal site in Hodgkin lymphoma. Rosenberg SA, Kaplan H. Evidence for an orderly progression in the spread of Hodgkin's disease. Cancer Res. 1966; 26:1225–31.

9. The correct answer is D. Bone marrow involvement at diagnosis is rare (<5 %) in Hodgkin lymphoma.

10. The correct answer is A. In children, nodular sclerosing is still the most common subtype of Hodgkin lymphoma, but mixed cellularity is seen more frequently in children < 10 years. Roberts KB, Hudson MM, Constine LS. Pediatric Hodgkin's lymphoma. In: Gunderson LL, Tepper JE, editors. Clinical radiation oncology. 3rd ed. Philadelphia: Elsevier Saunders; 2012. p.1489–503.

11. The correct answer is D. ABVD alone has not been well-established for early-stage favorable Hodgkin lymphoma. However, the NCIC HD6 trial investigated IA/IIA, non-bulky, disease limited to above the diaphragm Hodgkin lymphoma patients with 4 different treatment arms: STLI (favorable only), ABVD × 2 + STLI (unfavorable patients), ABVD × 2 → CR → ABVD × 2, and ABVD × 2 → PR → ABVD × 4. Results suggested that while RT improved FFP, OS was slightly better in the ABVD-alone arms. FFP was found to be much better in these ABVD-alone arms if a CR was obtained after 2 cycles of ABVD, which occurred in 40 % of patients on the HD6 trial. The criticisms of the HD6 trial include the following: the trial was stopped early in 2002 due to an outdated radiation technique of STLI to 35 Gy; the RT arm was considered to include the STLI-only patients and the patients who received ABVD × 2 and STLI which when broken down, OS was 98 % in the STLI with only 1 death from any cause while the ABVD × 2 and STLI arms included 5 deaths (difficult to relate directly to treatment or lack of efficacy); deaths from cardiac events were equivalent in both arms, death from Hodgkin lymphoma were equivalent in both arms, and 2nd malignancies included four in the ABVD-alone arms and nine in the radiation arms, six of which were pelvic malignancies and considered out of field with only 1 lung and 1 breast case in each for the chemo-alone arms and the

radiation arms. Meyer et al. Randomized comparison of ABVD chemotherapy with a strategy that includes radiation therapy in patients with limited-stage Hodgkin's lymphoma: National Cancer Institute of Canada Clinical Trials Group and the Eastern Cooperative Oncology Group. JCO 2005;23:4634–42.

12. The correct answer is B. The German Hodgkin Study Group (GHSG) HD10 trial is a 4-arm trial that compared (1) ABVD × 2 + 20 Gy, (2) ABVD × 4 + 20 Gy, (3) ABVD × 2 + 30 Gy, and (4) ABVD × 4 + 30 Gy for early-stage favorable patients with no risk factors based on the GHSG criteria which include the following: ESR > 50 with no B symptoms, ESR > 30 with B symptoms, Mediastinal Mass Ratio (MMR) > 0.33, # nodal sites > 2, and any E lesions. It is important to know the different unfavorable definitions including GHSG, EORTC, NCIC, Stanford, and NCCN. EORTC: age $\geq$ 50, ESR > 50 with no B symptoms, ESR > 30 with B symptoms, Mediastinal Tumor Ratio (MTR) > 0.35 (max width of the mass divided by the intrathoracic diameter at T5/6), and > 3 nodal sites; NCIC: age $\geq$ 40, mixed cellularity or lymphocyte-depleted histology, ESR > 50, any B symptoms, MMR > 0.33 or any site > 10 cm, > 3 nodal sites; Stanford: any B symptoms, MMR > 0.33; NCCN: ESR > 50, any B symptoms, MMR > 0.33 or any site > 10 cm, > 3 nodal sites. It is also important to know that the GHSG considers all hilar disease as part of the mediastinum as well as all infraclavicular disease as part of supraclavicular/cervical disease and these don't count as separate nodal sites. The GHSG also divides abdominal disease into upper and lower sites. Therefore, B is the correct answer because the disease includes > 2 nodal sites. Based on the GHSG criteria, A involves only 2 nodal sites, C includes B symptoms but with an ESR of 25 this is acceptable, and D meets all the criteria as laid out by the GHSG for favorable disease. Engert A et al. Reduced treatment intensity in patients with early-stage Hodgkin's lymphoma. N Engl J Med 2010;363:640–52.

13. The correct answer is C. The German HD10 trial randomized 1,370 (1,163 in ITT analysis) patients with non-bulky, stage I/II Hodgkin lymphoma to one of 4 arms: (1) ABVD × 2 + 20 Gy, (2) ABVD × 4 + 20 Gy, (3) ABVD × 2 + 30 Gy, and (4) ABVD × 4 + 30 Gy. Patients were stratified by age (<50 vs. $\geq$50), systemic symptoms, albumin level (<4 vs. $\geq$4 g/dL), and supradiaphragmatic versus infradiaphragmatic disease. Radiotherapy consisted of IFRT. Grade III/IV toxicity was increased in those receiving 4 versus 2 cycles of ABVD (51.7 % vs. 33.2 %, $p < 0.001$). Grade III/IV toxicity was increased in those receiving 30 Gy versus 20 Gy (8.7 % vs. 2.9 %, $p < 0.001$). No differences between secondary neoplasms or mortality were seen between the combined chemotherapy and combined radiation groups. Intent to treat analysis showed no difference in overall survival or progression-free survival between chemotherapy arms and between radiation arms. This trial established 2 cycles ABVD and 20 Gy IFRT as the new standard for early-stage, favorable Hodgkin disease. Engert, A. et al. Reduced treatment intensity in patients with early-stage Hodgkin's lymphoma. N Engl J Med 2010;363:640–652.

14. The correct answer is D. The German HD10 trial randomized 1370 (1163 in ITT analysis) patients with non-bulky, stage I/II Hodgkin lymphoma to one of 4 arms: (1) ABVD × 2 + 20 Gy, (2) ABVD × 4 + 20 Gy, (3) ABVD × 2 + 30 Gy, and (4) ABVD × 4 + 30 Gy. Patients were stratified by age (<50 vs. ≥50), systemic symptoms, albumin level (<4 vs. ≥4 g/dL), and supradiaphragmatic versus infradiaphragmatic disease. Radiotherapy consisted of IFRT. Grade III/IV toxicity was increased in those receiving 4 versus 2 cycles of ABVD (51.7 % vs. 33.2 %, $p < 0.001$). Grade III/IV toxicity was increased in those receiving 30 Gy versus 20 Gy (8.7 % vs. 2.9 %, $p < 0.001$). No differences between secondary neoplasms or mortality were seen between the combined chemotherapy and combined radiation groups. Intent to treat analysis showed no difference in overall survival or progression-free survival between chemotherapy arms and between radiation arms. This trial established 2 cycles ABVD and 20 Gy IFRT as the new standard for early-stage, favorable Hodgkin disease. Engert A et al. Reduced treatment intensity in patients with early-stage Hodgkin's lymphoma. N Engl J Med 2010;363:640–52.

15. The correct answer is A. The German HD8 trial sought to determine optimal field size in treatment of early-stage unfavorable Hodgkin lymphoma. 1064 patients with stage I/II with 1+ risk factors and IIIA without risk factors were treated with COPP/ABVD × 2 cycles and then randomized to (1) EFRT 30 Gy or (2) IFRT 30 Gy. A 10 Gy boost was given to bulky disease. Risk factors: large mediastinal mass, extranodal involvement, massive splenic involvement, elevated ESR, >2 lymph node groups involved. The initial report in 2003 showed no difference in 5-year freedom from treatment failure between the arms (86 % EFRT vs. 84 % IFRT, NS) nor was there a difference in overall survival. Toxicity (nausea/vomiting, pharyngitis, leucopenia) were worse in the EFRT arm. A subset analysis of elderly patients (>60 years) treated with EFRT was published in 2007, and in these patients, EFRT was found to worsen survival (59 % EFRT vs. 81 % IFRT). Engert A et al. Involved-field radiotherapy is equally effective and less toxic compared with extended-field radiotherapy after 4 cycles of chemotherapy in patients with early-stage unfavorable Hodgkin's lymphoma: results of the HD8 trial of the German Hodgkin's Lymphoma Study Group. J Clin Oncol. 2003;21(19):3601–8. Klimm B et al. Poorer outcome of elderly patients treated with extended-field radiotherapy compared with involved-field radiotherapy after chemotherapy for Hodgkin's lymphoma: an analysis from the German Hodgkin Study Group. Ann Oncol. 2007;18(2):357–63. Epub 27 Oct 2006.

16. The correct answer is C. Involved nodal radiation therapy (INRT) is beginning to replace involved-field radiation therapy (IFRT) in clinical trials. The EORTC H10U and H10F trials utilized INRT to 30 Gy in both arms of both these trials. It is important to note that both trials were closed early due to increased events in the chemotherapy-alone arms relative to the combined modality arms, but this presumably has nothing to do with the selection of INRT as all remaining

patients in the chemotherapy-alone arms were transitioned to the CMT arms consisting of INRT. Additionally, the GHSG HD17 trial is testing INRT to 30 Gy in the chemotherapy-alone arm without complete response by PET/CT after BEACOPPesc × 2 + ABVD × 2 which will be compared to the standard arm of BEACOPPesc × 2 + ABVD × 2 + IFRT to 30 Gy. Therefore, C is the correct answer.

17. The correct answer is D. Escalated BEACOPP is typically reserved as first-line therapy for patients with stage III/IV disease with an IPS of ≥ 4 per the NCCN guidelines (Version 2.2012). IPS is not utilized for patients with stage I and II disease. GHSG HD9 determined that BEACOPP esc improved FFP, FFF, and OS compared to COPP/ABVD and BEACOPP baseline, which did include bulky IIB, III, and IV patients. Engert et al. Escalated-dose BEACOPP in the treatment of patients with advanced-stage Hodgkin's lymphoma: 10 years of follow-up of the HGSH HD9 study. JCO. 2009;27:4548–54.

18. The correct answer is B. Stanford V can be given over 8 weeks or 12 weeks depending on stage and risk factors. Advani et al. reported the results of the Stanford G4 trial which suggested that stage I and II patients with an elevated ESR and > 3 sites of disease could still be managed with the 8-week regimen but that patients with bulky mediastinal disease or any disease > 10 cm and/or with B symptoms should be managed with the 12-week regimen, as would patients with low IPS stage III/IV disease. Therefore, B is the correct answer, as 11 cm disease would be classified as bulky disease. 5 % weight loss over 6 months does not qualify as a B symptom in answer choice D (10 % is required). The 8-week regimen is followed by 30 Gy of IFRT. Advani et al. Efficacy of abbreviated Stanford V chemotherapy and involved-field radiotherapy in early stage Hodgkin's disease: mature results of the G4 trial. Blood 2009;114:1670.

19. The correct answer is D. Waldeyer's ring is a circle of protective lymphoid tissue at the proximal portion of the aerodigestive tract that includes bilateral palatine tonsils, the lingual tonsil in the base of tongue, the nasopharynx (adenoid), and some intervening lymphatic tissue. The soft palate and uvula are not a part of this structure. Waldeyer's ring is commonly involved in lymphomas and must be inspected carefully on physical examination both by direct oral cavity inspection and by indirect mirror exam and/or nasopharyngoscopy.

20. The correct answer is C. 12 weeks of Stanford V is an option for patients with low IPS (<3) stage III/IV disease and patients with stage IB/IIB and/or bulky I/II disease. Patients with non-bulky IA/IIA disease and patients with >3 sites of disease and/or elevated ESR can be treated with the 8-week regimen. The 8-week regimen is followed by 30 Gy to all involved sites. Patients with unfavorable stage I/II disease (bulky and/or B symptoms) can be treated with 30 Gy to all involved sites with 36 Gy reserved for bulky disease. In patients with low

IPS stage III/IV disease, 36 Gy is given to initial sites > 5 cm, residual PET positive disease, and for macroscopic spleen involvement. Therefore, C is the correct answer. Note that the ECOG 2496 trial showed no difference in response, FFS, OS, or toxicity between ABVD and Stanford V for bulky stage I/II and III/IV patients. Horning, SJ et al. Efficacy and late effects of Stanford V chemotherapy and radiotherapy in untreated Hodgkin's disease: mature data in early and advanced stage patients. Blood 2004;104:308.

21. The correct answer is A. Autologous stem cell transplant remains the best option for relapsed patients. Randomized trials by the British National Lymphoma Investigation and the GHSG compared autologous stem cell transplant to conventional systemic therapy for relapsed Hodgkin lymphoma and showed an improvement in PFS with transplant though the OS appeared similar. Induction chemotherapy and radiation (in radiation-naïve patients) should be given, as there is data that decreased disease burden prior to transplant improves both 5-year OS and 5-year PFS. Radiation in the relapsed setting is best utilized in patients who were initially treated with chemotherapy alone. Allogeneic transplant is generally avoided given the high rate of mortality, but there is some evidence that it provides improved outcomes over autologous transplant. Linch DC et al. Dose intensification with autologous bone-marrow transplantation in relapsed and resistant Hodgkin's disease: results of a BNLI randomised trial. Lancet 1993;341(8852):1051–4. Schmitz N et al. Aggressive conventional chemotherapy compared with high-dose chemotherapy with autologous haemopoietic stem-cell transplantation for relapsed chemosensitive Hodgkin's disease: a randomised trial. Lancet 2002;359(9323):2065–71. Sirohi B et al. Long-term outcome of autologous stem-cell transplantation in relapsed or refractory Hodgkin's lymphoma. Ann Oncol 2008;19:1312–9.

22. The correct answer is C. ABVD= doxorubicin, bleomycin, vinblastine, dacarbazine. BEACOPP= bleomycin, etoposide, doxorubicin, cyclophosphamide, vincristine, prednisone, procarbazine. Stanford V= mechlorethamine, vincristine, prednisone, doxorubicin, bleomycin, vinblastine, etoposide. MOPP= mechlorethamine, vincristine, procarbazine, prednisone. Ng AK, Weiss L, LaCasce AS. Hodgkins lymphoma. In: Gunderson LL, Tepper JE, editors. Clinical radiation oncology. 3rd ed. Philadelphia: Elsevier Saunders; 2012. p. 1527–43.

23. The correct answer is A. Combination chemotherapy and radiation regimens reduce the risk of secondary malignancies when compared to extended-field radiation-alone regimens. A meta-analysis suggests that breast cancer risk is reduced by changing from extended-field techniques to involved-field techniques and the NCCN (*Version 2.2012*) recommends excluding uninvolved axillae in all women even if traditionally included in involved-field radiation. Colorectal cancer has been associated with chemotherapy-alone regimens, and lung cancers have been associated with both chemotherapy-alone and combined

modality regimens. Franklin et al. Second malignancy risk associated with treatment of Hodgkin's lymphoma: meta-analysis of the randomized trials. Ann Oncol. 2006;17:1749–60.

24. The correct answer is C. Lymphocyte-predominant Hodgkin lymphoma expresses CD20 antigen and multiple small series have demonstrated 100 % response rates to single-agent and combined regimens including rituximab, an anti-CD20 antibody. The duration of drug delivery and duration of response have not been standardized, and rituximab is often combined with traditional chemotherapy regimens including ABVD, ESHAP, and CHOP. Maeda et al. The emerging role for rituximab in the treatment of nodular lymphocyte-predominant Hodgkin lymphoma. Curr Opin Oncol. 2009;21:397–400.

25. The correct answer is B. Diffuse large B-cell is the most common subtype of non-Hodgkin lymphoma (1/3 of cases), with follicular lymphoma being the 2nd most common subtype. Tsang RW, Gospodarowicz MK. Non-Hodgkin's lymphoma. In: Gunderson LL, Tepper JE, editors. Clinical radiation oncology. 3rd ed. Philadelphia: Elsevier Saunders; 2012. p.1545–72.

26. The correct answer is D. Follicular lymphoma is characterized by the CD5−, CD10+, CD43− immunophenotype. Those rare follicular lymphomas that are CD43+ tend to be large-cell type with focally diffuse areas +/− t(14:18) fusion gene product. Lai R et al. Frequency of CD43 expression in non-Hodgkin lymphoma. A survey of 742 cases and further characterization of rare CD43+ follicular lymphomas. Am J Clin Pathol. 1999;111(4):488–94.

27. The correct answer is B. Mantle-cell lymphoma is characterized by the CD5+, CD10−, CD23− immunophenotype. Tsang RW, Gospodarowicz MK. Non-Hodgkin's Lymphoma. In Gunderson LL, Tepper JE, editors. Clinical radiation oncology. 3rd ed. Philadelphia: Elsevier Saunders; 2012. p. 1545–72).

28. The correct answer is D. MALT lymphoma is characterized by the CD5−, CD10−, CD23− immunophenotype. Tsang RW, Gospodarowicz MK. Non-Hodgkin's lymphoma. In: Gunderson LL, Tepper JE, editors. Clinical radiation oncology. 3rd ed. Philadelphia: Elsevier Saunders; 2012. p. 1545–72.

29. The correct answer is C. t(11;18) is associated with gastric MALT lymphoma and is more frequently associated with advanced presentations. Presence of t(11;18) is also predictive of decreased response to antibiotics even in *H. pylori*-positive patients and is an indication to consider up-front radiation in these patients. Liu et al. t(11;18) is a marker for all stage gastric MALT lymphomas that will not respond to *H. pylori* eradication. Gastroenterology. 2002;122:1286–94.

30. The correct answer is D. The majority of patients (>50 %) diagnosed with follicular lymphoma present at an advanced stage with bone marrow involvement.

Armitage JO, Weisenburger DD. New approach to classifying non-Hodgkin's lymphomas: clinical features of the major histologic subtypes. Non-Hodgkin's Lymphoma Classification Project. J Clin Oncol. 1998;16:2780–95.

31. The correct answer is C. The majority of follicular lymphoma cases present at an advanced stage with the risk of bone marrow being positive at diagnosis approximately 50 %. Stage I/II patients are generally treated with radiation alone to a dose of 30–36 Gy. Combination regimens with sequential chemotherapy and radiation have not shown a convincing benefit in early-stage disease. Fifteen-year OS is 40 % and 15-year relapse-free survival is 40 % for early-stage disease but appears to be better for stage I than stage II patients. Standard doses are in the range of 30–36 Gy with 2 Gy × 2 fractions to 4 Gy typically reserved for palliation of symptomatic disease in advanced-stage patients, as good response can be achieved with very low doses of radiation. Guadagnolo et al. Long-term outcome and mortality trends in early-stage, Grade 1–2 follicular lymphoma treated with radiation therapy. Int J Radiat Oncol Biol Phys. 2006;64:928–34.

32. The correct answer is D. The FLIPI predicts 5-year progression-free survival (PFS) by stratifying patients into three risk groups – low, intermediate, and high based on the following: age $\geq$ 60, Ann Arbor Stage of III or IV, hemoglobin < 12 g/dL, serum LDH > upper limit of normal, and number of nodal sites $\geq$ 5. 0–1 = low risk, 2 = intermediate, and $\geq$ 3 = high. Approximate PFS are: low = 90 %, intermediate = 70 %, and high = 50 %. Updated 10-year OS: low = 70 %, intermediate = 50 %, and high = 30 %. It is important to note that the FLIPI represents pre-rituximab data. The FLIPI-2 is prognostic after rituximab-based treatment and includes bone marrow positivity, largest involved lymph node > 6 cm, age > 60, hemoglobin < 12 g/dL, and elevated beta-2 microglobulin with predicted 3-year PFS ranging from 57 % to 89 % after rituximab. Solal-Celigny et al. Follicular lymphoma international prognostic index. Blood. 2004;104:1258–65.

33. The correct answer is D. Follicular lymphoma transforms to diffuse large B-cell lymphoma at a rate of approximately 3% per year for 15 years. Al-Tourah et al., Population-based analysis of incidence and outcome of transformed non-Hodgkin's lymphoma. J Clin Oncol. 2008;26:5165–9.

34. The correct answer is B. EBV DNA viral load has been found to offer prognostic and diagnostic information and may be a useful tool for monitoring of NK/T-cell lymphoma. A threshold has been identified as 6.1×10^7 copies/mL, with poorer survival seen in patients with EBV viral loads above this value. Additionally, patients with a decrease of EBV DNA viral load levels to undetectable levels had a better median OS than those with residual detectable levels. Au et al. Quantification of circulating Epstein-Barr virus (EBV) DNA in the diagnosis and monitoring of natural killer cell and EBV-positive lymphomas in immunocompetent patients. Blood. 2004;104:243–9.

35. The correct answer is A. Early-stage non-bulky DLBCL is often treated with 3 cycles of R-CHOP followed by 30–36 Gy of IFRT assuming complete response after chemotherapy and before radiation. SWOG 8736 demonstrated 3 cycles of CHOP followed by IFRT improved 5-year PFS and OS, though this benefit did disappear with longer follow-up, when compared with 8 cycles of CHOP alone. SWOG 0014 revealed a 4-year PFS of 88 % and OS of 92 % for R-CHOP × 3 followed by IFRT. Randomized data has failed to show a benefit to dose dense R-CHOP, though there does appear to be a benefit for dose dense CHOP alone. Standard doses of 30–36 Gy are recommended with the exception of certain patients that have an incomplete response to initial chemotherapy in which case 45 Gy can be considered, particularly in patients who are not transplant candidates. R-EPOCH is first-line chemotherapy option and is used particularly in patients with impaired left ventricular function who may not be able to tolerate the doses of doxorubicin used in CHOP. Miller et al. Chemotherapy alone compared with chemotherapy plus radiotherapy for localized intermediate- and high-grade non-Hodgkin's lymphoma. N Engl J Med. 1998;339:21–6.

36. The correct answer is B. The ECOG 1482 trial randomized patients with stage I/II non-bulky non-Hodgkin lymphoma after CHOP × 8 to subsequent IFRT or observation. Those sustaining a complete response to chemotherapy received 30 Gy; those sustaining a partial response received 40 Gy. Those in the IFRT arm with a complete response had better disease-free survival, failure free survival, and time to progression, though there was no overall survival difference. Conversion to complete response with IFRT did not significantly influence the outcome of patients with an initial partial response from chemotherapy. Horning SJ et al. Chemotherapy with or without radiotherapy in limited-stage diffuse aggressive non-Hodgkin's lymphoma: Eastern Cooperative Oncology Group study 1484. J Clin Oncol. 2004;22(15):3032–8. Epub 2004 Jun 21.

37. The correct answer is C. The ECOG 1482 trial randomized patients with stage I/II non-bulky non-Hodgkin lymphoma after CHOP × 8 to subsequent IFRT or observation. Those sustaining a complete response to chemotherapy received 30 Gy; those sustaining a partial response received 40 Gy. Those in the IFRT arm with a complete response had better disease-free survival, failure free survival, and time to progression, though there was no overall survival difference. Conversion to complete response with IFRT did not significantly influence the outcome of patients with an initial partial response from chemotherapy. Horning SJ et al. Chemotherapy with or without radiotherapy in limited-stage diffuse aggressive non-Hodgkin's lymphoma: Eastern Cooperative Oncology Group study 1484. J Clin Oncol. 2004;22(15):3032–8. Epub 2004 Jun 21.

38. The correct answer is C. The SWOG 8736 trial randomized patients with stage I/II non-bulky non-Hodgkin lymphoma to (1) CHOP × 8 versus (2) CHOP × 3 + IFRT (50 Gy partial responders; 40 Gy complete responders). The addition of IFRT was found to improve 5-year progression-free and overall survival, though

this benefit disappeared with longer follow-up as the CHOP × 3 arm later sustained increased relapses. Miller TP et al. Chemotherapy alone compared with chemotherapy plus radiotherapy for localized intermediate- and high-grade non-Hodgkin's lymphoma. N Engl J Med. 1998;339(1):21–6. Miller TP et al. CHOP alone compared to CHOP plus radiotherapy for early stage aggressive non-Hodgkin's lymphomas: update of the SWOG Randomized Trial. Blood. 2001;98:724A. Abstr 3024.

39. The correct answer is C. Restaging with PET/CT at 8 weeks minimizes the risk of false positives after radiation for follow-up of disease status. The NCCN reports that the ideal timing of follow-up PET/CT imaging is not known but recommends 8 weeks. NCCN Guidelines. Non-Hodgkin's Lymphoma. Version 2.2012

40. The correct answer is B. The IPI for non-Hodgkin lymphoma is a prognostic index based on the following features: age > 60 years, elevated serum LDH, performance status ECOG 2–4, stage III or IV disease, and >1 site of extranodal involvement. 0–1 = low risk, 2 = low intermediate risk, 3 = high intermediate risk, and 4–5 = high risk. 5-yr OS: low= 75 %, low intermediate = 51 %, high intermediate = 43 %, and high = 25 %. The International non-Hodgkin lymphoma prognostic factors project. A predictive model for aggressive non-Hodgkin's lymphoma. N Engl J Med. 1993;329:987–94.

41. The correct answer is C. The FIT trial randomized 414 patients with CD20+ stage III/IV follicular lymphoma with either a complete or partial response after first-line induction treatment to observation versus consolidation yttrium-90-ibritumomab. Consolidation with yttrium-90-ibritumomab improved progression-free survival in all patients, regardless of degree of response to induction therapy (complete vs. partial), or Follicular Lymphoma International Prognostic Index risk subgroup. With yttrium-90-ibritumomab consolidation, 77 % of those in partial response after induction subsequently achieved a complete response, bringing the final complete response rate to 87 %. Morschhauser et al. Phase III trial of consolidation therapy with yttrium-90-ibritumomab tiuxetan compared with no additional therapy after first remission in advanced follicular lymphoma. J Clin Oncol. 2008;26:5156–64.

42. The correct answer is D. Early-stage gastric MALT lymphoma that is *H. pylori* positive will often respond well to antibiotics in combination with a proton pump inhibitor. A currently accepted regimen includes metronidazole, tetracycline, omeprazole, and bismuth. Durable disease response has been seen and reported to antibiotic therapy. Presence of the t(11;18) translocation predicts for poorer response to antibiotic therapy alone, even in *H. pylori*-positive patients and alternative treatments, including radiation, should be considered as first-line therapy in these patients. Wundisch et al. Long-term follow-up of gastric MALT lymphoma after Helicobacter pylori eradication. J Clin Oncol. 2005;23: 8018–24. NCCN Guidelines. Non-Hodgkin's Lymphomas. Version 2.2012.

43. The correct answer is C. Patients with early-stage limited plaque disease are most appropriately treated with local skin-directed therapies which can include topical steroids, topical nitrogen mustard, topical carmustine, topical bexarotene, and local radiation to 24–36 Gy. Radiation is especially suited for patients who present with a single lesion. Generalized skin-directed therapies are more appropriate for patients with widespread disease and include UVA combined with psoralen, UVB and total skin electron beam therapy. NCCN Guidelines. Non-Hodgkin's Lymphomas. Version 2.2012.

44. The correct answer is A. Sezary syndrome appears to be an aggressive variant of cutaneous T-cell lymphoma, typically presenting with erythroderma, lymphadenopathy, and the presence of circulating leukemic cells in the peripheral blood. It accounts for approximately 5% of cutaneous T-cell lymphomas. Willemze et al. WHO-EORTC classification for cutaneous lymphomas. Blood. 2005;105:3768–85.

45. The correct answer is A. Cutaneous B-cell lymphomas represent approximately 30 % of all primary cutaneous lymphomas with three subtypes identified: primary cutaneous marginal zone lymphoma, primary cutaneous follicle center cell lymphoma, and primary cutaneous diffuse large B-cell, leg type. Approximate 5-year OS based on subtype is 97 %, 96 %, and 73 %, respectively. Primary cutaneous follicle center cell lymphoma is the most common type and primary cutaneous diffuse large B-cell, leg type, is the least common and also carries the worst prognosis of the three. Of note, primary cutaneous diffuse large B-cell, leg type, also is associated with the highest incidence of extracutaneous relapse at 47 % versus approximately 10 % for each of the other subtypes. Senff et al. Reclassification of 300 primary cutaneous B-cell lymphomas according to the new WHO-EORTC classification for cutaneous lymphomas: comparison with previous classifications and identification of prognostic markers. J Clin Oncol. 2007;25:1581–7.

46. The correct answer is B. Approximately 15 % of patients with primary CNS lymphoma will also have concurrent ocular involvement. This is why ocular involvement needs to be ruled out at diagnosis with slit lamp exam. Chan CC et al., Primary vitreoretinal lymphoma: a report from an International Primary Central Nervous System Lymphoma Collaborative Group symposium. Oncologist. 2011;16(11):1589.

47. The correct answer is C. Of those with isolated ocular lymphoma, approximately half will subsequently develop primary CNS lymphoma. Grimm et al. reported their findings from 83 patients with primary ocular lymphoma. Forty-seven percent of patients relapsed in the brain at a median time to progression of 19 months. Hormigo A et al. Ocular presentation of primary central nervous system lymphoma: diagnosis and treatment. Br J Haematol. 2004;126(2): 202–8. Grimm SA et al. Primary intraocular lymphoma: an International

Primary Central Nervous System Lymphoma Collaborative Group Report. Ann Oncol. 2007;18(11):1851–5. Epub 2007 Sep 5.

48. The correct answer is A. Of the listed prognostic factors, age is the most important in primary CNS lymphoma. Age >60 and performance status (ECOG ≥ 2) are generally the two most universally accepted negative prognostic factors. A study published by Ferreri et al. confirmed the prognostic value of age and performance status but also established the value of elevated LDH serum level, elevated CSF protein concentration, and involvement of deep structures as negative predictors of survival. This study analyzed data from 378 patients with primary CNS lymphoma from 23 centers, found these five factors, and identified three different risk groups, based on the presence of 0–5 of these risk factors. Two-year overall survival significantly correlated by risk group: 0–1 (RF: 80 % ± 8 %), 2–3 (RF: 48 % ± 7 %), 4–5 (RF: 15 % ± 7 %), ($p < 0.000$). Corry J et al. Primary central nervous system lymphoma: age and performance status are more important than treatment modality. Int J Radiat Oncol Biol Phys. 1998;41:615–20. Ferreri AJM et al. Prognostic scoring system for primary CNS lymphomas: the international extranodal lymphoma study group experience. J Clin Oncol. 2003;21(2):266–72.

49. The correct answer is C. Methotrexate is highly effective against primary CNS lymphoma and is commonly combined with cytarabine and/or vincristine, procarbazine, and rituximab. Addition of intrathecal methotrexate to high-dose systemic methotrexate is generally not helpful and increases toxicity. Steroids should always be used once histologic confirmation has been obtained but due to rapid and impressive responses, should be used cautiously prior to biopsy as it can make diagnosis difficult. Whole brain radiation is effective for consolidation, but patients over the age of 60 can suffer debilitating neurologic side effects with radiation and it is recommended to reserve it for salvage particularly after a complete response to chemotherapy. Blood–brain barrier disruption with mannitol and intra-arterial chemotherapy has been demonstrated to have excellent response and survival, but is currently offered in few centers and does not represent a realistic treatment approach at this time, according to the NCCN guidelines for Central Nervous System cancers, version 2.2012. Batchelor et al. Treatment of primary CNS lymphoma with methotrexate and deferred radiotherapy: a report of NABTT 96-07. J Clin Oncol. 2003;21:1044–9.

50. The correct answer is C. A retrospective study by Haas and colleagues revealed high rates of response (92 % overall response rate) to 4 Gy in 2 fractions. Most patients had grade 1 or 2 follicular lymphoma; a very small number of patients had extranodal marginal zone lymphoma. Median time to local progression was 25 months and was 42 months for those patients who achieved a CR (61 % of patients). This suggests that 2 Gy × 2 fractions is a useful regimen for indolent lymphomas and the NCCN version 2.2012 guidelines suggest its use as palliation for follicular lymphomas, SLL, marginal zone lymphoma, and mantle-cell

lymphoma. Haas et al. High response rates and lasting remissions after low-dose involved-field radiotherapy in indolent lymphomas. J Clin Oncol. 2003;21: 2474–80.

51. The correct answer is D. Mantle-cell lymphoma tends to be a systemic disease, but for the uncommon patient with localized presentation, there is no accepted standard of care. Inclusion of radiation has retrospectively been demonstrated to improve PFS. Current trends outside of a clinical trial include IFRT with or without chemotherapy for early-stage, localized disease, and rituximab is frequently added, as it seems to improve response rates. Therefore, all of the presented regimens would be considered acceptable for this uncommon scenario. Leitch et al. Limited-stage mantle-cell lymphoma. Ann Oncol. 2003;14:1555–61.

52. The correct answer is B. Anaplastic large-cell lymphoma has been associated with development in the fibrous capsule surrounding a breast implant in rare cases. A number of cases have been reported and a matched case–control study from the Netherlands identified 11 patients with ALCL of the breast, and when matched to subjects with other lymphomas of the breast, breast implant was found to be a risk factor for development of ALCL. Optimal treatment is unclear, but it seems that in the majority of cases, removal of the implant and capsule may be curative and systemic involvement is uncommon. de Jong et al. Anaplastic large-cell lymphoma in women with breast implants. JAMA. 2008;300:2030–5.

53. The correct answer is B. Primary mediastinal B-cell lymphoma appears to be a distinct clinical entity from diffuse large B-cell lymphoma with mediastinal disease with or without other sites of disease, though the histology is indistinct from diffuse large B-cell lymphoma. It occurs most commonly in the fourth decade with a female predilection. Gene expression profiling suggests a similarity to classical Hodgkin lymphoma and is distinct from DLBCL. Standard-of-care regimens have not been established, but there seems to be a benefit to more intensive chemotherapy regimens over CHOP; however, with the addition of rituximab, this is uncertain. The role of radiation is less clear than in DLBCL. Faris et al. Primary mediastinal large B-cell lymphoma. Clin Adv Hematol Oncol. 2009;7:125–33.

54. The correct answer is D. Approximately, 10–15 % of orbital lymphomas are bilateral. Bhatia S. Curative radiotherapy for primary orbital lymphoma. Int J Radiat Oncol Biol Phys. 2002;54(3):818–23. Stafford SL et al. Orbital lymphoma: radiotherapy outcome and complications. Radiother Oncol. 2001;59(2): 139–44.

55. The correct answer is A. Approximately two thirds of orbital lymphomas are marginal zone in histology. Tsang RW, Gospodarowicz MK. Non-Hodgkin's

Lymphoma. In: Gunderson LL, Tepper JE, editors. Clinical radiation oncology. 3rd ed. Philadelphia: Elsevier Saunders; 2012. p. 1545–72.

56. The correct answer is C. A radiotherapy dose of 30 Gy is typically employed for orbital lymphomas and in multiple series has yielded local control >95 %. Bhatia S et al. Curative radiotherapy for primary orbital lymphoma. Int J Radiat Oncol Biol Phys. 2002;54(3):818–23. Chao CKS et al. Radiation therapy for primary orbital lymphoma. Int J Radiat Oncol Biol Phys. 1995;31(4):929–34.

57. The correct answer is D. Diagnosis of solitary plasmacytoma requires extensive workup for multiple myeloma, as underlying systemic disease will frequently be found. Smoldering myeloma is defined as M protein in serum $\geq$ 30 g/L and/or bone marrow plasma cells $\geq$ 10 % without any symptomatic or end organ impairment (no related anemia, renal failure, hypercalcemia, or bony lesions outside of the primary lesion). Active myeloma requires at least one of the following: hypercalcemia >11.5 mg/dL, creatinine > 2 g/dL, anemia with a hemoglobin < 10 g/dL (or 2 g/dL < normal), or bone disease. NCCN Guidelines. Multiple Myeloma. Version 1.2012.

58. The correct answer is C. Plasma cells are characterized by the following immunophenotype: CD5–, CD20–, CD38+.

59. The correct answer is B. Despite a negative serum protein electrophoresis, Bence Jones proteins will be seen on urine protein electrophoresis in approximately 20 % of patients with multiple myeloma. Kyle RA et al. Review of 1027 patients with newly diagnosed multiple myeloma. Mayo Clin Proc. 2003;78(1):21–33. Smith A, Wisloff F, Samson D, for the UK Myeloma Forum, Nordic Myeloma Study Group, and British Committee for Standards in Haematology. Guidelines on the diagnosis and management of multiple myeloma 2005. Br J Haematol. 2006;132(4):410–51

60. The correct answer is D. Approximately, 1–2 % of monoclonal gammopathy of undetermined significance (MGUS) will progress to a B-cell neoplasm yearly. Ucci G et al. Cooperative Group for the Study and Treatment of Multiple Myeloma: Presenting features of monoclonal gammopathies: an analysis of 684 newly diagnosed cases. J Intern Med. 1993;24:165–73

61. The correct answer is B. POEMS syndrome (polyneuropathy, organomegaly, endocrinopathy, M protein, and skin changes) is a variant of multiple myeloma, associated with a solitary or a limited number of sclerotic bone lesions. Bone marrow involvement is limited to <5 %, and M protein levels are usually <3g/dL. Bence Jones proteinuria is rare. This variant form is important because local radiotherapy to a dominant sclerotic lesion can substantially improve the polyneuropathy component of this disease in more than 50 % of patients. Delauch

MC et al. Peripheral neuropathy and plasma cell neoplasias: a report of 10 cases. Br J Haematol. 1981;48:383–92. Kelly Jr JJ et al. Osteosclerotic myeloma and peripheral neuropathy. Neurology. 1983;33:202–10.

62. The correct answer is B. False. The risk of progression to multiple myeloma within 10 years is approximately 60–70 % for solitary osseous plasmacytoma and approximately 30–40 % for solitary extraosseous plasmacytoma. Correlation of post-radiation disappearance of paraprotein has been observed in patients that experience less frequent systemic relapse. Pre-radiation level does not appear predictive. Mendenhall et al. Solitary plasmacytoma of bone and soft tissues. Am J Otolaryngol. 2003;24;(6):395–9. Holland JM. Plasmacytoma. Treatment results and conversion to myeloma. Cancer. 1992;69(6):1513–7.

63. The correct answer is A. Extramedullary plasmacytoma is most commonly found in the head and neck region (>80 %). Kotner LM, Wang CC. Plasmacytoma of the upper air and food passages. Cancer. 1972;30:414–8.

64. The correct answer is D. Solitary osseous plasmacytoma should be treated to a total of 50 Gy. Extramedullary plasmacytoma can be treated to 45–50 Gy, with good resulting local control. Frassica DA et al. Solitary plasmacytoma of bone: Mayo Clinic experience. Int J Radiat Oncol Biol Phys. 1989;16:43–8. Holland JM. Plasmacytoma. Treatment results and conversion to myeloma. Cancer. 1992;69(6):1513–7.

65. The correct answer is C. Bortezomib-based regimens have been associated with a higher incidence of herpes zoster; prophylaxis with acyclovir is recommended for these patients. Hepatitis B reactivation is a concern for rituximab-containing regimens. Bisphosphonates have been associated with osteonecrosis of the jaw. Thalidomide and lenalidomide with dexamethasone have been associated with thrombotic events with prophylactic anticoagulation recommended in these patients. Long-term steroid use is associated with *pneumocystis* pneumonia (PCP) and prophylaxis is recommended, commonly with trimethoprim and sulfamethoxazole for nonallergic patients. NCCN Guidelines. Multiple Myeloma. Version 1.2012.

Chapter 13
Sarcoma

Celine Bicquart Ord and Arthur Y. Hung

Questions

1. All of the following are true regarding soft tissue sarcoma, except:
   A. They are derived from mesenchymal tissue.
   B. Median age of onset is 55–55 years.
   C. Five-year survival for all sites and stages combined is 50–60 %.
   D. Local progression is the mode of death for extremity and torso sarcomas.

2. What syndrome is associated with the development of intra-abdominal desmoid tumors?
   A. Gardner's syndrome
   B. Cowden's syndrome
   C. Ataxia telangiectasia
   D. Nelson's syndrome

3. What translocation is characteristic of synovial cell sarcoma?
   A. t(9;22)
   B. t(12;16)
   C. t(2;13)
   D. t(X: 18)

C.B. Ord, MD (✉)
Department of Radiation Oncology, Scott & White Memorial Hospital,
2401 S. 31st Street, Temple, TX 76508, USA
e-mail: celineord@gmail.com

A.Y. Hung, MD
Department of Radiation Medicine, Oregon Health Science University,
3181 SW Sam Jackson Park Rd, KPV4, Portland, OR 97239-3098, USA
e-mail: hunga@ohsu.edu

C.B. Ord et al. (eds.), *Radiation Oncology Study Guide*,
DOI 10.1007/978-1-4614-6400-6_13, © Springer Science+Business Media New York 2013

4. What translocation is characteristic of Ewing's sarcoma?
   A. t(11;22)
   B. t(12;16)
   C. t(9;22)
   D. t(X: 18)

5. All are true regarding Li-Fraumeni syndrome, except:
   A. It results from a germ-line mutation of p53.
   B. There is a 50 % risk of malignancy by age 70.
   C. There is a risk of developing breast cancer.
   D. There is a risk of developing osteosarcoma.

6. Which is the most common malignancy associated with hereditary retinoblastoma?
   A. Osteosarcoma
   B. Pineoblastoma
   C. Hepatocellular carcinoma
   D. Colorectal cancer

7. Which is the most common site of soft tissue sarcoma?
   A. Trunk
   B. Upper extremity
   C. Head and neck
   D. Lower extremity

8. All of the following are true regarding angiosarcoma, except:
   A. It is not staged by the TNM system.
   B. Fifty percent of cases occur in the head and neck.
   C. Local recurrence is frequent but distant metastases are not.
   D. Regional lymph node metastases are more frequent than in other soft tissue sarcomas.

9. All of the following are true regarding dermatofibrosarcoma protuberans, except:
   A. It exhibits slow, indolent growth.
   B. It stains for CD 34+.
   C. It rarely recurs after simple local excision.
   D. Those with the t(17;22) translocation respond to imatinib.

10. Regarding the NCI soft tissue sarcoma trial of amputation versus limb-sparing surgery + radiation, which of the following is not true?
    A. Local control in the amputated arm was 100 %.
    B. Total radiation dose was 45–50 Gy.
    C. All patients received postoperative chemotherapy.
    D. 15 % of limb-sparing patients had positive surgical margins.

11. Regarding the NCI soft tissue sarcoma trial of amputation versus limb-sparing surgery + radiation, which of the following is not true?
    A. There was no difference in local control between arms.
    B. Most recurrences in the limb-sparing arm were isolated local failures.
    C. There was no difference in disease-free survival between the arms.
    D. There was no difference in overall survival between the arms.

12. What is the local recurrence rate with a planned positive margin after resection?
    A. 4 %
    B. 8 %
    C. 12 %
    D. 16 %

13. What is the local recurrence rate with an unplanned resection elsewhere with a positive margin on re-excision?
    A. 20 %
    B. 30 %
    C. 40 %
    D. 50 %

14. What is the expected local control rate of a sarcoma after surgery and adjuvant radiation?
    A. 75 %
    B. 80 %
    C. 85 %
    D. 90 %

15. In the NCI trial of limb-sparing surgery +/− adjuvant therapy for sarcomas of the extremities, all of the following are true, except:
    A. No chemotherapy was used in any patients.
    B. Local control for those receiving radiation was improved.
    C. There was no difference in local control in low- versus high-grade tumors.
    D. Those with low-grade tumors were randomized to adjuvant radiation versus observation.

16. In the Memorial Sloan-Kettering Cancer Center trial of limb-sparing surgery +/− adjuvant brachytherapy, which of the following is not true?
    A. Complications were reduced with loading of catheters on post-op day 5 as opposed to immediately postoperatively.
    B. Total brachytherapy dose was 45 Gy.
    C. Positive surgical margins predicted for local recurrence.
    D. A local control benefit for brachytherapy was found only for high-grade tumors.

17. In the NCI-Canada trial of pre- versus postoperative EBRT, all of the following are true, except:
    A. There was no local control difference between the arms.
    B. Positive surgical margins predicted for local recurrence.
    C. Size and grade of the primary tumor did not predict for recurrence-free survival.
    D. Positive surgical margins were treated with a 16–20 Gy boost.

18. All of the following situations preclude brachytherapy as the sole adjuvant therapeutic modality for soft tissue sarcoma, except:
    A. The CTV cannot be adequately encompassed in implant geometry.
    B. Proximity of treatment volume near a critical structure precludes delivery of a meaningful dose.
    C. Resection margins are positive.
    D. Skin ulceration is not present.

19. Which of the following radiation dose recommendations is incorrect?
    A. Preoperative external beam radiation—50 Gy
    B. Postoperative external beam radiation for negative margins—50–60 Gy
    C. Postoperative HDR brachytherapy alone—45 Gy
    D. Boost dose for positive margins—16–20 Gy

20. All of the following are true regarding radiation target volumes for soft tissue sarcoma, except:
    A. Tumor cells are generally found at a maximum of 4 cm from the primary tumor.
    B. The deep margin still needs to include deep muscle for a superficial tumor.
    C. Longitudinal margins are longer than radial margins.
    D. Soft tissue sarcoma generally respects anatomical fascial planes.

21. What translocation is associated with alveolar rhabdomyosarcoma?
    A. t(2;13)
    B. t(X;17)
    C. t(12;22)
    D. t(X;18)

22. All of the following are true regarding the sequential chemotherapy and radiation neoadjuvant treatment approach described by DeLaney et al., except:
    A. Five-year overall survival was significantly improved versus historical controls.
    B. The improvement in overall survival was due to improved local control.
    C. Radiotherapy consisted of two split courses of 22 Gy.
    D. Positive margins were treated with a radiotherapy boost.

23. All of the following are true regarding isolated limb perfusion for soft tissue sarcomas, except:
    A. Chemotherapy consists of melphalan and TNF-α.
    B. Overall response rates are in excess of 95 %.
    C. Limb-preservation rates are in excess of 80 %.
    D. Most appropriate in patients of resection with probable sacrifice of important function.

24. Which of the following was not a finding from the landmark meta-analysis of adjuvant chemotherapy in soft tissue sarcoma by the Sarcoma Meta-analysis Collaboration (Lancet 1997)?
    A. Distant relapse-free interval was improved with chemotherapy.
    B. Overall recurrence-free survival was improved with chemotherapy.
    C. Overall survival was improved with chemotherapy.
    D. Local recurrence-free interval was improved with chemotherapy.

25. All of the following are true regarding retroperitoneal sarcomas, except:
    A. These tumors typically present larger in size due to late presentation of symptoms.
    B. Adjuvant radiation can be easily delivered with the use of IMRT.
    C. Preoperative radiation does not increase wound complications.
    D. Intraoperative radiotherapy may improve local control and overall survival.

26. Which of the following is false regarding primary sarcomas of the stomach?
    A. Gastrointestinal stromal tumors frequently recur with lung metastases.
    B. Gastrointestinal stromal tumors respond well to imatinib.
    C. Half of gastrointestinal stromal tumor recurrences are in the liver.
    D. Complete excision is one of the most important factors for improvement of disease-specific survival.

27. All of the following are true regarding phyllodes tumors of the breast, except:
    A. Malignancy is determined by the stroma.
    B. Treatment of choice is surgical excision with wide margins.
    C. Breast conservation is contraindicated.
    D. Compared to epithelial breast cancers, phyllodes tumors do not frequently metastasize to lymph nodes.

28. Which of the following is false regarding giant cell tumors?
    A. The majority are not malignant.
    B. There is >90 % local control with surgery alone.
    C. Local control rates with radiation alone are poor.
    D. These occur most commonly at the epiphysis.

29. Osteosarcoma most commonly occurs in which part of the bone?
    A. Metaphysis.
    B. Diaphysis.
    C. Epiphysis.
    D. There is equal distribution throughout the bone.

30. Which is the second most common sarcoma in children?
    A. Osteosarcoma
    B. Ewing's sarcoma
    C. Rhabdomyosarcoma
    D. Leiomyosarcoma

31. Which is the most important prognostic factor in clear cell sarcoma?
    A. Margin status
    B. Lymphovascular invasion
    C. Grade
    D. Size

32. Any node positive sarcoma is AJCC 7th edition stage:
    A. IIA
    B. IIB
    C. III
    D. IV

33. A 3 cm soft tissue sarcoma with invasion of the superficial fascia is not found
    on CT scan to involve the deep musculature. By AJCC 7th edition staging, this
    would be considered:
    A. T1a
    B. T1b
    C. T2a
    D. T2b

Answers and Rationales

1. The correct answer is D. Soft tissue sarcomas are rare malignancies, comprising 1 % of adult malignancies yearly. They are derived from mesenchymal cells and present at one of three sites: (1) extremity and torso (50 %), (2) retroperitoneal (35 %), and (3) head and neck (10 %). The median age of presentation is 50–55 years, and 5-year survival for all sites and stages is 50–60 %. While retroperitoneal sarcomas have aggressive local and recurrent behaviors, the mode of death for extremity and truncal sarcomas is predominately distant (lung metastases). Jemal A, et al. Cancer statistics. CA Cancer J Clin. 2004;54:8–29. Pollock R et al. The National Cancer Data Base report on soft tissue sarcoma. Cancer. 1996;78:2247–57.

2. The correct answer is A. Gardner's syndrome, a subset of familial adenomatous polyposis, is associated with the development of intra-abdominal desmoids tumors. Posner MC et al. The desmoids tumor. Not a benign disease. Arch Surg. 1989;124:191–6.

3. The correct answer is D. The t(X;18) translocation is characteristic of synovial cell sarcomas. This translocation involves the SSX1 or SSX2 gene and the SYT gene from chromosome 18q11. t(12;16) is characteristic of classical myxoid liposarcoma. t(2;13) is characteristic of alveolar rhabdomyosarcoma. Kawai A et al. SYT-SSX gene fusion as a determinant of morphology and prognosis in synovial sarcoma. N Engl J Med. 1998;338:153–60. Ladanyi M et al. Impact of SYT-SSX fusion type of the clinical behavior of synovial sarcoma: A multi-institutional retrospective study of 243 patients. Cancer Res. 2002;62:135–40.

4. The correct answer is A. Ewing's sarcoma is associated with the t(11;22) translocation. Schuck A, Paulussen M. Pediatric sarcomas of bone. In: Gunderson LL, Tepper JE, editors. Clinical radiation oncology. 3rd ed. Philadelphia: Elsevier Saunders; 2012. p. 1435–42.

5. The correct answer is B. Li-Fraumeni syndrome results from a germ-line mutation of p53 on chromosome 17. It is inherited in an autosomal dominant fashion and carries a 50 % risk of malignancy by age 30 % and 90 % risk by age 70. Associated malignancies include breast cancer, soft tissue sarcoma, rhabdomyosarcoma, osteosarcoma, ALL, glioma, and adrenal tumors. O'Sullivan B, Dickie C, Chung P, Catton C. Soft tissue sarcoma. In: Gunderson LL, Tepper JE, editors. Clinical radiation oncology. 3rd ed. Philadelphia: Elsevier Saunders; 2012. p. 1355–91.

6. The correct answer is A. In those with hereditary retinoblastoma, there is a several-hundredfold risk of developing osteosarcoma in the early years, melanoma or a brain tumor through middle age, and epithelial malignancies in later age. Friend SH et al. A human DNA segment with properties of the gene that

predisposes to retinoblastoma and osteosarcoma. Nature. 1986;323:643. Bookstein R et al. Suppression of a tumorigenicity of human prostate carcinoma cell by replacing a mutation RB gene. Science. 1990;247:643.

7. The correct answer is D. Soft tissue sarcomas are most commonly found in the lower extremity (45 %), with 75 % of these above the knee. The second most common site is the trunk. O'Sullivan B, Dickie C, Chung P, Catton C. Soft tissue sarcoma. In: Gunderson LL, Tepper JE, editors. Clinical radiation oncology. 3rd ed. Philadelphia: Elsevier Saunders; 2012. p. 1355–91.

8. The correct answer is C. Angiosarcomas have an unusual behavior that precludes their staging using the TNM system. Superficial angiosarcomas occur half of the time in the head and neck region. Unfortunately, regional metastases are common in this tumor type, as is both local and distant recurrence. Sobin L et al. TNM classification of malignant tumours. 6th ed. New York:Wiley-Liss; 2002. Fletcher CDM. Pleomorphic malignant fibrous histiocytomas: fact or fiction? A reappraisal based on 159 tumors diagnosed as pleomorphic sarcoma. Am J Surg Pathol. 1992;16:213–28. Mark RJ et al. Angiosarcoma of the head and neck. The UCLA experience 1955 through 1990. Arch Otolaryngol Head Neck Surg. 1993;119:973–8. Holden CA et al. Angiosarcoma of the face and scalp, prognosis and treatment. Cancer. 1987;59:1046–57.

9. The correct answer is C. Dermatofibrosarcoma protuberans (DFSP) is a superficial tumor of the dermis with neural differentiation (given CD 34+). It grows slowly, with a propensity for local recurrence after local excision alone. As such, resection can be supplanted with adjuvant radiation to improve local control. Given its slow growth, it is not staged within the TNM system. Those DFSP with the t(17;22) translocation respond well to imatinib. Sobin L et al. TNM classification of malignant tumours. 6th ed. New York:Wiley-Liss; 2002. Greene FL et al. AJCC cancer staging manual, 6th ed. New York: Springer; 2002. McArthur GA et al. Molecular and clinical analysis of locally advanced dermatofibrosarcoma protuberans treated with imatinib: imatinib target exploration consortium study B2225. J Clin Oncol. 2005;23:866–73. Ballo MT et al. The role of radiation therapy in the management of dermatofibrosarcoma protuberans. Int J Radiat Oncol Biol Phys. 1998;40:823–7. Suit H et al. Radiation in the management of patients with dermatofibrosarcoma protuberans. J Clin Oncol. 1996;14:2365–9. Sun M et al. Dermatofibrosarcoma protuberans: treatment results of 35 cases. Radiother Oncol. 2000;57:175–81.

10. The correct answer is B. The NCI trial reported by Rosenberg et al. randomized 43 patients with high-grade soft tissue sarcoma of the extremity to amputation versus wide local excision with generous margins + post-op radiation (45–50 Gy, followed by boost to 60–70 Gy). Positive margins were allowed at critical structures and were present in 15 % of the limb-sparing patients. All patients received postoperative chemotherapy with Adriamycin + Cytoxan, then methotrexate. There was no difference in local control between the arms (100 % vs.

85 %, $p=0.06$), 5-year disease-free survival (78 % vs. 71 %, NS), or overall survival (88 % vs. 83 %, NS). Notably, of the 4 local recurrences in the limb sparing arm, only 1 was an isolated local recurrence; 3 had simultaneous distant metastases. Rosenberg SA et al. The treatment of soft-tissue sarcomas of the extremities: prospective randomized evaluations of (1) limb-sparing surgery plus radiation therapy compared with amputation (2) the role of adjuvant chemotherapy. Ann Surg. 1982;196(3):305–15.

11. The correct answer is B. The NCI trial reported by Rosenberg et al. randomized 43 patients with high-grade soft tissue sarcoma of the extremity to amputation versus wide local excision with generous margins + post-op radiation (45–50 Gy, followed by boost to 60–70 Gy). Positive margins were allowed at critical structures and were present in 15 % of the limb-sparing patients. All patients received postoperative chemotherapy with Adriamycin + Cytoxan, then methotrexate. There was no difference in local control between the arms (100 % vs. 85 %, $p=0.06$), 5-year disease-free survival (78 % vs. 71 %, NS), or overall survival (88 % vs. 83 %, NS). In those with local failures, most also had simultaneous distant failure. Rosenberg SA et al. The treatment of soft-tissue sarcomas of the extremities: Prospective randomized evaluations of (1) limb-sparing surgery plus radiation therapy compared with amputation (2) the role of adjuvant chemotherapy. Ann Surg. 1982;196(3):305–15.

12. The correct answer is A. In excisions planned from the outset by a multidisciplinary team to have a positive margin to spare a critical anatomic structure, local recurrence is 3.6 %. In unplanned excisions elsewhere with a positive margin on re-excision, local recurrence is 31.6 %. Gerrand CH et al. Classification of positive margins after resection of soft-tissue sarcoma of the limb predicts the risk of local recurrence. J Bone Joint Surg Br. 2001;83-B:1149–55.

13. The correct answer is B. In excisions planned from the outset by a multidisciplinary team to have a positive margin to spare a critical anatomic structure, local recurrence is 3.6 %. In unplanned excisions elsewhere with a positive margin on re-excision, local recurrence is 31.6 %. Gerrand CH et al. Classification of positive margins after resection of soft-tissue sarcoma of the limb predicts the risk of local recurrence. J Bone Joint Surg Br. 2001;83-B:1149–55.

14. The correct answer is D. Strander et al. reported data on 4,579 patients with soft tissue sarcoma and found that adjuvant radiation improved local control after surgery in trunk/extremity sarcomas with negative, close, or microscopically positive margins, expected to be 90 %. The role of radiation for improving local control in retroperitoneal, head and neck, breast, and uterine sarcomas is less certain. Strander H et al. A systematic overview of radiation therapy effects in soft tissue sarcoma. Acta Oncol. 2003;42:516–31.

15. The correct answer is A. The NCI trial reported by Yang et al. sought to determine the benefit of adjuvant radiation. One hundred forty-one patients with extremity sarcomas were randomized after surgery to +/− RT alone (low-grade) or chemoRT (high-grade) versus observation (low-grade) or chemo alone (high-grade). Chemotherapy was doxorubicin + cyclophosphamide; radiation was 63 Gy. In the high-grade tumors, local control was improved with chemoRT (100 % vs. 81 %), though there was no difference in disease-free or overall survival. In low-grade tumors, local control was also improved with adjuvant RT (96 % vs. 66 %), though there was no difference in overall survival. Yang JC et al. Randomized prospective study of the benefit of adjuvant radiation therapy in the treatment of soft tissue sarcomas of the extremity. J Clin Oncol. 1998;16(1):197–203.

16. The correct answer is C. One hundred sixty-four patients with extremity soft tissue sarcoma were randomized after limb-sparing surgery to +/− brachytherapy with Ir^{192} (42–45 Gy). A 2 cm margin around the surgical bed defined the CTV, and catheters were placed 1 cm apart. While initially loaded right away, due to complications, this shifted to 5 days postoperatively. There was a local control benefit seen with brachytherapy only in high-grade tumors (89 % vs. 66 %, $p=0.0025$). On multivariate analysis, age >60 was the only factor that predicted local recurrence. Margin status (positive margins) did not predict for recurrence. Pisters PW, et al. Long-term results of a prospective randomized trial of adjuvant brachytherapy in soft tissue sarcoma. J Clin Oncol. 1996;14(3):859–68.

17. The correct answer is C. The NCI-Canada trial of pre- versus post-op EBRT randomized 190 of 266 planned patients to (1) pre-op radiation 50 Gy/25 fractions, with additional 16–20 Gy boost if positive surgical margins or (2) post-op radiation 50 Gy/25 fractions + 16–20 Gy boost. Five-year results presented at ASCO in 2004 showed no difference in local control, recurrence-free survival, or overall survival between the arms. Positive surgical margins were found to predict for local recurrence, while size/grade of the primary tumor were found to predict for recurrence-free and overall survival. Late effects of RT included worse fibrosis, edema, and joint stiffness in post-op RT, though not statistically significant. O'Sullivan B et al. Five-year results of a randomized phase III trial of pre-operative versus post-operative radiotherapy in extremity soft tissue sarcoma. J Clin Oncol. 2004 ASCO Annual Meeting Proceedings. Vol 22, No 14S (July 15 Supplement), 2004; 9007. Davis AM et al. Late radiation morbidity following randomization to preoperative versus postoperative radiotherapy in extremity soft tissue sarcoma. Radiother Oncol. 2005;75(1):48–53.

18. The correct answer is D. Per the American Brachytherapy Society, all of the listed reasons preclude the use of brachytherapy as the sole adjuvant modality after surgery except the last choice—the lack of skin ulceration. The first three scenarios would require supplementary EBRT. Nag S et al. The American Brachytherapy Society recommendations for brachytherapy of soft tissue sarcomas. In J Radiat Oncol Biol Phys. 2001;49:1033–43.

19. The correct answer is C. Preoperative radiotherapy dose is typically 50 Gy/25 fractions, with a postoperative boost of 16–20 Gy for positive margins. Postoperative radiotherapy is typically 50–60 Gy for negative margins and 66 Gy for positive margins (boost of 16 Gy). Brachytherapy delivered by LDR is given as 45 Gy in 4–6 days with 0.45 Gy/h. Brachytherapy delivered by HDR is given as 36 Gy in BID fractions of 3.6 Gy in 5 days. Pisters PW et al. Long-term results of a prospective randomized trial of adjuvant brachytherapy in soft tissue sarcoma. J Clin Oncol. 1996;14:859–68. O'Sullivan B et al. Preoperative versus postoperative radiotherapy in soft-tissue sarcoma of the limbs: A randomised trial. Lancet. 2002;359:2235–41. Nag S et al. The American Brachytherapy Society recommendations for brachytherapy of soft tissue sarcomas. In J Radiat Oncol Biol Phys. 2001;49:1033–43. Arthur DW et al. Partial breast brachytherapy after lumpectomy: Low dose-rate and high-dose-rate experience. Int J Radiat Oncol Biol Phys. 2003;56:681–9.

20. The correct answer is B. Soft tissue sarcoma generally follows anatomical fascial planes, which has implications in postsurgical management. Radiotherapy volumes follow this behavior, with longer longitudinal margins than axial margins. Superficial tumors are resected with the deep fascia as the deep margin; as such, postoperative radiation does not need to extend into the deeper muscle compartment. A radiological-pathological series of 15 patients from Mt. Sinai and Princess Margaret Hospital in Canada showed that tumor cells are found at a maximum of 4 cm from the primary tumor, suggesting that the longitudinal CTV margin can be 4 rather than 5 cm. White LM et al. Histological assessment of peritumoral edema in soft tissue sarcoma. Int J Radiat Oncol Biol Phys. 2005;61(5)1439–45. O'Sullivan B et al. Target description for radiotherapy of soft tissue sarcoma. In: Gregoire V, Scalliet P, Ang KK, editors. Clinical target volumes in conformal radiotherapy and intensity modulated radiotherapy. Heidelberg: Springer; 2003. p. 205–27.

21. The correct answer is A. Alveolar rhabdomyosarcoma is characterized by the t(2;13) and t(1;13) translocations. The t(X;18) translocation is characteristic of synovial cell sarcomas. t(12;22) is characteristic of myxoid liposarcoma. t(X;17) is characteristic of alveolar sarcoma of soft parts. Kawai A et al. SYT-SSX gene fusion as a determinant of morphology and prognosis in synovial sarcoma. N Engl J Med. 1998;338:153–60. Ladanyi M et al. Impact of SYT–SSX fusion type of the clinical behavior of synovial sarcoma: A multi-institutional retrospective study of 243 patients. Cancer Res. 2002;62:135–40.

22. The correct answer is B. DeLaney et al. described their experience of treating 48 patients with localized, high-grade, large (>8 cm) soft tissue sarcomas with sequential chemotherapy (doxorubicin, ifosfamide, mesna, and dacarbazine × 3), sandwiched between two courses of 22 Gy/11 fractions radiotherapy, followed by surgery. Positive margins were treated with a subsequent 16 Gy boost. Five-year overall survival compared to historical cohorts was 87 % versus 58 %, with the difference attributed to the vastly improved distant metastasis-free rate

of 75 % versus 44 % historically ($p=0.0016$). DeLaney TF et al. Neoadjuvant chemotherapy and radiotherapy for large extremity soft-tissue sarcomas. Int J Radiat Oncol Biol Phys. 2003;56:1117–27.

23. The correct answer is C. Isolated limb perfusion uses a heart-lung machine to deliver chemotherapy (melphalan and TNF-α) to the solely affected limb. A multicenter trial in Europe showed overall response rates of 76 % in initially unresectable soft tissue sarcomas, with 71 % of limbs preserved. The patients chosen for isolated limb perfusion are those in whom conventional resection would have left a marked functional loss or amputation. One series reports overall response rates of 95 % for soft tissue sarcoma with a 61 % complete response rate. Amputation was avoided in all cases. Grunhagen DJ et al. Isolated limb perfusion with tumor necrosis factor and melphalan prevents amputation in patients with multiple sarcomas in arm or leg. Ann Surg Oncol. 2005;12:473–9. Eggermont AM et al. Current uses of isolated limb perfusion in the clinic and a model system for new strategies. Lancet Oncol. 2003;4:429–37. Grunhagen DJ et al. TNF-based isolated limb perfusion in unresectable extremity desmoid tumors. Eur J Surg Oncol. 2005;31:912–6.

24. The correct answer is C. The Sarcoma Meta-analysis Collaboration showed that adjuvant doxorubicin-based chemotherapy improved both distant recurrence-free and local recurrence-free intervals, as well as overall recurrence-free survival, but did not improve overall survival. The hazard ratio for overall survival with chemotherapy was 0.89 (0.76–1.03), and not significant ($p=0.12$), but represented a 4 % absolute benefit at 10 years. A subsequent meta-analysis was published by the Sarcoma Meta-analysis Collaboration in 2000 and showed that in 14 trials of 1,568 patients, doxorubicin-based adjuvant therapy improved both local recurrence-free interval and overall recurrence-free survival—corresponding to a significant absolute benefit of 6–10 % at 10 years. As in the previous meta- analysis, overall survival improved by 4 %, though the hazard ratio for overall survival was still not significant (HR 0.89 95 % CI 0.76–1.03). The largest benefit for adjuvant chemotherapy was shown in patients with sarcoma of the extremities. More recently, a new meta-analysis including 1,953 patients in 18 trials was published. Doxorubicin-based adjuvant chemotherapy for localized, resectable soft tissue sarcoma continues to show a local recurrence, distant recurrence, and overall recurrence benefit. The OR for overall survival with doxorubicin alone was 0.84 (95 % CI 0.68–1.03, $p=0.09$), though it was 0.56 (95 % CI 0.36–0.85, $p=0.01$) when doxorubicin was combined with ifosfamide. Sarcoma Meta-analysis Collaboration: Adjuvant chemotherapy for localized resectable soft-tissue sarcoma of adults: meta-analysis of individual data. Lancet 1997;350:1647–54. Sarcoma Meta-analysis Collaboration: Adjuvant chemotherapy for localized resectable soft-tissue sarcoma of adults. Cochrane Database Syst Rev. 2000;(4):CD001419. Pervaiz N et al. A systematic meta-analysis of randomized controlled trials of adjuvant chemotherapy for localized resectable soft-tissue sarcoma. Cancer. 2008;113(3):573–81.

25. The correct answer is B. Retroperitoneal sarcomas comprise 10–15 % of all sarcomas and, unlike extremity sarcomas, present much later and larger in size due to the absence of symptoms. The most common histologies are liposarcoma and leiomyosarcoma. Primary therapy is surgical resection with a less clear role for adjuvant or neoadjuvant therapy. The difficulty with adjuvant radiotherapy is the dose-limiting adjacent bowel now in a poorly defined treatment volume. IMRT does not change this. An advantage of preoperative radiotherapy is that the tumor in place displaces the dose-limiting bowel. Intraoperative radiotherapy has been an approach at Massachusetts General, delivering an electron boost after preoperative external beam. With this nonrandomized approach, both local control and overall survival are improved (83 % vs. 74 %) and (61 % vs. 30 %), respectively. Gieschen HL et al. Long-term results of intra-operative electron beam radiotherapy for primary and recurrent retroperitoneal soft tissue sarcoma. Int J Radiat Oncol Biol Phys. 2001;50:127–31.

26. The correct answer is A. Primary sarcomas of the stomach are rare and are comprised of two major types: gastrointestinal stromal tumors (GIST) and leiomyosarcoma. Complete excision is one of the most important factors for improved disease-specific survival. While local recurrence as the initial recurrence occurs in ~40 % of both tumor types, pulmonary metastases are much more common in leiomyosarcoma than GIST tumors. Conversely, GIST tumors present with hepatic metastases as the first site of recurrence in half of cases, compared to only 20 % for leiomyosarcoma. A phase II trial of imatinib mesylate × 2 doses in patients with metastatic or unresectable GIST showed partial response rates of 68 %. Clary BM et al. Gastrointestinal stromal tumors and leiomyosarcoma of the abdomen and retroperitoneum: a clinical comparison. Ann Surg Oncol. 2001;8:290–9. Demetri GD et al. Efficacy and safety of imatinib mesylate in advanced gastrointestinal stromal tumors. N Engl J Med. 2002;347:472–80.

27. The correct answer is C. Phyllodes tumors of the breast are tumors of both epithelial and stromal elements, with the stromal environment (cellular polymorphism, nuclear atypia, increased mitotic activity, stromal overgrowth) determining malignancy. Contrasted to epithelial breast tumors, these rarely metastasize to regional lymph nodes. Treatment of choice is surgical excision with wide margins; breast-conserving surgery is a reasonable option. In the cases of close/positive margins, adjuvant radiation can be used to reduce the chance of local recurrence (the predominant mode of failure). Mangi AA et al. Surgical management of phyllodes tumors. Arch Surg. 1999;134:487–92; discussion 292–483. Rowell MD et al. Phyllodes tumors. Am J Surg. 1993;165:76–379. Kapiris I et al. Outcome and predictive factors of local recurrence and distant metastases following primary surgical treatment of high-grade malignant phyllodes tumours of the breast. Eur J Surg Oncol. 2001;27:723–30.

28. The correct answer is C. Giant cell tumors are most commonly (98–90 %) nonmalignant and occur in the epiphysis. Surgery alone is the primary initial management and has excellent local control (>90 %). Radiation alone (54 Gy) can also be

used for inoperable or margin positive tumors, with excellent control rates. These occur more commonly in those aged 20–30. O'Sullivan B, Dickie C, Chung P, Catton C. Soft tissue sarcoma. In: Gunderson LL, Tepper JE, editors. Clinical radiation oncology. 3rd ed. Philadelphia: Elsevier Saunders; 2012. p. 1355–91.

29. The correct answer is A. Osteosarcoma most frequently occurs in the metaphysis of the bone. Ewing's sarcoma most frequently occurs in the diaphysis of the bone. O'Sullivan B, Dickie C, Chung P, Catton C. Soft tissue sarcoma. In: Gunderson LL, Tepper JE, editors. Clinical radiation oncology. 3rd ed. Philadelphia: Elsevier Saunders; 2012. p. 1355–91.

30. The correct answer is B. While rhabdomyosarcoma is the most common sarcoma in children, the second most common is Ewing's sarcoma. Krasin MJ. Pediatric soft tissue sarcomas. In: Gunderson LL, Tepper JE, editors. Clinical radiation oncology. 3rd ed. Philadelphia: Elsevier Saunders; 2012. p. 1425–42.

31. The correct answer is D. Size is the most important prognostic factor in clear cell sarcoma. In Kawai A et al. Clear cell sarcoma of tendons and aponeuroses: An analysis of 75 cases. J Clin Oncol. 2006 ASCO Meeting Proceedings Part I. Vol 24, No. 18S (June 20 Supplement): 9572.

32. The correct answer is C. In the 7th edition of AJCC staging, nodal positivity constitutes stage III disease. Edge SB, Byrd DR, Compton CC, et al., editors. Soft tissue sarcoma. AJCC cancer staging handbook. 7th ed. New York: Springer; 2010.

33. The correct answer is B. A 3 cm tumor is T1 (≤5 cm), but invasion of the superficial fascia constitutes a deep tumor, denoted by "b". Edge SB, Byrd DR, Compton CC, et al, editors. Soft tissue sarcoma. AJCC cancer staging handbook. 7th ed. New York: Springer; 2010.

Chapter 14
Pediatric Non-central Nervous System Cancers

Celine Bicquart Ord and Carol Marquez

Questions

1. Rhabdomyosarcoma is most frequently associated with abnormalities of which organ system?
   A. Genitourinary
   B. Central nervous system
   C. Gastrointestinal
   D. Cardiovascular

2. Which subtype of rhabdomyosarcoma is characterized by "spindle-shaped rhab-domyoblasts, small round cells with hyperchromatic nuclei on a background of a myxoid stroma"?
   A. Botryoides
   B. Extraosseous Ewing's
   C. Alveolar
   D. Embryonal

3. Botryoid tumors commonly occur in all of the following sites, except:
   A. Extremity
   B. Genitourinary region
   C. Nasopharynx
   D. External auditory canal

C.B. Ord, MD (✉)
Department of Radiation Oncology, Scott & White Memorial Hospital,
2401 S. 31st Street, Temple, TX 76508, USA
e-mail: cord@sw.org

C. Marquez, MD
Department of Radiation Medicine, Oregon Health Science University,
3181 SW Sam Jackson Park Rd, KPV4, Portland, OR 97239, USA

C.B. Ord et al. (eds.), *Radiation Oncology Study Guide*,
DOI 10.1007/978-1-4614-6400-6_14, © Springer Science+Business Media New York 2013

4. Which one of the following primary sites of rhabdomyosarcoma has a 5-year overall survival of over 80 %?
   A. Bladder
   B. Parameningeal
   C. Orbit
   D. Extremity

5. What percentage of patients with rhabdomyosarcoma presents with metastatic disease at diagnosis?
   A. 20 %
   B. 25 %
   C. 30 %
   D. 35 %

6. Gross residual disease after biopsy would be classified in which International Rhabdomyosarcoma Study (IRS) Clinical Group?
   A. I
   B. II
   C. III
   D. IV

7. Lymph node involvement of a 4-cm rhabdomyosarcoma of the prostate is classified as what stage?
   A. 1
   B. 2
   C. 3
   D. 4

8. What was the 5-year overall survival rate in the International Rhabdomyosarcoma Study 1 (IRS-1)?
   A. 50 %
   B. 55 %
   C. 60 %
   D. 65 %

9. All of the following are true regarding International Rhabdomyosarcoma Study I (IRS-I), except:
   A. The risk of distant recurrence was greater than the risk of local recurrence.
   B. The addition of cyclophosphamide to clinical group II showed no benefit.
   C. The addition of doxorubicin to clinical group III improved overall survival.
   D. The orbit was found to be a more favorable site of disease.

10. All of the following are true regarding International Rhabdomyosarcoma Study II (IRS-II), except:
    A. Clinical group I did not receive radiation.
    B. The addition of cyclophosphamide did not improve outcomes in clinical groups I and II.
    C. Whole brain irradiation did not improve meningeal recurrence rates for parameningeal sites of disease.
    D. Five-year overall survival improved from IRS-I.

11. Regarding radiation of parameningeal sites of rhabdomyosarcoma, which of the following is not true?
    A. Meningeal recurrence rates were improved with the use of whole brain radiotherapy in IRS-II.
    B. IRS-IV recommends a radiation CTV of gross tumor + 2 cm.
    C. The reduction in treated radiotherapy volume from IRS-II to IRS-IV was associated with an increased risk of meningeal failure.
    D. Radiotherapy starts at day 0 in patients with meningeal impingement.

12. Regarding orbital rhabdomyosarcoma, all of the following are true, except:
    A. IRS-III showed that progression-free survival was improved with the addition of cyclophosphamide to vincristine + actinomycin.
    B. Most patients with orbital tumors have clinical group III disease.
    C. Radiation treatment volume is gross tumor volume +2 cm, not exceeding the bony orbit if there is no bony erosion.
    D. Cataracts are a frequent side effect of radiation.

13. All are true regarding the treatment of rhabdomyosarcoma of the paratesticular region, except:
    A. Surgery consists of radical inguinal orchiectomy with high spermatic cord ligation.
    B. Retroperitoneal lymph node dissection is no longer indicated.
    C. Radiation is indicated if the scrotum has been violated from transscrotal biopsy.
    D. Children <10 years old only undergo lymph node evaluation if there are positive or concerning findings on CT scan.

14. All of the following are true regarding Ewing's sarcoma, except:
    A. There is a predilection for whites.
    B. It is more common among males than females.
    C. Cytokeratin and neuron-specific enolase can be positive.
    D. Half of patients present with localized disease at diagnosis.

15. What is the most common site of osteosarcoma?
    A. Tibia
    B. Femur
    C. Fibula
    D. Humerus

16. All of the following are true regarding Ewing's sarcoma, except:
    A. Ewing's sarcoma exhibits chromosomal translocation t(11:22).
    B. Codman's triangle can be observed on radiography.
    C. Presents more commonly with localized disease than osteosarcoma.
    D. Radiation plays a prominent role in therapy.

17. All of the following are true regarding the Intergroup Ewing's Sarcoma (IESS-I) Study in which adriamycin was added to vincristine, actinomycin, and cyclophosphamide, except:
    A. The addition of adriamycin improved overall survival.
    B. The addition of adriamycin improved disease-free survival.
    C. Pelvic disease sites fared no worse than nonpelvic disease sites.
    D. Local recurrence did not differ by treatment.

18. All of the following are true regarding the Intergroup Ewing's Sarcoma (IESS-II) Study in which intermittent high dose was compared to continuous moderate-dose chemotherapy, except:
    A. High-dose chemotherapy improved overall survival.
    B. High-dose chemotherapy improved disease-free survival.
    C. The high-dose chemotherapy arm also had etoposide.
    D. Cardiac toxicity was worse in the high-dose arm.

19. All of the following are true regarding the Intergroup Ewing's Sarcoma (IESS-III) Study in which ifosfamide and etoposide were added to VAC + ADR chemotherapy, except:
    A. The addition of IE improved overall survival in patients with both metastatic and nonmetastatic disease.
    B. There was a greater reduction in local recurrence than in distant metastases.
    C. A quarter of the enrolled patients had metastatic disease.
    D. There was a greater benefit seen in pelvic tumors.

20. All of the following are true regarding the role of radiation in Ewing's sarcoma, except:
    A. Local control is equivalent with either surgery or radiation.
    B. Whole lung irradiation can be used for Ewing's with lung metastases.
    C. Actinomycin D and adriamycin given in conjunction with whole lung irradiation increase the risk of pneumonitis.
    D. Debulking prior to radiation of inoperable Ewing's tumors does not improve local control.

21. Which of the following is true regarding radiation volumes in the treatment of Ewing's sarcoma?
    A. Radiation to the tumor plus margin yields similar control to radiation of the whole tumor-bearing compartment.
    B. Pre-chemotherapy volumes are employed when treating pelvic/thoracic tumors without infiltration.
    C. Scars and drain sites do not need to be included in the radiation field.
    D. Circumferential radiation of the extremities is required to avoid marginal misses.

22. All of the following are true regarding the management of osteosarcoma, except:
    A. Surgical resection is the mainstay of local treatment of the primary.
    B. Surgical resection of a limited number of metastases results in improved survival.
    C. Whole lung irradiation as prophylaxis for metastatic disease improves outcomes in osteosarcoma.
    D. Palliative radiotherapy of inoperable metastases is associated with improved survival compared to no local therapy.

23. All of the following are true regarding Wilms' tumors, except:
    A. The peak incidence is between 3 and 4 years of age.
    B. It is more common in boys than girls.
    C. It can arise as both a hereditary or sporadic tumor.
    D. Children at risk for Wilms' tumors can be screened with ultrasound.

24. Beckwith-Wiedemann syndrome is most commonly associated with which of the following chromosomal abnormalities?
    A. WT1
    B. WT2
    C. FWT1
    D. FWT2

25. Denys-Drash syndrome is most commonly associated with which of the following chromosomal abnormalities?
    A. WT1
    B. WT2
    C. FWT1
    D. FWT2

26. All of the following are true regarding Wilms' tumors, except:
    A. The majority of tumors are solitary lesions.
    B. Anaplasia is the most important prognostic factor.
    C. Nearly half of presenting Wilms' tumors are of unfavorable histology.
    D. The most common presentation is an asymptomatic mass.

27. All of the following are the cell types that comprise Wilms' tumors, except:
    A. Blastemal
    B. Stromal
    C. Epithelial
    D. Basal

28. All of the following are true regarding less common childhood kidney tumors, except:
    A. Resected mesoblastic nephroma has an excellent prognosis.
    B. Clear cell sarcoma most frequently metastasizes to the lung.
    C. Rhabdoid tumor of the kidney predominantly affects infants.
    D. Renal cell carcinoma is rare in children.

29. Wilms' tumor presents most commonly at which stage?
    A. Stage I
    B. Stage II
    C. Stage III
    D. Stage IV

30. All are true regarding primary management of Wilms' tumor with surgery, except:
    A. Radical en bloc resection is the procedure of choice.
    B. Preoperative chemotherapy can be used to shrink large or unresectable tumors.
    C. Primary resection of tumor extension into the inferior vena cava is associated with increased morbidity.
    D. Tumor spillage during surgery can increase the risk for local and abdominal recurrence.

31. All are true regarding the NWTS 1 trial using age-adjusted radiotherapy dose schedules, except:
    A. No patients in group I derived a survival benefit from flank irradiation.
    B. Abdominal relapse rate in groups II and III was 5 %.
    C. The addition of vincristine improved survival in groups II and III.
    D. Radiation dose schedules ranged from 18 to 40 Gy.

32. All are true regarding the NWTS 2 trial using age-adjusted radiotherapy and chemotherapy dose schedules, except:
    A. The addition of vincristine was found to improve overall survival in group I patients.
    B. Group I patients were randomized to 6 versus 15 months of chemotherapy.
    C. There was a survival benefit associated with the longer chemotherapy course.
    D. Abdominal recurrence rate in groups II and III was 5 %.

33. All are true regarding the NWTS 3 trial using stage and histology adjusted radiotherapy and chemotherapy dose schedules, except:
    A. Stage I patients were randomized to 6 months versus 10 weeks of actinomycin D + vincristine.
    B. There was no benefit for the addition of adriamycin in stage II patients.
    C. There was no benefit for flank irradiation in stage II patients.
    D. There was a survival benefit for the addition of cyclophosphamide in stage IV patients.

34. All are true regarding the NWTS 4 trial which sought to determine optimal chemotherapy regimens, except:
    A. Stage I patients were randomized to standard versus pulse-intense chemotherapy.
    B. Stage II patients underwent a 2×2 randomization.
    C. Pulse-intense chemotherapy was found to yield inferior outcomes.
    D. Pulse-intense chemotherapy was less toxic than standard chemotherapy.

35. Which of the following is not true regarding the NWTS 5 trial looking at chromosomal prognostic factors?
    A. Patients were assayed for loss of heterozygosity of *1p* and *16q*.
    B. The loss of heterozygosity of either *1p* or *16q* was associated with an increased risk of relapse in stage I patients.
    C. The loss of heterozygosity of either *1p* or *16q* was associated with an increased risk of relapse in stage II patients.
    D. The loss of heterozygosity of either *1p* or *16q* was associated with increased risk of relapse in stage III patients.

36. A child undergoes resection of a large Wilms' tumor that extends beyond the kidney but is completely excised with negative margins. What is the correct National Wilms' Tumor Study (NWTS) stage?
    A. Stage I
    B. Stage II
    C. Stage III
    D. Stage IV

37. A child is found to have an unresectable Wilms' tumor. What is the correct National Wilms' Tumor Study (NWTS) stage?
    A. Stage II
    B. Stage III
    C. Stage IV
    D. Stage V

38. A child is found to have bilateral Wilms' tumors. What is the correct National Wilms' Tumor Study (NWTS) stage?
    A. Stage II
    B. Stage III
    C. Stage IV
    D. Stage V

39. All are true regarding the epidemiology of retinoblastoma, except:
    A. It is the most common intraocular tumor in children.
    B. It is the second most common intraocular tumor in all age groups.
    C. Ninety percent of cases are diagnosed before the first year of age.
    D. There is no difference in incidence between the left and right eyes.

40. All are true regarding retinoblastoma, except:
    A. The sporadic form of the disease is more common.
    B. The heritable form presents earlier than the sporadic form.
    C. There is an increased risk of also developing osteosarcoma.
    D. Multiple tumors in both eyes are rare, even in the heritable form.

41. Which is the least common tumor growth pattern of retinoblastoma?
    A. Endophytic
    B. Exophytic
    C. Combination of endophytic and exophytic
    D. Diffusely infiltrative

42. What is the second most common presenting sign of retinoblastoma?
    A. Leukocoria
    B. Strabismus
    C. Rubeosis iridis
    D. Decreased visual acuity

43. What is the eye preservation rate of International Classification for Intraocular Retinoblastoma group B tumors?
    A. >99 %
    B. 95 %
    C. 70–80 %
    D. 50–70 %

44. What is the treatment of choice for an International Classification for Intraocular Retinoblastoma group E tumor?
    A. Preoperative chemotherapy, then enucleation
    B. Enucleation
    C. Neoadjuvant chemotherapy, then external beam radiation
    D. Neoadjuvant chemotherapy, then cryotherapy

45. What is the treatment of choice for bilateral International Classification for Intraocular Retinoblastoma group D tumors?
    A. Enucleation of one eye, followed by chemotherapy and local therapy in the other
    B. Enucleation of both eyes
    C. Chemotherapy, then local therapy to both eyes
    D. Chemotherapy, then salvage of the better responding eye

46. All of the following are true regarding chemotherapy for retinoblastoma, except:
    A. Complete responses have been seen after 2 cycles of combination chemotherapy.
    B. Almost three-quarters of patients will experience recurrence with just 2 cycles of combination chemotherapy.
    C. Event-free survival after 6 cycles of combination chemotherapy is at best 90 %.
    D. Development of acute myelogenous leukemia is the most serious complication of chemotherapy for retinoblastoma.

47. All of the following are true regarding the use of radiation in treatment of retinoblastoma, except:
    A. Radiation is used mainly as a salvage treatment for progression after local laser or cryotherapy.
    B. The probability of retinopathy increases with increasing dose above 45 Gy.
    C. The probability of retinopathy increases with fraction size above 2.5 Gy.
    D. Diminished facial bone growth has been observed with doses over 30 Gy.

48. All of the following are true regarding neuroblastoma, except:
    A. Derived from adrenergic neuroblasts of neural crest tissue.
    B. The adrenal gland is the most common site of primary tumor.
    C. Median age of diagnosis is 3 years.
    D. It is the most common extracranial solid tumor in children.

49. All of the following are associated with unfavorable outcomes in neuroblastoma, except:
    A. *MYCN* amplification
    B. Near-diploid or pseudodiploid tumors
    C. Hyperdiploid or near-triploid tumors
    D. Deletion of *1p*

50. All of the following are common sites of metastatic neuroblastoma, except:
    A. Para-aortic lymph nodes
    B. Brain
    C. Posterior orbital bones
    D. Bone marrow

51. All of the following are true regarding the clinical presentation of neuroblastoma, except:
    A. Children <1 year of age typically present with localized disease.
    B. Children >1 year of age typically present with metastatic disease.
    C. Catecholemines secreted from neuroblastoma do not typically cause symptoms.
    D. Opsomyoclonus is a frequent symptom.

52. Regarding work-up of neuroblastoma, all of the following are true, except:
    A. Primary tumor and lymph nodes should be imaged with CT or MRI.
    B. Bone metastases can be detected with metaiodobenzylguanidine (MIBG) scan.
    C. Urinary catecholamines are typically measured.
    D. Bone marrow biopsy is usually unnecessary.

53. What would be the correct stage for a neuroblastoma found to be metastatic only to the bone marrow with 15 % involvement in a 9-month-old child?
    A. Stage 2B
    B. Stage 3
    C. Stage 4
    D. Stage 4S

54. What is the most appropriate postoperative radiation dose for stage I neuroblastoma?
    A. 21 Gy
    B. 18 Gy
    C. 10.8 Gy
    D. 0 Gy

55. All of the following are true regarding management of stage 2 neuroblastoma, except:
    A. Surgery is a mainstay of therapy.
    B. Chemotherapy is given either before or after surgery.
    C. 21 Gy of radiation is given immediately after surgery.
    D. 21 Gy of radiation is given only at the time of progression.

56. All of the following are true regarding the epidemiology of Hodgkin's lymphoma, except:
    A. The childhood form is associated with a male predominance.
    B. The young adult form is lower in individuals with multiple older siblings.
    C. The childhood form is associated with decreasing socioeconomic status.
    D. Mixed cellularity is the most common subtype in affluent societies.

57. All of the following are true regarding pathologic subtypes of Hodgkin's, except:
    A. Nodular-lymphocyte predominant is more common in younger patients.
    B. Mixed-cellularity subtype frequently presents with localized disease.
    C. Nodular sclerosing is the most common subtype in pediatric cases.
    D. Epstein-Barr virus associated lymphocyte-depleted Hodgkin's is more common in patients with HIV.

58. Which is the most common presentation of Hodgkin's lymphoma?
    A. Painless cervical or supraclavicular lymphadenopathy
    B. Tracheal compression
    C. Inguinal lymphadenopathy
    D. B symptoms

59. What percentage of patients with Hodgkin's lymphoma has B symptoms?
    A. 25 %
    B. 35 %
    C. 45 %
    D. 55 %

60. What percentage of patients with Hodgkin's lymphoma has splenic involvement?
    A. 10–20 %
    B. 30–40 %
    C. 50–60 %
    D. 70–80 %

61. All of the following are acceptable for staging Hodgkin's lymphoma, except:
    A. Bone marrow aspirate
    B. CT
    C. PET scan
    D. Technetium-99 bone scan

62. All of the following are true regarding MOPP chemotherapy for Hodgkin's lymphoma, except:
    A. The "M" in MOPP stands for nitrogen mustard.
    B. Secondary acute myelogenous leukemia is higher with MOPP than COPP-based therapy.
    C. Germ cell function is not affected by the number of cycles of MOPP.
    D. The "O" in MOPP stands for vincristine.

63. All of the following are true regarding ABVD chemotherapy for Hodgkin's lymphoma, except:
    A. Superior disease-free survival to MOPP.
    B. No excess risk of secondary cancers or infertility.
    C. Excess risk of pulmonary and cardiac toxicity.
    D. The "V" in ABVD stands for vincristine.

64. All are true regarding CCG 521 comparing ABVD + MOPP versus ABVD + radiation for unfavorable Hodgkin's, except:
    A. There were 6 cycles ABVD given with radiation.
    B. There were 6 cycles ABVD given with MOPP.
    C. Radiation dose was 21 Gy/12 fractions.
    D. There was no difference in event-free or overall survival between the two arms.

65. Which of the following is true regarding POG 8725 comparing MOPP/ABVD +/− total nodal irradiation for advanced Hodgkin's?
    A. Total radiation dose was 36 Gy.
    B. Event-free survival was improved with radiation.
    C. Overall survival was improved with radiation.
    D. Ninety percent of patients experienced complete response after chemotherapy.

66. All of the following are true regarding CCG 5942 randomizing Hodgkin's patients with a complete response to COPP/ABV × 4 to +/− radiation, except:
    A. There was an improvement in event-free survival in all groups with the addition of radiation.
    B. There was an improvement in overall survival in only the high-risk group with the addition of radiation.
    C. Radiation dose was 21 Gy.
    D. Infield recurrence was higher in the chemotherapy alone arm.

67. The GPOH-HD 95 trial of risk-adapted chemotherapy and radiation therapy showed all of the following, except:
    A. Disease-free survival was improved in all risk groups with the addition of radiation.
    B. Overall survival was not improved with the addition of radiation.
    C. Those in the low-risk group had disease-free survival >95 %.
    D. 20 Gy may be adequate in combination with chemotherapy.

68. Acute leukemias and lymphomas represent what percentage of childhood malignancies?
    A. 30 %
    B. 40 %
    C. 50 %
    D. 60 %

69. All of the following are true regarding the incidence of ALL, except:
    A. It is more common in girls.
    B. The peak age of incidence is between 2 and 5 years.
    C. It accounts for the majority of cases of childhood leukemia.
    D. T-cell ALL tends to be more common in boys.

70. All of the following are chromosomal abnormalities associated with ALL, except:
    A. Trisomy 21
    B. Klinefelter's
    C. Trisomy G
    D. Trisomy 11

71. Which one of the cytogenetic abnormalities seen in ALL has the worst prognosis?
    A. High ploidy with over 50 chromosomes
    B. Higher hyperdiploid with 56–67 chromosomes
    C. Near-tetraploid with 82–94 chromosomes
    D. Near-haploid with 24–28 chromosomes

72. Which one of the following translocations is associated with a favorable prognosis of ALL?
    A. t(8;14)
    B. t(9;22)(q34;q11)
    C. t(12;21)
    D. t(4;11)

73. All of the following are common presenting signs and symptoms of ALL, except:
    A. Fever
    B. Hepatomegaly
    C. Lymphadenopathy
    D. CNS symptoms

74. Which one of the following subgroups of ALL has the worst prognosis?
    A. 2-year-old with WBC count > 50,000/μL
    B. 8-month-old with WBC count < 50,000/μL
    C. 11-year-old with WBC count < 50,000/μL
    D. 4-year-old with WBC count > 100,000/μL

75. All of the following are true regarding treatment of ALL, except:
    A. The addition of L-asparaginase and/or an anthracycline to vincristine/glucocorticoid improves induction remission rates to >95 %.
    B. Prophylactic cranial irradiation is still indicated for high initial white count, T-cell phenotype, Ph+ chromosome, and CNS-3 disease.
    C. Intrathecal chemotherapy has successfully replaced spinal radiation as part of CNS preventive therapy.
    D. Maintenance regimens include methotrexate and 6-mercaptopurine.

76. All of the following high-risk groups will be treated with prophylactic cranial irradiation, except:
    A. T-cell subtype
    B. Ph + chromosome
    C. <1-year-old with 11q23 abnormalities
    D. t(4;11) translocation

77. What radiation dose did the Berlin-Frankfurt-Munster group find was adequate for CNS prophylaxis for CNS-1 disease?
    A. 1,000 cGy
    B. 1,200 cGy
    C. 1,500 cGy
    D. 1,800 cGy

78. All of the following are major conclusions from the Berlin-Frankfurt-Munster group trials for ALL, except:
    A. Reduced dose cranial RT is adequate for CNS prophylaxis.
    B. Those with a poor initial response to prednisone have a higher risk of relapse.
    C. Re-intensification is important for all risk patients.
    D. Longer (24 months) maintenance therapy is not better than standard 18 months.

79. All of the following are true regarding testicular leukemia, except:
    A. Overt testicular involvement manifests as painless enlargement.
    B. Occult testicular involvement is found in 50 % of cases.
    C. Bilateral testicular radiation is delivered in 2 Gy fractions to 24 Gy.
    D. Testicular relapse occurs in <5 % of cases.

80. All of the following are true regarding acute myelogenous leukemia, except:
    A. Fever and bone pain are frequent symptoms.
    B. Hepatosplenomegaly occurs in 50 % of children at diagnosis.
    C. Ara-C is used in induction AND postremission intensification therapy.
    D. With the use of Ara-C and IT-MTX, CNS relapse is <1 %.

81. All of the following are associated with an increased risk for development of non-Hodgkin's lymphoma in children, except:
    A. Wiskott-Aldrich syndrome
    B. Down's syndrome
    C. X-linked lymphoproliferative syndrome
    D. Ataxia- telangiectasia

82. All of the following are true regarding the epidemiology of non-Hodgkin's lymphoma in children, except:
    A. Presents more commonly with aggressive, diffuse tumors compared to NHL in adults.
    B. The frequency increases with increasing age.
    C. Like Hodgkin's lymphoma, there is a bimodal incidence.
    D. Incidence is higher in males than females.

83. All of the following are characteristic of the endemic type of Burkitt's lymphoma, except:
    A. B-cell phenotype
    B. Typically present in the abdomen or head and neck, with frequent jaw involvement
    C. Epstein-Barr virus associated
    D. Older age at diagnosis than the sporadic type

84. What is the biggest distinguishing factor between lymphoblastic lymphoma and ALL?
    A. Bone marrow involvement
    B. Precursor cell type
    C. Multi-agent chemotherapy regimen
    D. Antigen expression

85. All of the following are true regarding Langerhans cell histiocytosis, except:
    A. Birbeck cells are seen on electron microscopy.
    B. The most common single-organ presentation is bone.
    C. Radiotherapy is reserved for recurrent or unresectable disease.
    D. When used, radiotherapy doses in excess of 20 Gy are needed for control.

86. All of the following are true regarding juvenile nasopharyngeal angiofibroma, except:
    A. It is most common in adolescent boys.
    B. Its behavior is locally aggressive.
    C. Resection is the treatment of choice for less advanced tumors.
    D. Complete response to radiotherapy occurs frequently by the end of the treatment course.

87. In a patient with Ewing's sarcoma that has gross residual disease after chemotherapy and surgery, what is the correct radiation dose and volume?
    A. 45 Gy to the pre-chemo bone and post-chemo soft tissue tumor
    B. 45 Gy to the post-chemo bone and post-chemo soft tissue tumor
    C. 55.8 Gy to the pre-chemo bone and pre-chemo soft tissue tumor
    D. 55.8 Gy to the pre-chemo bone and post-chemo soft tissue tumor

Answers and Rationales

1. The correct answer is A. Although rhabdomyosarcoma is associated with all the listed organ systems, genitourinary abnormalities are most common. Ruymann FB et al. Congenital anomalies associated with rhabdomyosarcoma: an autopsy of 115 cases. A report from the intergroup rhabdomyosarcoma study committee. Med Pediatr Oncol. 1988;16:33.

2. The correct answer is D. Embryonal rhabdomyosarcoma is comprised of "spindle-shaped rhabdomyoblasts, small round cells with hyperchromatic nuclei on a background of a myxoid stroma." Alveolar subtype has tumors arranged in cords with pseudolining cleft-like spaces. Botryoides (a subset of embryonal) has grapelike clusters of small round cells surrounding a polypoid tumor. Maurer HM et al. Rhabdomyosarcoma. In: Fernbach D, Vietti T, editors. Clinical pediatric oncology. St. Louis: Mosby-Year Book; 1991. p. 491.

3. The correct answer is A. While it occurs in the genitourinary region, biliary tract, nasopharynx, and external auditory canal, botryoid tumor does not typically occur in the extremities. Alveolar subtype of rhabdomyosarcoma more frequently occurs in the extremities and trunk. Ruymann FB et al. Introduction and epidemiology of soft tissue sarcomas. In: Maurer HM et al., editors. Rhabdomyosarcoma and related tumors in children and adolescents. Boca Raton: CRC Press; 1991. p. 3.

4. The correct answer is C. A 5-year OS of over 80 % is seen in rhabdomyosarcoma of the orbit. The other listed sites have a 5-year OS of 50–70 %. Maurer HM, et al. The intergroup rhabdomyosarcoma study – II. Cancer. 1993;71:1904. Newton WA et al. Histopathology of childhood sarcomas. Intergroup rhabdomyosarcoma studies I and II: clinicopathologic correlation. J Clin Oncol. 1988;6:67.

5. The correct answer is A. Twenty percent of children present with metastatic disease at diagnosis, with the lung being the most common site of DM. Lymph node metastasis is infrequent, though it is seen with paratesticular and extremity primaries. Neville HL et al. Preoperative staging, prognostic factors, and outcome for extremity rhabdomyosarcoma: a preliminary report from the intergroup rhabdomyosarcoma study IV (1991–1997). J Pediatr Surg. 2000;35:317–21.

6. The correct answer is C. *Gross* residual disease after biopsy would be classified in International Rhabdomyosarcoma Study (IRS) clinical group III. Group I indicates complete resection of disease. Clinical group II indicates *microscopic* residual disease. Clinical group IV indicates metastatic disease.

Table 14.1 Five-year overall
survivals for IRS trials I–IV

	Five-year overall survival
IRS-I	55 %
IRS-II	63 %
IRS-III	71 %
IRS-IV	86 %

7. The correct answer is C. Stage 3 rhabdomyosarcoma includes unfavorable site tumors either <5 cm (A) with clinically involved lymph nodes or tumors >5 cm (B) with or without clinically involved lymph nodes. Stage 2 rhabdomyosarcoma includes unfavorable site tumors without lymph node involvement. Stage 1 includes all favorable site tumors. Stage 4 rhabdomyosarcoma includes all tumors with metastatic disease.

8. The correct answer is B. Five-year overall survival in IRS-I was 55 %. Five-year OS for IRS studies I–IV (Table 14.1). Maurer HM et al. The intergroup rhabdomyosarcoma study I-: a final report. Cancer. 1988;61:209–20. Maurer HM et al. The intergroup rhabdomyosarcoma study II. Cancer. 1993;71:1904. Crist WM et al. The third intergroup rhabdomyosarcoma study. J Clin Oncol. 1995;13:610. Crist WM et al. Intergroup rhabdomyosarcoma study IV: results for patients with non-metastatic disease. J Clin Oncol. 2001;19:3091–102.

9. The correct answer is C. IRS-I randomized 686 patients with rhabdomyosarcoma to chemotherapy alone versus chemotherapy + radiation. Overall, 5-year OS was 55 %. In Clinical group I, there was no benefit initially seen with the addition of radiation to VAC chemotherapy, though a later analysis did show a benefit in alveolar/undifferentiated histology. In clinical group II, there was no difference with the addition of cyclophosphamide to VA + radiation. Clinical groups III and IV showed no difference with the addition of doxorubicin to VAC + radiation. In all groups, the risk of distant metastasis was greater than the risk of local recurrence. Tumor sites in the orbit and genitourinary tract had a better prognosis than tumors in the retroperitoneum. Maurer HM et al. The intergroup rhabdomyosarcoma study I-: a final report. Cancer. 1988;61:209–20.

10. The correct answer is C. IRS-II randomized 999 patients with rhabdomyosarcoma to different treatments by clinical group, histology, and site. Building from IRS-I, clinical group I received no radiation but were randomized to receive VA versus VAC (excluding alveolar histology). Clinical groups II and III received 40–45 Gy and clinical group IV received 50–55 Gy. As in IRS-I, there was no benefit for the addition of cyclophosphamide for clinical groups I and II. In clinical group III (excluding pelvic sites), there was no benefit for the addition of doxorubicin. Whole brain radiation was given to parameningeal tumors with cranial nerve deficits, base of skull erosion, or intracranial extent and was found to improve meningeal recurrence rates and survival in high-risk patients (67 % vs. 45 % in IRS-I). Five-year OS for the entire cohort was 63 %. Maurer HM et al. The intergroup rhabdomyosarcoma study II. Cancer. 1993;71:1904–22.

11. The correct answer is C. While the rates of meningeal recurrence were improved in IRS-II with the additional of WBRT, IRS-IV showed no compromise in meningeal control with reduction of radiation clinical treatment volume to gross tumor + 2 cm. In IRS-IV, radiation for parameningeal sites of disease typically starts at week 12, except for those with meningeal impingement, for which radiation starts on day 0. Maurer HM et al. The intergroup rhabdomyosarcoma study II. Cancer. 1993;71:1904–22. Fryer C et al. Parameningeal rhabdomyosarcoma: a comparative analysis of IRS-I, -II, -III, and -IV with emphasis on changes in radiation volume. IRSG Abstracts from the 3rd international congress on soft tissue sarcoma in children and adolescents; 1997. p. 9–120.

12. The correct answer is A. Orbital rhabdomyosarcoma is a favorable site tumor, with 5-year OS of 95 %. As most tumors are biopsied only, most are clinical group III with gross residual disease. IRS-III showed that progression-free survival was not improved with the addition of cyclophosphamide to vincristine + actinomycin. As such, only two agents (vincristine and actinomycin) are needed for treatment. Radiation treatment volume is gross tumor volume + 2 cm, not exceeding the bony orbit if there is no bony erosion. While cataracts, dry eye, and decreased visual acuity are frequent side effects of radiation to the orbit, serious complications are infrequent. Crist WM et al. The third intergroup rhabdomyosarcoma study. J Clin Oncol. 1995;13:610. Oberlin O et al. Treatment of orbital rhabdomyosarcoma: survival and late effects of treatment- results of an international workshop. J Clin Oncol. 2001;19:197–204.

13. The correct answer is B. Rhabdomyosarcoma of the paratesticular region is treated with radical inguinal orchiectomy with high spermatic cord ligation, ipsilateral retroperitoneal lymph node dissection for patients >10 years, and radiotherapy if there is violation of the scrotum from transscrotal biopsy. Children <10 years old do not undergo lymph node evaluation unless there are positive lymph nodes or concerning findings on CT scan. Wiener ES et al. Controversies in the management of paratesticular rhabdomyosarcoma: is staging retroperitoneal lymph node dissection necessary for adolescents with resected paratesticular rhabdomyosarcoma? Semin Pediatr Surg. 2001;10:146–52.

14. The correct answer is D. Ewing's sarcoma is an undifferentiated blue round cell tumor, which can be cytokeratin and neuron-specific enolase positive. It presents more commonly in whites than Asians and males. Three-quarters of patients present with localized disease, and it most commonly presents during the adolescent growth spurt. Dorfman H et al. Bone cancers. Cancer. 1995;75:2186.

15. The correct answer is B. The femur is the most common site of osteosarcoma, with the tibia as the second most common site. Schuck A, Paulussen M. Pediatric sarcomas of bone. In: Gunderson LL, Tepper JE, editors. Clinical radiation oncology. 3rd ed. Philadelphia: Elsevier Saunders; 2012. p. 1435–42.

16. The correct answer is C. Ewing's sarcoma exhibits the t(11:22) chromosomal translocation and presents with localized disease 75 % of the time. Osteosarcoma presents with localized disease in 90 % of cases. While radiation plays a prominent role in the treatment of Ewing's, it does not play a prominent role in the treatment of osteosarcoma. Codman's triangle is an area of new subperiosteal bone formation created when tumor raises periosteum away from the bone. Truc-Carl C et al. Chromosomes in Ewing's sarcoma: I. An evaluation of 85 cases of remarkable consistency of t(11;22)(q24;q12). Cancer Genet Cytogenet. 1988;32:229.

17. The correct answer is C. The Intergroup Ewing's Sarcoma Study (IESS-I) randomized 335 patients to receive adriamycin in addition to VAC (vincristine, actinomycin, cyclophosphamide) + RT (45–55 Gy, followed by a 10 Gy boost). The addition of adriamycin to VAC improved both disease-free and overall survival. Pelvic disease sites had poorer survival than nonpelvic sites (34 % vs. 57 %, $p < 0.001$). Local recurrence did not differ by treatment. Nesbit ME et al. Multimodal therapy for the management of primary, nonmetastatic Ewing's sarcoma of bone: a long-term follow-up of the first intergroup study. J Clin Oncol. 1990;8(10):1664–74.

18. The correct answer is C. The Intergroup Ewing's Sarcoma Study (IESS-II) randomized 214 patients to receive VAC + ADR by either a moderate-dose continuous or a high-dose intermittent regimen. The more aggressive high-dose chemotherapy improved survival 77 % versus 63 %, $p < 0.05$, but was associated with greater cardiac toxicity. Burgert EO et al. Multimodal therapy for the management of nonpelvic, localized Ewing's sarcoma of bone: intergroup study IESS-II. J Clin Oncol. 1990;8(9):1514–24.

19. The correct answer is A. The Intergroup Ewing's Sarcoma Study (IESS-III) randomized 518 patients to receive ifosfamide and etoposide or not in addition to VAC + ADR. Twenty-three percent of patients had metastatic disease. In nonmetastatic patients, the addition of ifosfamide + etoposide improved event-free survival and overall survival. There was a greater reduction in local recurrence than in distant metastases and a greater benefit for large or pelvic tumors. Patients with metastatic disease did show not show a benefit for overall survival or event-free survival with the addition of IE. Grier HE et al. Addition of ifosfamide and etoposide to standard chemotherapy for Ewing's sarcoma and primitive neuroectodermal tumor of bone. N Engl J Med. 2003;348(8):694–701.

20. The correct answer is A. Radiation plays a myriad of roles of the treatment of Ewing's sarcoma. In the definitive setting, it can be used as the local therapy for inoperable or large tumors. However, it has been shown that local and systemic failures are higher (26 %) than the recurrence rates after surgery with or without radiation (4–10 %), even in patients with favorable, small extremity tumors. In the metastatic setting, with lung metastases as the only site of metastatic

disease, the addition of whole lung irradiation has been shown to improve event-free survival compared to receiving chemotherapy alone (47 % vs. 24 %). Whole lung irradiation with concurrent actinomycin D or adriamycin has been shown to increase the risk of pneumonitis. Paulssen M et al. Primary metastatic (stage IV) Ewing tumor: survival analysis of 171 patients from the EICESS studies. Ann Oncol. 1998;(9):275. Bacci F et al. Role of surgery in local treatment of Ewing's sarcoma of the extremities in patients undergoing adjuvant and neoadjuvant chemotherapy. Oncol Rep. 2004;11:111. Schuck A et al. Local therapy in localized Ewing tumors: results of 1,058 patients treated in the CESS 81, CESS 86, and EICESS 92 trials. Int J Radiat Oncol Biol Phys. 2003;55:168. Schuck A et al. Radiotherapy in Ewing's sarcoma and PNET of the chest wall: results of the trial CESS 81, CESS 86, and EICESS 92. Int J Radiat Oncol Biol Phys. 1988;42:1001.

21. The correct answer is A. Radiation to the tumor plus margin yields similar control to radiation of the whole tumor-bearing compartment. Local failures tend to occur within the high-dose radiation region. As such, planning target volume is defined as initial tumor extent on MRI of 2–3 cm longitudinally and 2 cm axially. Post-chemotherapy volumes are used for tumors protruding into the thorax/pelvis, and scar and drain sites must be included in the field. A strip of the extremity must be preserved to reduce the risk of lymphedema. When treating vertebral bodies, they should be either fully included or fully excluded. Donaldson S et al. The Pediatric Oncology Group (POG) experience in Ewing's sarcoma of bone. Med Pediatr Oncol. 1989;17:283. Donaldson S et al. A multidisciplinary study investigating radiotherapy in Ewing's sarcoma: end results of POG #8346. Pediatric Oncology Group. Int J Radiat Oncol Biol Phys. 1998;42:125.

22. The correct answer is C. The role of radiation therapy in treatment of osteosarcoma is limited. Therapy typically consists with neoadjuvant chemotherapy, surgery, and adjuvant chemotherapy. Radiation is used only in patients for whom complete resection cannot be obtained, either at the primary site or metastatic sites. Surgical resection of a limited number of metastatic sites has been shown to improve survival. Similarly, palliative radiotherapy of inoperable metastatic sites has also been shown to improve survival compared to receipt of no local therapy. Prophylactic whole lung irradiation has not been shown to be of benefit in the United States. Karger L et al. Primary metastatic osteosarcoma: presentation and outcome of patients treated on neoadjuvant Cooperative osteosarcoma study group protocols. J Clin Oncol. 2003;21:2011. Temeck B et al. Metastasectomy for sarcomatous pediatric histologies: results and prognostic factors. Ann Thorac Surg. 1995;59:1385. Rab GY et al. Elective whole lung irradiation in the treatment of osteogenic sarcoma. Cancer. 1976;38:939. Kempf-Bielack B et al. Osteosarcoma of the limbs. Report of the EORTC-SIOP 03 Trial 20781 investigating the value of adjuvant treatment with chemotherapy and/or prophylactic lung irradiation. Cancer. 1988;61:124.

23. The correct answer is B. Wilms' tumor is the most common childhood renal tumor, with a peak incidence between 3 and 4 years of age. It is more common in girls than boys. Wilms' tumor can arise either sporadically or as part of a hereditary tumor. Congenital anomalies such as WAGR syndrome, Beckwith-Wiedemann, and Denys-Drash are associated with the development of Wilms' tumors. Children at high risk for development of Wilms' tumors can be screened with ultrasound every 3 months for the first 5 years and then yearly. Coppes MJ et al. Principles of Wilms' tumor biology. Urol Clin North Am. 2000;27:423–33. Coppes MJ et al. Bilateral Wilms' tumor: long-term survival and some epidemiological features. J Clin Oncol. 1989;7:310–15. Little MH et al. Evidence that WT1 mutations in Denys-Drash syndrome patients may act in a dominant negative fashion. Hum Mol Genet. 1993;2:259–64.

24. The correct answer is B. Beckwith-Wiedemann syndrome is characterized by large birth weight, macroglossia, organomegaly, hemihypertrophy, neonatal hypoglycemia, abdominal wall defects, ear abnormalities, and a predisposition to Wilms' tumor, occurring in 5 %. Beckwith-Wiedemann maps to the WT2 locus at chromosome 11p15. Koufos A et al. Familial Wiedemann-Beckwith syndrome and a second Wilms' tumor locus both map to 11p15.5. Am J Hum Genet. 1989;44:711–9.

25. The correct answer is A. Denys-Drash syndrome is characterized by pseudohermaphroditism, glomerulopathy, renal failure, and a 95 % chance of Wilms' development and point mutations in the WT1 gene at 11p13. Little MH et al. Evidence that WT1 mutations in Denys-Drash syndrome patients may act in a dominant negative fashion. Hum Mol Genet. 1993;2:259–64.

26. The correct answer is C. Wilms' tumors are generally characterized as favorable (87 %) or unfavorable histology. The majority of tumors are solitary and present as an asymptomatic mass. One-third of patients present with abdominal pain, anorexia, vomiting, and malaise. Renal hypertension can be present in a quarter of patients, as can congenital anomalies. Anaplasia, the presence of greatly enlarged polypoid nuclei, is the most important prognostic factor and correlates with patient age. Beckwith JB et al. Histopathology and prognosis of Wilms' tumor: results from the national Wilms' Tumor study. Cancer. 1978;41:1937–48. Bonadio JR et al. Anaplastic Wilms' tumor: clinical and pathologic studies. J Clin Oncol. 1985;3:513–20. Bardeesy N et al. Anaplastic Wilms' tumor, a subtype displaying poor prognosis, harbors p53 gene mutations. Nat Genet. 1994;7:91–7. Faria P et al. Focal versus diffuse anaplasia in Wilms' tumor-new definitions with prognostic significance: a report from the National Wilms' Tumor study group. Am J Surg Pathol. 1996;20:909–20.

27. The correct answer is D. All of the listed cell types can comprise Wilms' tumors except the basal type, though not all Wilms' tumors consist of all three cell types. Some biphasic or monophasic tumors are seen. Beckwith JB et al.

Histopathology and prognosis of Wilms' tumor: results from the national Wilms' Tumor study. Cancer. 1978;41:1937–48.

28. The correct answer is B. Mesoblastic nephroma can be seen in the first month of life, with a median age of presentation of 3 months. Survival after resection is excellent, with rare local or distant recurrences. Clear cell sarcoma frequently metastasizes to bone (23 %), which contrasts to the other renal tumors, which more frequently metastasize to the lung. Rhabdoid tumor of the kidney can present with hypercalcemia and predominantly affects infants. Metastases to the lung are frequent, as are infradiaphragmatic relapses. Renal cell carcinoma is rare in children. Beckwith JB et al. Histopathology and prognosis of Wilms' tumor: results from the national Wilms' Tumor study. Cancer. 1978;41:1937–48. Beckwith JB et al. Wilms' tumor and other renal tumors of childhood: a selective review from the national Wilms' Tumor study pathology center. Hum Pathol. 1983;14:481–92. Beckwith JB et al. Wilms' tumor and other renal tumors in childhood. In: Feingold M,editor. Pathology of neoplasia in children and adolescents. Philadelphia: WB Saunders; 1986. p. 313–32. Marsden HB et al. Bone metastasizing renal tumor of childhood: morphological and clinical features and differences from Wilms' tumor. Cancer. 1978;42:1922–8.

29. The correct answer is A. The majority of Wilms' tumor presents at stage I (43 %). Kalapurakal JA, Dome JS. Wilms' tumor. In: Gunderson LL, Tepper JE, editors. Clinical radiation oncology. 3rd ed. Philadelphia: Elsevier Saunders; 2012. p. 1443–53).

30. The correct answer is A. Surgery is the mainstay of therapy for Wilms' tumors, with a transabdominal-transperitoneal approach utilized to provide adequate exposure for locoregional staging. Radical en bloc resection is associated with increased surgical complications and is unnecessary as most Wilms' tumor compress but do not invade adjacent structures. In the case of invasion, wedge resection of infiltrating disease can be performed with little operative morbidity. Intraoperative tumor spillage can increase the risk for local and abdominal recurrence but does not appear to worsen survival. In the case of large or unresectable tumors, preoperative chemotherapy can be used for downstaging to render subsequent resectability. Blakely ML et al. Controversies in the management of Wilms' tumor. Semin Pediatr Surg. 2001;10:127–31. Shamberger RC et al. Surgery-related factors and local recurrence of Wilms' tumor in national Wilms' Tumor study – 4. Ann Surg. 1999;229:292–7.

31. The correct answer is A. NWTS 1 randomized 259 patients after surgery to flank irradiation given on an age-adjusted dose schedule, ranging from 18 to 40 Gy and different chemotherapy regimens depending on tumor group. The most important finding was that children <24 months with group I tumors that received 15 months of dactinomycin derived no benefit from flank irradiation. Those children >24 months in group I had more infradiaphragmatic failures

without radiation, with worse survival, 77 % versus 58 %. Group II and III tumors showed an abdominal relapse rate of 5 %, with no observed dose response to radiation but improved survival with combination actinomycin D and vincristine, 81 % versus 55 %. D'Angio GJ et al. The treatment of Wilms' tumor: results of the national Wilms' Tumor study. Cancer. 1976;38(2): 633–46.

32. The correct answer is C. NWTS 2 randomized 513 patients after surgery to radiation within 10 days of surgery according to the same age-adjusted dose schedule, excluding group 1. Patients with pulmonary metastases were treated with 12 Gy whole lung irradiation. Chemotherapy in group I consisted of actinomycin D + vincristine × 6 months then randomization to an additional 9 months versus observation. Chemotherapy in groups II–IV consisted of 15 months of actinomycin D + vincristine +/− doxorubicin. The continuation of chemotherapy in group I did not improve recurrence-free or overall survival, though the addition of vincristine did improve 2-year overall survival compared to NWTS 1, 89 % versus 77 % (NWTS 1 with RT) versus 51 % (NWTS 1 without RT). As such, doublet chemotherapy with actinomycin and vincristine precluded the need for flank irradiation. In groups II–IV, the addition of doxorubicin was found to improve disease-free survival, 77 % versus 62 %. Abdominal relapse rates were <5 %. D'Angio GJ et al. The treatment of Wilms' tumor: results of the second national Wilms' Tumor study. Cancer. 1981;47(9):2302–11.

33. The correct answer is D. NWTS 3 randomized 1,439 patients to treatment adapted by stage and histology. Stage I patients were randomized to 6 months versus 10 weeks of actinomycin D + vincristine; no radiation was utilized. There was no difference in recurrence-free survival between the arms. Stage II patients were randomized in a 2×2 design to 20 Gy versus no radiation and actinomycin D + vincristine + adriamycin versus actinomycin D + vincristine, both for 15 months. There was no benefit for radiation or the more intense chemotherapy. Stage III patients were randomized in a 2×2 design to 20 Gy versus 10 Gy and actinomycin D + vincristine + adriamycin versus actinomycin D + vincristine, both for 15 months. There was no difference between the radiation dose regimens or between the chemotherapy regimens. Stage IV patients were randomized after radiation to receive actinomycin D + vincristine + adriamycin +/− cyclophosphamide, both for 15 months. The addition of cyclophosphamide did not improve outcomes. D'Angio GJ et al. Treatment of Wilms' tumor. Results of the third national Wilms' Tumor study. Cancer. 1989;64(2):349–60.

34. The correct answer is C. NWTS 4 randomized 1,638 patients to various chemotherapy randomizations. Stage I patients were randomized to standard versus pulse-intensive actinomycin D + vincristine. Stage II patients were randomized in a 2×2 chemotherapy randomization to standard versus pulse-intensive and short (5–6 months) versus long course (15 months) actinomycin D + adriamycin.

Stage III/IV patients randomized in a 2×2 chemotherapy randomization to standard versus pulse-intensive and short (5–6 months) versus long course (15 months) actinomycin D + adriamycin + vincristine. Pulse-intense chemotherapy was found to be equivalent to standard fractionated chemotherapy, was less toxic, and logistically easier. Green DM et al. Comparison between single-dose and divided-dose administration of dactinomycin and doxorubicin for patients with Wilms' tumor: a report from the national Wilms' Tumor study group. J Clin Oncol. 1998;16(1):237–45.

35. The correct answer is D. NWTS 5 was a prospective non-randomized study to risk-adapt treatment in an attempt to reduce toxicity for low-risk patients. Patients were assayed for loss of heterozygosity on chromosomes *1p* and *16q* and treated by risk. Loss of heterozygosity of *either* chromosomes *1p* or *16q* was associated with a risk of increased relapse and death in stage I and II patients. Loss of heterozygosity of *both* chromosomes *1p* and 16q was associated with a significantly increased risk of relapse and death in stage III and IV patients. Grundy PE et al. Loss of heterozygosity on chromosomes *1p* and *16q* is an adverse prognostic factor in favorable-histology Wilms tumor: a report from the national Wilms' Tumor study group. J Clin Oncol. 2005;23(29):7312–21.

36. The correct answer is B. A Wilms' tumor that extends beyond the kidney but is completely excised with negative margins is NWTS stage II. Stage II also includes tumors that involve blood vessels of the renal sinus, were biopsied prior to removal, or locally spill (confined to the flank). Kalapurakal JA, Dome JS. Wilms' tumor. In: Gunderson LL, Tepper JE, editors. Clinical radiation oncology. 3rd ed. Philadelphia: Elsevier Saunders; 2012. p. 1443–53.

37. The correct answer is B. Unresectable Wilms' tumor is NWTS stage III. Stage III also includes lymph node metastasis, positive surgical margins, or tumor spillage involving the peritoneal surfaces or transected tumor thrombus. Kalapurakal JA, Dome JS. Wilms' tumor. In: Gunderson LL, Tepper JE, editors. Clinical radiation oncology. 3rd ed. Philadelphia: Elsevier Saunders; 2012. p. 1443–53.

38. The correct answer is D. Bilateral renal involvement of Wilms' tumor at the time of initial diagnosis is stage V. However, each tumor should be staged based on the extent of disease prior to surgery. Kalapurakal JA, Dome JS. Wilms' tumor. In: Gunderson LL, Tepper JE, editors. Clinical radiation oncology. 3rd ed. Philadelphia: Elsevier Saunders; 2012. p. 1443–53.

39. The correct answer is C. Retinoblastoma is a poorly differentiated neuroectodermal tumor of the sensory retina, resulting from inactivation of both alleles of the *RB* tumor suppressor gene. Ninety percent of cases are diagnosed before age 5, and 7–10 % of patients have a positive family history. It is the most

common intraocular tumor in children and second most common in all age groups (uveal melanoma is most common). There is no difference in incidence between eyes, race, and gender. Kingston JE et al. Retinoblastoma. In: Plowman PN, Pinkerton CR, editors. Paediatric oncology: clinical practice and controversies. London: Chapman & Hall; 1992. p. 268–90. Rubenfeld M et al. Unilateral versus bilateral retinoblastoma. Correlations between age at diagnosis and stage of ocular disease. Ophthalmology 1986;93:1016. Shields CL et al. Retinoblastoma in older children. Ophthalmology 1991;98:395.

40. The correct answer is D. Retinoblastoma can present in one of two forms: heritable (40 %) or sporadic. The heritable form is less common and presents earlier (median 12 months) than the sporadic form (median 24 months). The heritable form often presents with multiple tumors in both eyes and can be associated with development of osteosarcoma, soft tissue sarcoma, melanoma, or bladder/lung cancer later in life. Francois J et al. Genesis and genetics of retinoblastoma. Ophthalmologica 1975;170:405. Green DM et al. Diagnosis and management of solid tumors in infants and children. Boston: Martinus Nijhoff; 1985. Knudson AG Jr, Mutation and Cancer: Statistical study of retinoblastoma. Proc Natl Acad Sci USA. 1971;68:820. Friend SH et al. A human DNA segment with properties of the gene that predisposes to retinoblastoma and osteosarcoma. Nature. 1986;323:643. Bookstein R et al. Suppression of tumorigenicity of human prostate carcinoma cell by replacing a mutated RB gene. science 1990;247:643.

41. The correct answer is D. Retinoblastoma can grow endophytically from the retina into the vitreous chamber; exophytically from the retina into the subretinal space; a combination of both endophytic and exophytic growth; and least commonly, by diffuse infiltration which resembles inflammation without a dominant mass, thus usually presenting at a later age. Rodriguez-Galindo C., Buchsbaum JC Retinoblastoma. In: Gunderson LL, Tepper JE, editors. Clinical radiation oncology. 3rd ed. Philadelphia: Elsevier Saunders; 2012. p. 1455–69. Philadelphia: Elsevier Saunders.

42. The correct answer is B. Leukocoria (white pupil) is the most common (56 %) presenting sign of retinoblastoma, with strabismus as the second most common (20 %) presenting sign. *Rubeosis iridis* (neovascularization of the iris) is seen in 17 % of patients. Decreased visual acuity, cloudy cornea, and glaucoma are less common presenting signs. Abramson DH et al. Presenting signs of retinoblastoma. J Pediatr. 1998;132:505. Shields J et al. In: Shields J, Shields C, editors. Intraocular tumors. A text and atlas. Philadelphia: WB Saunders; 1992. p. 305–32.

43. The correct answer is B. Choices A through D list the eye preservation rates of International Classification for Intraocular Retinoblastoma groups A–D, respectively. Group E tumors have a poor (2 %) eye preservation rate. Grabowski EF et al. Intraocular and extraocular retinoblastoma. Hematol Oncol Clin North

Am. 1987;1:721–35. Schvartzman E et al. Results of a stage-based protocol for the treatment of retinoblastoma. J Clin Oncol. 1996;14:1532–6.

44. The correct answer is B. Given the diffuse nature of growth of group E tumors, visual preservation is poor, and these tumors should undergo immediate enucleation to reduce the risk of tumor metastasis. In cases of optic nerve invasion, three preoperative cycles of chemotherapy followed by enucleation is reasonable. Schvartzman, E et al. Results of a stage-based protocol for the treatment of retinoblastoma. J Clin Oncol. 1996;14:1532–6.

45. The correct answer is D. In the case of bilateral advanced disease, it is reasonable to proceed with preoperative chemotherapy, followed by salvage of the better responding eye. Rodriguez-Galindo C, Buchsbaum J.C. Retinoblastoma. In: Gunderson LL, Tepper JE, editors. Clinical radiation oncology. 3rd ed. Philadelphia: Elsevier Saunders; 2012. p. 1455–69.

46. The correct answer is C. Chemotherapy is now the primary therapy for lower group retinoblastomas. A report from the Philadelphia group showed that more than half of patients experienced a complete response after 2 cycles of carboplatin, etoposide, and vincristine (CEV); however, 70 % recurred on repeat examination 6 weeks later. As such, after an increase of the number of cycles of CEV to 6 cycles, event-free survival in groups I–III was 100 %. While very effective, the most serious complication of CEV chemotherapy is development of acute myelogenous leukemia. Freire J et al. Retinoblastoma after chemoreduction and irradiation: preliminary results. In: Wiegel T, Bornfeld N, Foerster MH, Hinkelbein W, editors.Radiotherapy of ocular disease. Basel: Karger; 1997;30:88–92. Friedman DL et al. Chemoreduction plus focal therapy for retinoblastoma: factors predictive of need for treatment with external beam radiotherapy or enucleation. Am J Opthalmol. 2002;133:657–64.

47. The correct answer is B. With the success of chemotherapy and focal therapies such as laser or cryotherapy, radiation is now primarily used as a salvage treatment after progression, as adjuvant therapy for tumors at high risk for recurrence after enucleation, or for palliation of metastatic disease. Total radiation doses range from 36 to 50 Gy, with an observed risk of retinopathy above 50 Gy or with fraction sizes greater than 2.5 Gy. Diminished facial bone growth has been reported with radiation doses >30 Gy, with a significant risk >35 Gy. Krasin MJ et al. Intensity-modulated radiation therapy for children with intraocular retinoblastoma: potential sparing of the boy orbit. Clin Oncol. 2004;16:215–22. Pradhan DG et al. Radiation therapy for retinoblastoma: A retrospective review of 120 patients. Int J Radiat Oncol Biol Phys. 1997;39: 3–13. Kaste SC et al. Orbital development in long-term survivors of retinoblastoma. J Clin Oncol. 1997;1183–89. Peylan-Ramu N et al. Orbital growth retardation in retinoblastoma survivors: work in progress. Med Pediatr Oncol. 2001;37:465–70. Abramson DH et al. Second non-ocular tumors in survivors of bilateral retinoblastoma. Ophthalmology. 1998;105:573–80.

48. The correct answer is C. Neuroblastoma, a tumor derived from the adrenergic neural crest cells, is the most common extracranial solid tumor in children. It has a median age of diagnosis of 17 months, younger than the median age of diagnosis of Wilms' tumor. The most common site is in the adrenal gland (35 %). Brodeur G et al. Neuroblastoma. In: Pizzo P, Poplack D, editors. Principles and practice of pediatric oncology. 4th ed. Philadephia: Lippincott Williams and Wilkins; 2002. p. 895–937. Halperin E, Constine L, Tarbell N, Kun L. Neuroblastoma. In: Pediatric radiation oncology. 3rd ed. Philadelphia: Lippincott Williams and Wilkins; 1999. p. 163–203.

49. The correct answer is C. All of the listed abnormalities are associated with less favorable outcomes in neuroblastoma except hyperdiploid or near-triploid tumors. These typically lack *MYCN* amplification and are more likely to have a favorable outcome. Diploidy or pseudodiploidy frequently occurs with *MYCN* amplification. *MYCN* amplification has a strong correlation with less favorable outcomes and occurs in 25 % of neuroblastomas overall: in 5–10 % of low-stage neuroblastoma, but in 30–40 % of advanced disease. Deletion of *1p* is also found to be associated with worse prognosis. Fong CT et al. Loss of heterozygosity for the short arm of chromosome 1 in human neuroblastomas: correlation with *N-myc* amplification. Proc Natl Acad Sci USA. 1989;86:3753. Brodeur, GM et al. Amplification of *N-myc* in untreated neuroblastomas correlates with advanced disease stage. Science 1984;224:1121–4. Matthay KK, Neuroblastoma: biology and therapy. Oncology. 1997;11:1857–66.

50. The correct answer is B. Neuroblastoma frequently metastasizes to the lymph nodes, bone marrow, liver, and bone. It has a predilection for bones of the skull, such as the posterior orbit, giving the "raccoon eyes" from periorbital ecchymosis. Lung and brain metastases are rare. Wolden S, Neuroblastoma. In: Gunderson LL, Tepper JE, editors. Clinical radiation oncology. 3rd ed. Philadelphia: Elsevier Saunders; 2012. p. 1471–8.

51. The correct answer is D. Neuroblastoma in children <1 year tends to present with localized disease (57 %), whereas it presents more commonly (81 %) with disseminated disease in children >1 year. Opsomyoclonus, a paraneoplastic symptom of myoclonic jerking and random eye movements, is rare. Though they can secrete excess catecholamines (norepinephrine, vanillylmandelic acid, 3-methoxy-4-hydroxyphenylglycol, or homovanillic acid), these are rarely symptomatic. Wolden S, Neuroblastoma. In: Gunderson LL, Tepper JE, editors. Clinical radiation oncology. 3rd ed. Philadelphia: Elsevier Saunders; 2012. p. 1471–8.

52. The correct answer is D. Work-up for neuroblastoma includes CT or MRI to image the primary site, lymph nodes, and rule out distant metastatic disease in other organs (liver). Bone metastases are frequently assessed with MIBG scan, as well as technetium bone scan. Excess catecholamines are frequently measured in the urine, and complete staging includes bilateral iliac crest

bone marrow biopsy. If one result is positive, that is sufficient for bone marrow involvement documentation. Golding SJ et al. The role of computed tomography in the management of children with advanced neuroblastoma. Br J Radiol. 1984;57:661. Fletcher BD et al. Abdominal neuroblastoma: magnetic resonance imaging and tissue characterization. Radiology 1985;155:699. Heisel MA et al. Radionuclide bone scan in neuroblastoma. Pediatrics 1983;71:206. Voute PA et al. Detection of neuroblastoma with [I-131] metaiodobenzylguanidine. Prog Clin Biol Res. 1985;175:389–98. Brodeur GM et al. Revisions in the international criteria neuroblastoma diagnosis, staging, and response to treatment. J Clin Oncol. 1993;11:1466. LaBrosse EH et al. Catecholamine metabolism in neuroblastoma. J Natl Cancer Inst. 1976;57:633–43.

53. The correct answer is C. Neuroblastoma found to be metastatic only to the bone marrow with 15 % involvement in a 9-month-old child would be stage 4. Neuroblastoma metastatic to a child <1 year of age with either skin, liver, or bone marrow involvement <10 % is stage 4S.

54. The correct answer is D. In low-risk neuroblastoma, there is no role for adjuvant radiation. Event-free survival and overall survival are excellent with surgery alone, 93 % and 99 %, respectively. Brodeur G, Maris J, In: Pizzo P, Poplack D, editors. Principles and practice of pediatric oncology. 4th ed. Philadelphia: Lippincott Williams & Wilkins; 2002. p. 895–937.

55. The correct answer is C. Stages 2 and 3 intermediate risk neuroblastomas do not include radiation as an initial component of therapy. If resectable, the tumor is removed, and chemotherapy follows. Unresectable tumors are preceded by chemotherapy. Both stages 2 and 3 tumors have been treated without radiotherapy, with excellent outcomes. Matthay KK, Neuroblastoma: biology and therapy. Oncology. 1997;11:1857–66. Castleberry RP et al. Radiotherapy improves the outlook for patients older than 1 year with pediatric oncology group stage C neuroblastoma. J Clin Oncol. 1991;9:789–95.

56. The correct answer is D. Hodgkin's lymphoma has two forms: The childhood form presents in children <15 years and is associated with a male predominance, increasing family size, decreasing economic status, and mixed-cellularity subtype. The young adult form presents in those ages 15–34 and is associated with higher socioeconomic status and nodular sclerosing subtype. Grufferman S et al. Epidemiology of Hodgkin's disease. Epidemiol Rev. 1984;6:76–106. Spitz MR et al. Ethnic patterns of Hodgkin's disease incidence among children and adolescents in the United States. 1973–82. J Natl Cancer Inst. 1986;76 (2):235–9. Westergaard T et al. Birth order, sibship size, and risk of Hodgkin's disease in children and young adults: A population based study of 31 million person-years. Int J Cancer. 1997;72(6):977–81. Chang ET et al. Childhood social environment and Hodgkin's lymphoma: New findings from a population-based case–control study. Cancer Epidemiol Biomarkers Prev. 2004;13(8): 1361–70.

57. The correct answer is B. Nodular-lymphocyte predominant accounts for 10 % of cases and is more common in younger patients and male patients. The nodular sclerosing subtype is the most common (70 %) and frequently involves the cervical and mediastinal lymph nodes. Mixed cellularity is more common in children <10 years and usually presents with advanced disease with extranodal involvement. Epstein-Barr virus associated lymphocyte-depleted Hodgkin's is more common in patients with HIV. Donaldson SS et al. Pediatric Hodgkin's disease. In Mauch PM, Armitage JO, Diehl V. et al., editors. Hodkgin's disease. Philadelphia: Lippincott Williams & Wilkins; 1999. p. 531–605. Uccini S et al. High frequency of Epstein-Barr virus genome detection in Hodgkin's disease of HIV-positive patients. Int J Cancer. 1990;46 (4):581–5.

58. The correct answer is A. Painless cervical or mediastinal lymphadenopathy is the most common presentation (66 %) of pediatric Hodgkin's. Tracheal compression is possible from large mediastinal masses. Axillary and inguinal lymphadenopathy as the initial presenting symptom is rare. B symptoms occur in one third of patients only. Roberts KB, Hudson MM, Constine, LS, Pediatric Hodgkin's Lymphoma. In: Gunderson LL, Tepper JE, editors. Clinical radiation oncology. 3rd ed. Philadelphia: Elsevier Saunders; 2012. p. 1489–1503).

59. The correct answer is B. B symptoms are prognostically significant constitutional symptoms: (1) unexplained fever >38 °C orally, (2) weight loss >10 % within the 6 months preceding diagnosis, and (3) drenching night sweats. These occur in one-third of patients. Ruhl U et al. Response-adapted radiotherapy in the treatment of pediatric Hodgkin's disease: An interim report at 5 years of the German GPOH-HD 95 trial. Int J Radiat Oncol Biol Phys. 2001;51(5):1209–18. Nachman JB et al. Randomized comparison of low-dose involved-field radiotherapy and no radiotherapy for children with Hodgkin's disease who achieve a complete response to chemotherapy. J Clin Oncol. 2002;20(18):3765–71.

60. The correct answer is B. Splenic involvement occurs in 30–40 % of pediatric patients with Hodgkin's lymphoma. Roberts KB, Hudson MM, Constine LS Pediatric Hodgkin's Lymphoma. In Gunderson LL, Tepper JE, editors. Clinical radiation oncology. 3rd ed. Philadelphia: Elsevier Saunders; 2012. p. 1489–503.

61. The correct answer is A. In the work-up of Hodgkin's, CT is used to evaluate nodal regions and the thoracic and abdominal cavities. PET is useful for only giving not only anatomical, but also functional tumor characteristics. PET response has also been found to be prognostic. Technetium-99 is not required but should be performed in those with bone pain or extranodal disease. Bone marrow biopsy is necessary only in those with clinical stage III/IV disease or in those with B symptoms. As bone marrow infiltration can be focal or diffuse, biopsy rather than aspirate is required. Jerusalem G et al. Whole-body positron emission tomography using 18F-fluorodeoxyglucose for post-treatment evaluation

in Hodgkin's disease and non-Hodgkin's lymphoma has higher diagnostic and prognostic value than classical computed tomography scan imaging. Blood. 1999;94(2):429–33.

62. The correct answer is C. MOPP chemotherapy (nitrogen mustard, oncovin (vincristine), procarbazine, prednisone) has been shown on follow-up studies to be associated with secondary acute myeloid leukemia, peaking at 5–10 years after treatment. COPP (cyclophosphamide for nitrogen mustard) chemotherapy has a 15-year cumulative incidence of s-AML of <1 % compared to 4–8 % with MOPP. Gonadal injury is common in those treated with MOPP and appears to be cycle-dependent; it is preserved with <3 cycles and irreversible with >6 cycles. De Vita VTJ et al. A decade of combination chemotherapy of advanced Hodgkin's disease. Cancer. 1972;30:1495–504. Longo DL et al. Twenty years of MOPP therapy for Hodgkin's disease. J Clin Oncol. 1986;4(9):1295–306. Bhatia S et al. Breast cancer and other second neoplasms after childhood Hodgkin's disease. N Engl J Med. 1996;33[12]:745–51. Schellong G et al. Low risk of secondary leukemias after chemotherapy without mechlorethamine in childhood Hodgkin's disease. German- Austrian pediatric Hodgkin's disease group. J Clin Oncol 1997;15(6);2247–53. Horning SJ et al. Female reproductive potential after treatment for Hodgkin's disease. N Engl J Med. 1981;304(23):1377–82. da Cunha MF et al. Recovery of spermatogenesis after treatment for Hodgkin's disease: Limiting dose of MOPP chemotherapy. J Clin Oncol. 1984;2(6):571–7.

63. The correct answer is D. ABVD chemotherapy (adriamycin, bleomycin, vinblastine, dacarbazine) has been shown to yield superior disease-free survival to MOPP without the excess risk of infertility and secondary malignancy. There is a risk of cardiotoxicity with adriamycin and pulmonary toxicity with bleomycin, especially in combination with thoracic radiotherapy. Fryer CJ et al. Efficacy and toxicity of 12 courses of ABVD chemotherapy followed by low-dose regional radiation in advanced Hodgkin's disease in children: A report from the children's cancer study group. J Clin Oncol. 1990;8(12):1971–80. Bonadonna G et al. Alternating non-cross-resistant combination chemotherapy or MOPP in stage IV Hodgkin's disease. A report of 8-year results. Ann Intern Med. 1986;104(6):739–46. Keefe DL. Anthracycline-induced cardiomyopathy. Semin Oncol. 2001;28(4 Suppl 12):2–7. Kreisman H et al. Pulmonary toxicity of antineoplastic therapy. Semin Oncol. 1992;19(5):508–20.

64. The correct answer is B. CCG 521 randomized 111 patients with stage III/IV Hodgkin's to either MOPP/ABVD × 12 cycles versus ABVD × 6 cycles + EFRT 21 Gy/12 fx. Residual disease was boosted with 14 Gy, for total of 35 Gy. There was no difference in 4-year event-free survival with radiation (87 %) versus (77 %) in the MOPP arm, $p = 0.09$, nor was there a difference in overall survival. There were more relapses in stage IV patients (27 %) than stage III (11 %). This trial showed that MOPP can be eliminated from front-line therapy.

Hutchinson RJ et al. MOPP or radiation in addition to ABVD in the treatment of pathologically staged advanced Hodgkin's disease in children: results of the children's cancer group phase III trial. J Clin Oncol. 1998;16(3):897–906.

65. The correct answer is D. POG 8725 randomized 183 patients with stages IIB–IV Hodgkin's after completion of 8 cycles MOPP/ABVD to +/– total nodal irradiation. After chemotherapy, 90 % of patients were in complete remission. Importantly, nine patients did not receive radiation despite randomization (major protocol violation). The addition of total nodal irradiation did not improve either event-free or overall survival. A later quality assurance review showed that radiation delivered without protocol deviations yielded a 5-year recurrence-free survival of 96 %, ten better than with protocol deviations (which have similar RFS to chemotherapy alone). Weiner MA et al. Randomized study of intensive MOPP-ABVD with or without low-dose total nodal radiation therapy in the treatment of stages IIB, IIIA2, IIIB, and IV Hodgkin's disease in pediatric patients: a pediatric oncology group study. J Clin Oncol. 1997;15(8):2769–79. FitzGerald TJ et al. Processes for quality improvements in radiation oncology clinical trials. Int J Radiat Oncol Biol Phys. 2008;71(1 Suppl):S76–9.

66. The correct answer is B. CCG 5942 sought to determine the value of radiation in patients with a complete response to chemotherapy. Of 829 enrolled patients, the 501 patients with a complete response to COPP/ABV × four were randomized to +/– 21 Gy involved-field radiation. Patient risk groups were as follows: stages I–II low risk 26 %, stages I–II high risk/stage III 47 %, stage IV 17 %. The study was closed prematurely due to inferior event-free survival in the chemotherapy alone arm (92 % vs. 87 %), though there was no overall survival difference. Radiation improved event-free survival in all risk groups. Local recurrences (as opposed to out of field recurrences) were more common in the chemotherapy alone arm. Nachman JB et al. Randomized comparison of low-dose involved-field radiotherapy and no radiotherapy for children with Hodgkin's disease who achieve a complete response to chemotherapy. J Clin Oncol. 2005;20(18):3765–71.

67. The correct answer is A. The GPOH-HD 95 trial prospectively randomized children with Hodgkin's to risk-adapted chemotherapy (OPPA (girls)/OEPA (boys)) depending on stage: stages I–IIA 2 cycles; stages IIEA, IIB, IIIA 2 cycles + 2 cycles COPP; and stages IIEB, IIIAE, IIIB, IV 2 cycles + 4 cycles COPP. Etoposide was substituted for procarbazine in boys to reduce testicular dysfunction. Those without a complete response (78 %) were randomized to one of three radiation regimens depending on extent of response: >75 % response 20 Gy; <75 % response 30 Gy; if >50 mL residual mass 35 Gy. In early stage (I–IIA), the addition of radiation did not improve disease-free survival (96 %). In the intermediate group, radiation did improve disease-free survival (92 % vs. 78 %). In the advanced group, radiation improved disease-free survival (91 % vs. 79 %). No overall survival difference was seen in any group.

The study suggests that radiation may be omitted for early stage but is needed for intermediate/advanced stage, but a lower dose (20 Gy) can be given. Dorffel W et al. Preliminary results of the multicenter trial GPOH-HD 95 for the treatment of Hodgkin's disease in children and adolescents: analysis and outlook. Klin Padiatr. 2003;215(3):139–45.

68. The correct answer is B. Childhood leukemias and lymphomas represent 40 % of childhood malignancies. Marcus KJ, Sandlund JT. Pediatric leukemias and lymphomas. In: Gunderson LL, Tepper JE, editors. Clinical radiation oncology. 3rd ed. Philadelphia: Elsevier Saunders; 2012. p. 1479–88).

69. The correct answer is A. Acute lymphoblastic leukemia accounts for 75 % of childhood leukemias. It has a peak incidence between 2 and 5 years and is more common in boys, especially in terms of incidence of T-cell subtype. Gurney J et al. Incidence of cancer in children in the United States: sex-, race-, and 1-year age-specific rates by histologic type. Cancer. 1995;75:2186. Greenlee RT et al. Cancer stat, 2000. CA Cancer J Clin. 2000;50:7–34. Fraumeni JF et al. Changing sex differentials in leukemia. Public Health Rep. 1974;79:1093.

70. The correct answer is D. All of the listed chromosomal abnormalities is associated with ALL, except Trisomy 11. Of these, Trisomy 21 (Down's syndrome) is the most common. Dordelmann M et al. Down's syndrome in childhood acute lymphoblastic leukemia: clinical characteristics and treatment outcomes in four consecutive BFM trial. Berlin- Frankfurt- Munster Group. Leukemia. 1998;12:645–51. Muts- Homshma s et al. Klinefelter's syndrome and acute non-lymphocytic leukemia. Blut. 1981;44:15.

71. The correct answer is D. In ALL, the higher the ploidy, the better the prognosis, except those with near-tetraploid (82–94) chromosomes, which have a poorer prognosis. The worst prognosis is in those with near-haploid (24–28 chromosomes) ALL. Chromosomal abnormalities and their clinical significance in acute lymphoblastic leukemia. Third international workshop on chromosomes in leukemia. Cancer Re. 1983 43:868–73. Pui CH et al. Near- triploid and near-tetraploid acute lymphoblastic leukemia of childhood. Blood. 1990;76:590–6. Heerema NA et al. Prognostic impact of trisomies of chromosomes 10, 17, and 5 among children with acute lymphoblastic leukemia and high hyperdiploidy (>50 chromosomes). J Clin Oncol. 1000;18:1876–87. Brodeur GM et al. Near-haploid acute lymphoblastic leukemia: a unique subgroup with a poor prognosis? Blood. 1981;58:14–19. Heerema NA et al. Hypodiploidy with less than 45 chromosomes confers adverse risk in childhood acute lymphoblastic leukemia: a report from the children's cancer group. Blood. 1999;94:4036–45.

72. The correct answer is C. The t(12;21) chromosomal translocation is the most commonly identified translocation (16–22 % of cases) and is associated with a favorable prognosis. In contrast, the other listed translocations are associated

with early treatment failure. The t(9;22)(q34;q11) translocation is the Ph chromosome, seen in 5 % of childhood ALL, and has the worst prognosis. Chromosomal abnormalities and their clinical significance in acute lymphoblastic leukemia. Third international workshop on chromosomes in leukemia. Cancer Res. 1983 43:868–73. Bloomfield CD et al. Chromosomal abnormalities identify high-risk and low- risk patients with acute lymphoblastic leukemia. Blood. 1986;68:205–12. Nowell P. Molecular monitoring of pre-B acute lymphoblastic leukemia. J Clin Oncol. 1987;5:692. Ribeiro RC et al. Clinical and biologic hallmarks of the Philadelphia chromosome in childhood acute lymphoblastic leukemia. Blood. 1987;70:948–53.

73. The correct answer is D. Presenting signs and symptoms of ALL relate to the degrees of extramedullary involvement and bone marrow infiltration. Fever, lymphadenopathy, and hepatomegaly (two thirds of patients) are common. CNS symptoms at presentation are rare, as less than 5 % of children present with CNS involvement. Bleyer WA Central nervous systemic leukemia. Pediatr Clin North Am. 1988;35:789–814.

74. The correct answer is B. Of the listed subgroups, the 8-month old has the worst prognosis. Age <1 year is a very high-risk feature and associated with the worst outcome event-free survival 10–20 %. While WBC >100,000/μL is a very high-risk feature, age 4 is not high risk. WBC >50,000/μL is high risk, as is age >10 years, but outcomes are still worst in infants <1 year. Simone JV et al. Initial features and prognosis in 363 children with acute lymphoblastic leukemia. Cancer. 1975;36:2099–108. Sather HN. Age at diagnosis in childhood acute lymphoblastic leukemia. Med Pediatr Oncol 1986;14:166–72. Reaman G et al. Acute lymphoblastic leukemia in infants less than one year of age: a cumulative experience of the Children's cancer study group. J Clin Oncol. 3:1985;1513–21. Crist W et al. Acute lymphoid leukemia in adolescents: clinical and biologic features predict a poor prognosis- a pediatric oncology group study. J Clin Oncol 1988;6:34–43.

75. The correct answer is B. Treatment of ALL occurs in four phases: remission induction, CNS preventive therapy, consolidation, and maintenance. Remission induction is achieved in 85 % of children with vincristine and glucocorticoid; this is improved to 95 % with the addition of L-asparaginase and/or anthracycline chemotherapy. After remission induction, CNS prophylaxis is achieved in standard risk patients with triple intrathecal chemotherapy, evolved from the previous craniospinal irradiation employed, with the benefit of avoiding neurocognitive sequelae from radiation. B is the correct answer because patients with high initial WBC count do not automatically get PCI. Those patients with CNS3 disease are still considered for PCI even though they have visible cells at presentation. Consolidation follows with intensified chemotherapy, frequently including L-asparaginase and doxorubicin. Maintenance includes methotrexate and 6-mercaptopurine. Ortega JA et al. L-Asparaginase, vincristine, and prednisone

for induction of first remission in acute lymphoblastic leukemia. Cancer Res. 1977;37:535–40. Rivera GK et al. Controversies in the management of childhood acute lymphoblastic leukemia: treatment intensification, CNS leukemia, and prognostic factors. Semin Hematol 1987;24:12–26. Rivera GK et al., Improved outcome in childhood acute lymphoblastic leukemia with reinforced early treatment and rotational combination chemotherapy. Lancet. 1991;337:61–6. Schorin MA et al. Treatment of childhood acute lymphoblastic leukemia: results of Dana- Farber cancer institute/children's hospital acute lymphoblastic leukemia consortium protocol 85-01. J Clin Oncol. 1994;12:740–7. Aur RJ et al. Childhood acute lymphocytic leukemia: study VIII. Cancer. 1978;42:2123–34. Holland JF et al. Chemotherapy of acute lymphoblastic leukemia of childhood. Cancer. 1972;30:1480–7.

76. The correct answer is C. All of the listed groups would receive cranial irradiation for CNS prophylaxis except the <1-year-olds due to their young age. They would instead receive intensified chemotherapy. Marcus KJ, Sandlund JT. Pediatric leukemias and lymphomas. In: Gunderson LL, Tepper JE, editors. Clinical radiation oncology. 3rd ed. Philadelphia: Elsevier Saunders; 2012. P. 1479–88.

77. The correct answer is B. Through four consecutive ALL trials of 4440 children, the Berlin-Frankfurt Munster group found an improvement in event-free survival, especially in those with an early response (90 % at 8 years). Isolated CNS relapse was very low (1.1 % in BFM-90), improved from 5.3 % in ALL-BFM 81. Four major conclusions were found from this study: (1) Re-intensification is crucial, even for low-risk patients. (2) Cranial RT can be reduced to 12 Gy or eliminated if replaced by intensive chemotherapy and IT-MTX. (3) Longer maintenance therapy is better (24 vs. 18 months). (4) Poor response to initial 7-day prednisone defines 10 % of patients with high risk of relapse. Other features of patients at high risk for relapse are hyperleukocytosis, age <1 year, Ph + chromosome. Schrappe M et al. Long-term results of four consecutive trials in childhood ALL performed by the ALL-BFM study group from 1981 to 1995. Berlin- Frankfurt- Munster. Leukemia 2000;14(12):2205–22.

78. The correct answer is D. Through four consecutive ALL trials of 4,440 children, the Berlin-Frankfurt Munster group found an improvement in event-free survival, especially in those with an early response (90 % at 8 years). Isolated CNS relapse was very low (1.1 % in BFM-90), improved from 5.3 % in ALL-BFM 81. Four major conclusions were found from this study: (1) Re-intensification is crucial, even for low-risk patients. (2) Cranial RT can be reduced to 12 Gy or eliminated if replaced by intensive chemotherapy and IT-MTX. (3) Longer maintenance therapy is better (24 vs. 18 months). (4) Poor response to initial 7-day prednisone defines 10 % of patients with high risk of relapse. Other features of patients at high risk for relapse are hyperleukocytosis, age <1 year, Ph + chromosome. Schrappe M et al. Long-term results of four consecutive trials in childhood ALL performed by the ALL-BFM study group from 1981 to 1995. Berlin- Frankfurt- Munster. Leukemia 2000;14(12):2205–22.

79. The correct answer is B. Overt testicular involvement is rare and manifests as painless enlargement. In 25 % of cases, there is occult testicular involvement. With current systemic therapy, testicular relapses occurs in <5 % of cases. Testicular relapse can be treated with bilateral testicular radiation, delivered in 2 Gy fractions to 24 Gy. Treatment is delivered to the bilateral testes with the legs in the supine frog-leg position. The penis is taped out of the field. Kim TH, Kay H et al. Testicular irradiation in leukaemia. (letter). Lancet. 1981;2:1115. Nesbit ME et al. Sanctuary therapy: a randomized trial of 724 children with previously untreated acute lymphoblastic leukemia: a report from children's cancer study group. Cancer Res. 1982;42:674–80. Cap J et al. Prognostic significance of testicular relapse in boys with acute lymphoblastic leukemia. Neoplasma. 1992;39:115–8. Dordelmann M et al. Intermediate dose methotrexate is as effective as high dose methotrexate in preventing isolated testicular relapse in childhood acute lymphoblastic leukemia. J Pediatr Hematol Oncol. 1998;20:444–50. Mirro J Jr et al. Testicular leukemic relapse: rate of regression and persistent disease after radiation therapy. J Pediatr. 1981;99:439–40.

80. The correct answer is D. AML represents 15–25 % of childhood leukemia, with seven different subtypes: M1–M7. Children often present with fever (33 %), bone pain, and hepatosplenomegaly in up to 50 % of cases. Disseminated intravascular coagulation can occur. Treatment includes induction of remission with chemotherapy, postremission consolidation, intensification, and maintenance. In AML, Ara-C plays a large role in therapy as the backbone for induction and intensification. It is also used in combination with IT-MTX for CNS prophylaxis. With the use of prophylaxis, CNS relapse is 5 %, with the highest risk in those that are M4 or M5 subtype. Creutzig U et al. Identification of two risk groups in childhood acute myelogenous leukemia after therapy intensification in study AML-BFM-83 as compared with study AML-BFM-78. AML-BFM study group. Blood. 1990;75:1932–40. Ravendranath Y et al. High-dose cytarabine for intensification of early therapy of childhood acute myeloid leukemia: a pediatric oncology group study. J Clin Oncol. 1991;9:572–80. Woods WG et al. Timed- sequential induction therapy improves postremission outcome in acute myeloid leukemia: a report from the children's cancer group. Blood. 1996;87:4979–89.

81. The correct answer is B. All of the listed syndromes are associated with an increased risk of non-Hodgkin's lymphoma in children except Down's syndrome, which is associated with ALL. Sandlung JT et al. Non- Hodgkin's lymphoma in childhood. N Engl J Med. 1996;334:1238–48.

82. The correct answer is C. Non-Hodgkin's in children, as opposed to in adults, presents more commonly with aggressive, diffuse tumors. The median age of diagnosis is 10 years old, with an increasing frequency with age. There is not a bimodal incidence as in Hodgkin's. The incidence is higher in African-Americans and in males by 2–3×. There are three main subtypes: (1) Burkitt's (39 %), (2) lymphoblastic (29 %), and (3) large cell (27 %). Ries LAG et al.

SEER cancer statistics review. 1973–1991. Bethesda MD. National institutes of health. 1994. Gurney JG et al. Incidence of cancer in children in the United States: sex-, race-, and 1-year age-specific rates by histologic type. Cancer. 1995;75:2186–95.

83. The correct answer is D. Burkitt's lymphoma has two types: endemic and sporadic. The endemic type, seen in Africa, is EBV associated, characterized by a younger age at diagnosis, and involves the jaw, orbit, abdomen, and paraspinal area. The sporadic type occurs more frequently in the United States and Western Europe, presents at an older age, and frequently involves the abdomen, bone marrow, and nasopharynx. The backbone of therapy is cyclophosphamide. Magrath IT et al. Pathogenesis of small noncleaved cell lymphoma (Burkitt's lymphoma). In: Magrath IT, editor. The non-Hodgkin's lymphomas. London: Arnold; 1997. p. 385–409.

84. The correct answer is B. Lymphoblastic leukemia and ALL are difficult to distinguish as they share many morphologic, immunophenotypic, and cytogenetic features. Both share similar antigen expression, and both frequently involve bone marrow. They are treated similarly with multi-agent chemotherapy using vincristine, prednisone, cytarabine, methotrexate, and cyclophosphamide. The biggest difference between them is the precursor cell type: 90 % of lymphoblastic lymphomas are of T-cell lineage, whereas most ALL is of B-cell lineage. Harris NL et al. A revised European-American classification of lymphoid neoplasms: a proposal from the international lymphoma study group. Blood. 2001;97:3370–9. Murphy SB. Classification, staging, and end results of treatment lymphomas in adults. Semin Oncol. 1980;7:332. Bernard A et al. Cell surface characterization of malignant T cells from lymphoblastic lymphoma using monoclonal antibodies. Evidence for phenotypic differences between malignant T cell from patients with acute lymphoblastic leukemia and lymphoblastic lymphoma. Blood. 1981;57:1105.

85. The correct answer is D. Langerhans cell histiocytosis (LCH) is a monoclonal proliferation of dendritic antigen-presenting cells normally found in mucosa, skin, spleen, and the lymphatic system. The characteristic cell on electron microscopy is the Birbeck granule. Single-organ presentation most commonly involves the bone, with the skin as the second most commonly involved organ. The role of radiation is limited to recurrent or unresectable disease. Bony LCH responds well to curettage and/or steroid injection. When used, radiotherapy doses are low, 9–10 Gy. For skin LCH, topical nitrogen mustards are first-line therapy. Single-organ presentations have a good prognosis. Banchereau J et al. Dendritic cells and the control of immunity. Nature. 1998;392:245–52. Valladeau J et al. Langerin, a novel C-type lectin specific to the Langerhans cell, is an endocytic receptor that induces the formation of Birbeck granules. Immunity 2000;12: 71–81. Broadbent V et al. Current therapy for Langerhans cell histiocytosis. Hematol Oncol Clin North Am. 1998;12:327–38. Ceci A

et al. Langerhans cell histiocytosis in childhood: Results from the Italian cooperative AIEOP-CNR-H.X'83 study. Med Pediatr Oncol. 1993;21:259–64. Gadner H et al. Treatment strategy for disseminated Langerhans cell histiocytosis. DAL HX-83 study group. Med Pediatr Oncol. 1994;23:72–80. Selch MT et al. Radiation therapy in the management of Langerhans cell histiocytosis. Med Pediatr Oncol. 1990;18:97–31. Chu T. Langerhans cell histiocytosis. Australia's J Dermatol. 2001;42:237–42.

86. The correct answer is D. Juvenile nasopharyngeal angiofibroma is a proliferation of vascular channels within a fibrous stroma and may represent a hamartomatous process versus neoplasm. It affects predominately adolescent males and presents with epistaxis and a locally aggressive behavior. Resection is the current treatment of choice for early-stage lesions, with radiation to 36–40 Gy as another alternative. Tumor response to radiation is delayed with a median time to complete response of 13 months (Reddy et al.). Mann WJ et al. Juvenile angiofibromas: Changing surgical concept over the last 20 years. Laryngoscope. 2004;114:291–93. Reddy KA et al. Long-term results of radiation therapy for juvenile nasopharyngeal angiofibroma. Am J Otolaryngol. 2001;22:172–5. Lee JT et al. The role of radiation in the treatment of advanced juvenile angiofibroma. Laryngoscope. 2002;112:1213–20.

87. The correct answer is D. In Ewing's sarcoma, radiation is delivered after chemotherapy and surgery, as indicated. 45 Gy is delivered to the pre-chemotherapy bone and soft tissue tumor involvement. The CTV is GTV + 1 cm and the PTV is CTV plus "institutional specified margin for setup variation" so can be as little as 0.5 cm. Subsequently, the pre-chemo bone disease and post-chemo soft tissue disease are treated to a total of 55.8 Gy, if there is gross residual disease. If the patient had only microscopic disease, then the dose would be 50.4 Gy. If radiation was delivered alone in the definitive setting, total dose would also be 55.8 Gy. Schuck A, Paulussen M. Pediatric Sarcomas of Bone. In: Gunderson LL, Tepper JE,editors. Clinical radiation oncology. 3rd ed. Philadelphia: Elsevier Saunders; 2012. p. 1435–42.

Chapter 15
Benign and Metastatic Disease

Celine Bicquart Ord and John M. Holland

Questions

1. Which of the following symptoms in metastatic non-small cell lung cancer is most likely to be palliated by radiation?
   A. Dyspnea
   B. Hemoptysis
   C. Chest wall pain
   D. Cough

2. Which is the most common site of bone metastases?
   A. Skull
   B. Femur
   C. Pelvis
   D. Vertebrae

3. Which of the following has the most functioning bone marrow?
   A. Thoracic spine
   B. Iliac crests
   C. Ribs
   D. Skull

C.B. Ord, MD (✉)
Department of Radiation Oncology, Scott & White Memorial Hospital, Temple,
TX 76508, USA
e-mail: cord@sw.org

J.M. Holland
Department of Radiation Oncology, Oregon Health and Science University,
3181 SW Sam Jackson Park Rd, KPV4, Portland, OR 97239-3098, USA
e-mail: hollanjo@ohsu.edu

C.B. Ord et al. (eds.), *Radiation Oncology Study Guide*,
DOI 10.1007/978-1-4614-6400-6_15, © Springer Science+Business Media New York 2013

4. Brain metastases are most likely to develop from which of the following malignancies?
   A. Breast cancer
   B. Prostate cancer
   C. Melanoma
   D. Lung cancer

5. Which one of the following histologies of brain metastases is least likely to present as or become hemorrhagic?
   A. Breast infiltrating ductal carcinoma
   B. Melanoma
   C. Renal cell carcinoma
   D. Choriocarcinoma

6. Whole brain radiation will improve neurologic symptoms in approximately what percentage of patients with brain metastases, as reported by Cairncross et al.?
   A. 25 %
   B. 50 %
   C. 75 %
   D. 90 %

7. Recursive partitioning analysis (RPA) of data from three consecutive RTOG brain metastases trials identified each of the following as factors in RPA class 1, except:
   A. Age <65 years
   B. Karnofsky performance status ≥ 70
   C. Controlled primary
   D. Controlled extracranial metastases

8. What is the median survival seen using recursive partitioning analysis (RPA) of data from three consecutive RTOG brain metastases trials in RPA class I patients?
   A. 9 months
   B. 7 months
   C. 4 months
   D. 2 months

9. Which of the following is false regarding RTOG 95-08, a phase III trial randomizing patients with brain metastases to whole brain radiation +/− stereotactic radiosurgery?
   A. Patients with 1–4 metastases were eligible for enrollment.
   B. The maximum eligible tumor diameter was 4 cm.
   C. Most patients had metastatic lung cancer.
   D. The whole brain radiation dose was 37.5 Gy.

10. RTOG 95-08, a phase III trial that randomized patients with brain metastases to whole brain radiation (WBRT) +/– stereotactic radiosurgery (SRS), showed:
    A. A median survival improvement with the addition of SRS
    B. No change in the use of steroids
    C. Improved survival in RPA class I patients
    D. No improvement in performance status with the addition of SRS

11. Which of the following is false regarding RTOG 97-14, a phase III trial randomizing patients with bone metastases to either 8 Gy or 30 Gy?
    A. There was no difference in complete response rates between the two arms.
    B. Acute toxicity was worse in the 8 Gy arm.
    C. Retreatment was more likely in the 8 Gy arm.
    D. Overall response rate was 66 %.

12. What percentage of patients with lung cancer will develop superior vena cava syndrome?
    A. <5 %
    B. 10 %
    C. 15 %
    D. 20 %

13. Which of the following is the most common malignancy associated with the development of superior vena cava syndrome?
    A. Lymphoma
    B. Lung cancer
    C. Germ cell tumors
    D. Colon cancer

14. Which of the following is true regarding RTOG 97-14, a phase III trial randomizing patients with bone metastases to either 8 Gy or 30 Gy?
    A. Retreatment rate was not different between the arms.
    B. Late toxicity was increased in the 8 Gy arm.
    C. Patients with breast, prostate, or non-small cell lung cancer were eligible for enrollment.
    D. Patients with 1–3 sites of bony involvement and moderate/severe pain were eligible for enrollment.

15. Approximately what percentage of patients with non-small cell lung cancer will experience palliation of symptoms from superior vena cava syndrome?
    A. 10 %
    B. 25 %
    C. 50 %
    D. 75 %

16. What is the approximate palliative response rate for hemoptysis using radiotherapy?
    A. 20 %
    B. 40 %
    C. 60 %
    D. 80 %

17. Which one of the following is most likely to predict the success of relieving obstruction from lung cancer?
    A. Adenocarcinoma versus squamous cell histology
    B. Overall stage of cancer
    C. Total radiotherapy dose delivered
    D. Duration of obstruction

18. What was the whole brain radiation dose used in Patchell's second study, a trial of patients with resected solitary brain metastasis randomized to whole brain radiation versus observation?
    A. 36 Gy
    B. 45 Gy
    C. 50.4 Gy
    D. 54 Gy

19. Which of the following is false regarding Patchell's second study, a trial of patients with resected solitary brain metastasis randomized to whole brain radiation versus observation?
    A. The addition of WBRT decreased all intracranial recurrences.
    B. The addition of WBRT decreased recurrence at the original site of metastasis.
    C. The addition of WBRT improved overall survival.
    D. The addition of WBRT decreased the likelihood from dying of neurologic causes.

20. Which of the following is false regarding Patchell's first study randomizing patients with a suspected single metastasis to either whole brain radiation (WBRT) alone or surgery + WBRT?
    A. Local recurrence was decreased with the addition of surgery.
    B. Time to recurrence was increased with the addition of surgery.
    C. Median survival improved with the addition of surgery.
    D. Duration of functional independence did not change with the addition of surgery.

21. What dose of whole brain radiation was utilized in Patchell's first study randomizing patients with a suspected single metastasis to either whole brain radiation (WBRT) alone or surgery + WBRT?
    A. 36 Gy
    B. 37.5 Gy

C. 45 Gy
D. 50.4 Gy

22. What was the median survival of those receiving surgery + WBRT in the first Patchell trial?
    A. 15 weeks
    B. 30 weeks
    C. 40 weeks
    D. 45 weeks

23. Which of the following is false regarding Patchell's third study - a randomized trial evaluating the role of surgery in patients with spinal cord compression from metastatic cancer?
    A. More patients regained the ability to walk with the addition of surgery.
    B. The addition of surgery did not increase the ability to walk in those unable to walk at the beginning of the trial.
    C. The addition of surgery helped retain the ability to walk longer.
    D. The radiation dose employed was 30 Gy.

24. Which of the following was not found to be a predictor of response in the treatment of metastatic spinal cord compression with radiotherapy alone, as reported by Maranzano et al.?
    A. Favorable histology
    B. Ability to walk prior to radiation
    C. Female sex
    D. Total radiotherapy dose

25. Approximately what percentage of patients with spinal cord compression treated with radiation will experience recurrent cord compression?
    A. 10 %
    B. 20 %
    C. 30 %
    D. 40 %

26. Which of the following is true regarding RTOG 85-02, in which patients were treated with BID fractions of palliative radiotherapy?
    A. BID fractions of 2.5 Gy were given for 3 days.
    B. Late toxicity was worse in those randomized to the shorter interval rest arm.
    C. Complete remission was seen in 10 % of patients.
    D. Tumor control was better in the shorter interval rest arm.

27. A 56-year-old male who has previously undergone open reduction internal fixation of the right hip after a traumatic fracture now presents with pain and immobility. An X-ray of the hip shows bone spurs on both the pelvis and proximal

end of the right femur, with a distance of 1.2 cm in between them. What is the correct Brooker classification for this stage of heterotopic ossification?
A. Brooker class I
B. Brooker class II
C. Brooker class III
D. Brooker class IV

28. Which of the following is the most appropriate radiation dose for heterotopic ossification prophylaxis?
A. 5 Gy
B. 7 Gy
C. 10 Gy
D. 12 Gy

29. A meta-analysis comparing radiotherapy to nonsteroidal anti-inflammatory drugs (NSAIDs) for the prevention of heterotopic ossification showed:
A. Radiation was more effective than NSAIDs in preventing Brooker class I–II ossification.
B. No difference between the groups.
C. NSAIDS were more effective than radiation in preventing Brooker class III–IV ossification.
D. There was a significant dose response with postoperative radiotherapy.

30. A double-blind randomized trial of radiation versus sham irradiation for Graves' orbitopathy showed all of the following, except:
A. There was no improvement seen in any of the patients that received sham irradiation.
B. The benefit seen in those that received radiation was in the grade of diplopia.
C. Despite improvements in orbitopathy, three-quarters of patients still needed strabismus surgery.
D. Elevation was the only variable to improve quantitatively.

31. Which of the following is false comparing samarium-153 and strontium-89, radioisotopes used in the palliation of bone metastases?
A. Typical response time is faster with Sm-153.
B. Typical response duration is longer with Sr-89.
C. Time to marrow nadir is faster in Sr-89.
D. Time to marrow recovery is faster in Sm-153.

32. The most common dose-limiting toxicity of either samarium-153 or strontium-89 is:
A. Thrombocytopenia
B. Pain flare
C. Cost
D. Neutropenia

33. Which of the following would not preclude radionuclide therapy?
    A. Spinal cord compression
    B. Index lesions with poor uptake on bone scan
    C. Platelet count of 50,000 per μL
    D. Painful blastic metastases that show uptake on bone scan

34. Which of the following is false regarding the ALSYMPCA trial of alpharadin versus placebo for symptomatic castration-resistant prostate cancer?
    A. Alpharadin targets bone metastases with high-energy protons of short range.
    B. Median survival was increased in those receiving alpharadin.
    C. Median time to skeletal-related events was increased with alpharadin.
    D. Bone pain was the most common grade III/IV toxicity.

35. Which of the following symptoms from recurrent rectal cancer is most likely to be palliated with radiotherapy?
    A. Bleeding
    B. Mass effect
    C. Pain
    D. Neuropathy

36. Which of the following symptoms from recurrent rectal cancer is least likely to be palliated with radiotherapy?
    A. Bleeding
    B. Mass effect
    C. Pain
    D. Neuropathy

37. According to Morganti et al., what is the approximate pain response rate with palliative radiotherapy for painful, unresectable pancreatic cancer?
    A. 10 %
    B. 25 %
    C. 50 %
    D. 75 %

38. As reported by Leibel et al. in an RTOG study, approximately what percentage of patients with hepatic metastases achieve complete pain relief after palliative radiotherapy?
    A. 25 %
    B. 50 %
    C. 75 %
    D. 90 %

Answers and Rationales

1. The correct answer is B. In a small prospective series, 65 patients with locally advanced and metastatic non-small cell lung cancer were assessed with EORTC quality of life questionnaires 2 weeks before, 6 weeks following, and 3 months following palliative radiotherapy. Quality of life response rates showed that of the symptoms seen in metastatic non-small cell lung cancer, hemoptysis was the best palliated with radiation (79 % response). Appetite loss (11 %) was the least palliated. Langendijk JA et al. Quality of life after palliative radiotherapy in non-small lung cancer: a prospective study. Int J Radiat Oncol Biol Phys. 2000;47(1):149–155.

2. The correct answer is D. The most common site of bony metastasis is in the vertebrae. Chow E, Finkelstein JA, Sahgal A, Coleman RE. Metastatic cancer to the bone. In: DeVita VT, Lawrence TS, Rosenberg SA, editors. DeVita, Hellman, and Rosenberg's cancer: principles and practice of oncology. 9th ed. Philadelphia: Lippincott Williams & Wilkins; 2011. p. 2192–204.

3. The correct answer is B. The iliac crests and upper femurs are the site of the most functioning bone marrow in the body. Hayman JA et al. Distribution of proliferating bone marrow in adult cancer patients determined using FLT-PET imaging. Int J Radiat Oncol Biol Phys. 2011;79(3):847–52.

4. The correct answer is D. Lung cancer is the most common histology of brain metastases. Barnholtz-Sloan J et al. Incidence proportions of brain metastases in patients diagnosed (1973–2001) in the Metropolitan Detroit Cancer Surveillance System. J Clin Oncol. 2004;22:2865–72.

5. The correct answer is A. Histologies that are most likely to be hemorrhagic: choriocarcinoma, renal cell carcinoma, melanoma, testicular cancer, hepatocellular carcinoma, thyroid cancer, and primitive neuroectodermal tumor.

6. The correct answer is C. Cairncross reported 74 % improvement of neurologic symptoms (such as headache) with 65 % improved for at least 9 months or duration of life. Cairncross, J.G. Radiation Therapy for Brain Metastases. Ann Neurol. 1980;7(6):529–41.

7. The correct answer is D. Recursive partitioning analysis was performed on data from 1,200 patients from three consecutive RTOG brain metastases trials and identified three classes. Class I included patients < 65 years of age, Karnofsky performance status ≥70, and controlled primary tumor with the brain as the only site of metastatic disease. No extracranial metastatic disease was permitted. Class III included those patients with Karnofsky performance status <70.

Gaspar L et al. Recursive portioning analysis (RPA) of prognostic factors in three Radiation Therapy Oncology Group (RTOG) brain metastases trials. Int J Radiat Oncol Biol Phys. 1997;37(4):745–51.

8. The correct answer is B. Recursive partitioning analysis was performed on data from 1,200 patients from three consecutive RTOG brain metastases trials and identified three classes. Class I included patients < 65 years of age, Karnofsky performance status ≥ 70, and controlled primary tumor with the brain as the only site of metastatic disease. No extracranial metastatic disease was permitted. Class III included those patients with Karnofsky performance status <70. Median survival in classes I–III were 7.1, 4.2, and 2.3 months, respectively. Gaspar L et al. Recursive portioning analysis (RPA) of prognostic factors in three Radiation Therapy Oncology Group (RTOG) brain metastases trials. Int J Radiat Oncol Biol Phys. 1997;37(4):745–51.

9. The correct answer is A. RTOG 95-08 randomized 331 patients with 1–3 brain metastases (maximum diameter 4 cm) to WBRT (37.5 Gy/15 fractions) +/– SRS (24 Gy vs. 18 Gy vs. 15 Gy, based on size). The majority (63 %) of patients had metastatic lung cancer and were RPA class II (74 %). There was no difference in median survival between the two arms, though the addition of SRS did improve 3-month response rate, 1-year intracranial control (81 % vs. 72 %), KPS, and decrease steroid use. Local recurrence was more likely with WBRT alone. On multivariate analysis, survival was improved with the addition in SRS both RPA class I ($p < 0.0001$) and those with favorable histology (squamous) ($p = 0.0121$). Andrews DW et al. Whole brain radiation therapy with or without stereotactic radiosurgical boost for patients with one to three brain metastases: phase III results of the RTOG 95-08 randomised trial. Lancet 2004;363(9422):1665–72.

10. The correct answer is C. RTOG 95-08 randomized 331 patients with 1–3 brain metastases (maximum diameter 4cm) to WBRT (37.5 Gy/15 fractions) +/– SRS (24 Gy vs. 18 Gy vs. 15 Gy, based on size). The majority (63 %) of patients had metastatic lung cancer and were RPA class II (74 %). There was no difference in median survival between the two arms, though the addition of SRS did improve 3-month response rate, 1-year intracranial control (81 % vs. 72 %), KPS, and decreased steroid use. Local recurrence was more likely with WBRT alone. On multivariate analysis, survival was improved with the addition of SRS in both RPA class I patients ($p < 0.0001$) and those with a favorable histological status ($p = 0.0121$). Andrews DW et al. Whole brain radiation therapy with or without stereotactic radiosurgical boost for patients with one to three brain metastases: phase III results of the RTOG 95-08 randomised trial. Lancet 2004;363(9422):1665–72.

11. The correct answer is B. RTOG 97-14 was a randomized trial that sought to compare two commonly used radiation fractionations. Eight hundred ninety-eight patients with painful metastases (1–3 sites) from either breast or prostate cancer were randomized to receive either 8 Gy in one fraction or 30 Gy in ten fractions over 2 weeks. Pain relief at 3 months was evaluated with the Brief Pain Inventory. Overall response rate was 66 %. There was no difference in complete response between the 30 Gy and 8 Gy arms: 18 % and 15 %, $p=0.6$. There was no difference in partial response between the 30 Gy and 8 Gy arms: 48 % versus 50 %, $p=0.6$. Retreatment rate was higher in the single fraction arm: 18 % versus 9 %, $p<0.001$. Grade II/IV acute toxicity was greater in the 30 Gy arm (17 %) versus the 8 Gy arm (10 %), $p=0.002$. Late toxicity was comparable between the arms. Hartsell WF et al. Randomized trial of short- versus long-course radiotherapy for palliation of painful bone metastases. J Natl Cancer Inst. 2005;97(11):798–804.

12. The correct answer is A. Though lung cancer is the most common etiology of superior vena cava syndrome, the minority of patients with lung cancer (<5 %) will actually develop superior vena cava syndrome. Wagner H. Non-small cell lung cancer. In: Gunderson LL, Tepper JE, editors. Clinical radiation oncology, 3rd ed. Philadelphia: Elsevier Saunders; 2012. p. 805–38.

13. The correct answer is B. Lung cancer accounts for 75 % of cases of superior vena cava syndrome, with other cancers (germ cell tumors, lymphoma, metastases) as other observed etiologies. Wagner H. Non-small cell lung cancer. In: Gunderson LL, Tepper JE, editors. Clinical radiation oncology, 3rd ed. Philadelphia: Elsevier Saunders; 2012. p. 805–38.

14. The correct answer is D. RTOG 97-14 was a randomized trial that sought to compare two commonly used radiation fractionations. Eight hundred ninety-eight patients with painful metastases (1–3 sites) from either breast or prostate cancer were randomized to receive either 8 Gy in one fraction or 30 Gy in ten fractions over 2 weeks. Pain relief at 3 months was evaluated with the Brief Pain Inventory. Overall response rate was 66 %. There was no difference in complete response between the 30 Gy and 8 Gy arms: 18 % and 15 %, $p=0.6$. There was no difference in partial response between the 30 Gy and 8 Gy arms: 48 % versus 50 %, $p=0.6$. Retreatment rate was higher in the single fraction arm: 18 % versus 9 %, $p<0.001$. Grade 2–4 acute toxicity was greater in the 30 Gy arm (17 %) versus the 8 Gy arm (10 %), $p=0.002$. Late toxicity was comparable between the arms. Hartsell WF et al. Randomized trial of short- versus long-course radiotherapy for palliation of painful bone metastases. J Natl Cancer Inst. 2005;97(11):798–804.

15. The correct answer is C. Approximately half of patients with non-small cell lung cancer will sustain palliation from radiotherapy for superior vena cava syndrome. Wagner H. Non-small cell lung cancer. In: Gunderson LL, Tepper

JE, editors. Clinical radiation oncology, 3rd ed. Philadelphia: Elsevier Saunders; 2012. p. 805–38. Urban T et al. Superior vena cava syndrome in small-cell lung cancer. Arch Int Med. 1993;153(3):384–7. Würschmidt F et al. Small cell lung cancer with and without superior vena cava syndrome: a multivariate analysis of prognostic factors in 408 cases. Int J Radiat Oncol Biol Phys. 1995;33(1):77–82.

16. The correct answer is D. Hemoptysis is well palliated by radiotherapy, with a response rate of 83 % reported by Slawson et al. Slawson RG, Scott RM. Radiation herapy in bronchogenic carcinoma. Radiology. 1979;132(1):175–6.

17. The correct answer is D. Duration of obstruction/lung collapse prior to initiation of radiotherapy best predicts response to palliative radiotherapy. Reddy et al. reported that 71 % treated within 2 weeks of radiographic obstruction had complete re-expansion of the lung versus 23 % of those treated after 2 weeks of collapse. Reddy SP, Marks JE. Total atelectasis of the lung secondary to malignant airway obstruction. Response to radiation therapy. Am J Clin Oncol. 1990;13(5):394–400.

18. The correct answer is C. The second Patchell study sought to determine the benefit of postoperative radiotherapy after complete surgical resection. Ninety-five patients s/p complete resection of a single brain metastasis were randomized to +/− adjuvant whole brain radiation (WBRT—50.4 Gy using 28 fractions of 1.8 Gy). Intracranial recurrence was less frequent with the addition of WBRT: 18 % versus 70 %, $p < 0.001$. Recurrence at the site of original metastasis was also decreased: 10 % versus 46 %, $p < 0.001$. The addition of WBRT also reduced the likelihood of dying from neurologic causes: 14 % versus 44 %, $p = 0.003$. There was no difference in overall survival or the length of time that patients remained functionally independent. Patchell RA et al. Postoperative radiotherapy in the treatment of single metastases to the brain: a randomized trial. JAMA. 1998;280(17):1485–9.

19. The correct answer is C. The second Patchell study sought to determine the benefit of postoperative radiotherapy after complete surgical resection. Ninety-five patients s/p complete resection of a single brain metastasis were randomized to +/− adjuvant whole brain radiation (WBRT—50.4 Gy). Intracranial recurrence was less frequent with the addition of WBRT: 18 % versus 70 %, $p < 0.001$. Recurrence at the site of original metastasis was also decreased: 10 % versus 46 %, $p < 0.001$. The addition of WBRT also reduced the likelihood of dying from neurologic causes: 14 % versus 44 %, $p = 0.003$. There was no difference in overall survival or the length of time that patients remained functionally independent. Patchell RA et al. Postoperative radiotherapy in the treatment of single metastases to the brain: a randomized trial. JAMA. 1998;280(17):1485–9.

20. The correct answer is D. The first Patchell study randomized 48 patients to either WBRT alone (36 Gy/12 fractions) or surgery + WBRT. The addition of surgery decreased local recurrence (52 % vs. 20 %, $p = 0.03$), increased median survival (40 weeks vs. 15 weeks, $p < 0.01$), and increased time of functional independence (38 weeks vs. 8 weeks, $p < 0.005$). Time to recurrence was also increased: 14 months versus 5 months. Patchell R.A. et al., A randomized trial of surgery in the treatment of single metastases to the brain. N Engl J Med 1990;322(8):494–500.

21. The correct answer is A. The first Patchell study randomized 48 patients to either WBRT alone (36 Gy/12 fractions) or surgery + WBRT. The addition of surgery decreased local recurrence (52 % vs. 20 %, $p = 0.03$), increased median survival (40 weeks vs. 15 weeks, $p < 0.01$), and increased time of functional independence (38 weeks vs. 8 weeks, $p < 0.005$). Time to recurrence was also increased: 14 months versus 5 months. Patchell RA et al. A randomized trial of surgery in the treatment of single metastases to the brain. N Engl J Med. 1990;322(8):494–500.

22. The correct answer is C. The first Patchell study randomized 48 patients to either WBRT alone (36 Gy/12 fractions) or surgery + WBRT. The addition of surgery decreased local recurrence (52 % vs. 20 %, $p = 0.03$), increased median survival (40 weeks vs. 15 weeks, $p < 0.01$), and increased time of functional independence (38 weeks vs. 8 weeks, $p < 0.005$). Time to recurrence was also increased: 14 months versus 5 months. Patchell RA et al. A randomized trial of surgery in the treatment of single metastases to the brain. N Engl J Med 1990;322(8):494–500.

23. The correct answer is B. The third Patchell study assessed the role of surgery in cord compression from metastatic cancer. One hundred one patients with cord compression from metastatic cancer were randomized to radiation (30 Gy) +/– surgery prior to radiation. The trial was stopped early due to meeting a predetermined stopping rule. More patients in the surgery group ($n = 42/50$, 84 %) regained the ability to walk after treatment and retained that ability longer (122 days vs. 13 days, $p = 0.003$). Of the 32 patients that entered the study unable to walk, more ($n = 10$) from the surgery group regained the ability to walk, $p = 0.01$. Patchell RA et al. Direct decompressive surgical resection in the treatment of spinal cord compression caused by metastatic cancer: a randomised trial. Lancet. 2005;366(9486):643–8.

24. The correct answer is D. Maranzano reported their series of 275 consecutive patients with metastatic spinal cord compression, of whom 255 were treated with radiation (30 Gy) and steroids alone. Total response rate was 82 %, with 54 % experiencing complete response. Three-quarters of patients either recovered or preserved walking ability. Early diagnosis of cord compression was the most important response predictor. With late diagnosis, tumors with favorable

histology (breast, myeloma, prostate) had a better response to radiation. Survival was longer in those able to walk before radiation, in those with favorable histology, and in females. Maranzano E, Latini P. Effectiveness of radiation therapy without surgery in metastatic spinal cord compression: final results from a prospective trial. Int J Radiat Oncol Biol Phys. 1995;32(4):959–67.

25. The correct answer is A. Loeffler et al. reported an 11.3 % incidence of recurrent cord compression in 80 patients with prior cord compression treated with radiation. One-quarter of patients experienced cord compression within the spinal canal, but out of the original treatment field. Loeffler JS et al. Treatment of spinal cord compression: a retrospective analysis. Med Pediatr Oncol. 1983; 11(5):347–51.

26. The correct answer is C. RTOG 85-02 began as a phase II trial in which 151 patients with various cancers (40 % gynecologic) were treated with 3.7 Gy BID × 2 days (14.8 Gy), to a total of 44.4 Gy, with an interval of 4 weeks between courses. Fifty-nine percent of the patients completed all three courses. Complete remission was seen in 10 % of patients, partial remission in 22 %, no change in 24 %, progression in 7 %, and unknown in 8 %. An additional 144 patients were subsequently randomized into a phase III trial to undergo an interval of either 2 or 4 weeks between courses. No difference in tumor control was noted between the randomized arms. No patients receiving <30 Gy developed late toxicity. There was no difference in late effects between the 2-week and 4-week rest arms, $p = 0.47$. Spanos WJ Jr. et al. Phase II study of multiple daily fractionations in the palliation of advanced pelvic malignancies: preliminary report of RTOG 8502. Int J Radiat Oncol Biol Phys. 1989;17(3):659–61. Spanos WJ Jr. et al. Late effect of multiple daily fraction palliation schedule for advanced pelvic malignancies (RTOG 8502). Int J Radiat Oncol Biol Phys. 1994;29(5):961–7.

27. The correct answer is B. A distance of 1.2 cm between bone spurs is consistent with Brooker class II, which has a distance >1 cm in between bone spurs. Brooker class I has islands of bone within the soft tissues. Brooker class III describes those bone spurs between opposing bone surfaces with <1 cm in between. Class IV shows apparent bone ankylosis of the hip. Brooker A et al. Ectopic ossification following total hip replacement: incidence and a method of classification. J Bone Joint Surg Am. 1973;55:1629.

28. The correct answer is B. Of the listed choices, the best choice of total radiation dose employed for heterotopic ossification prophylaxis is 7 Gy.

29. The correct answer is D. In a meta-analysis of seven randomized trials including 1,143 patients, radiation was found to be more effective than NSAIDs in preventing Brooker class III–IV ossification, though the absolute risk difference is only 1.8 %. In subgroup analysis, early (16–20 h preoperative) radiation was not effective. In postoperative radiotherapy, there was a significant dose-response

relationship, $p = 0.008$. While 6 Gy was found to be equally effective to NSAIDs, higher RT doses were found to be more effective. Pakos EE et al. Radiotherapy vs. nonsteroidal anti-inflammatory drugs for the prevention of heterotopic ossification after major hip procedures: a meta-analysis of randomized trials. Int J Radiat Oncol Biol Phys. 2004;60(3):888–95.

30. The correct answer is A. A double-blind randomized trial randomized 60 patients with moderately to severe Graves' orbitopathy to either radiation (20 Gy/10 fractions) or sham irradiation (0 Gy/10 fractions). Outcomes were measured both qualitatively and quantitatively (eyelid aperture, proptosis, eye movements) at 24 weeks. Qualitatively, successful outcomes were seen in 60 % of irradiated patients and 31 % of sham-irradiated patients. These benefits were seen in diplopia grade, but not proptosis reduction or eyelid swelling. Quantitatively, only elevation improved. Despite the benefit of radiation, 75 % of the patients that underwent radiation still needed additional strabismus surgery. Mourits, MP et al., Radiotherapy for Graves' orbitopathy: randomised placebo-controlled study. Lancet. 2000;355(9214):1505–9.

31. The correct answer is C. Samarium-153 and strontium-89 are radionuclides employed in the treatment of painful, blastic bone metastases. The typical response time is shorter with Sm-153 (2–7 days) versus 14–28 days with Sr-89, as is the time to nadir (2–4 weeks) versus 4 weeks in Sm-153 and the time to recovery (8–12 weeks) versus 12 weeks in Sr-89. Typical response duration is longer in Sr-89 (12–26 weeks) versus 8 weeks in Sm-153. U.S. Nuclear Regulatory Commission: Part 35- Medical use of byproduct material. http:// www.nrc.gov/reading-rm/doc-collections/cfr/part035/. Perez C, Brady L, Halperin E, et al., editors. Principles and practice of radiation oncology. Philadelphia: Lippincott, Williams, and Wilkins; 2004. Serafini AN. Therapy of metastatic bone pain. J Nucl Med. 2001;42:895–906. Bauman G et al. Radiopharmaceuticals for the palliation of painful bone metastases- a systematic review. Radiother Oncol. 2005;75:258–70.

32. The correct answer is A. While neutropenia and pain flare are toxicities seen with radionuclide therapy, thrombocytopenia is the most common dose-limiting toxicity. U.S. Nuclear Regulatory Commission: Part 35- Medical use of byproduct material. http://www.nrc.gov/reading-rm/doc-collections/cfr/part035/. Perez C, Brady L, Halperin E, et al., editors. Principles and practice of radiation oncology. Philadelphia: Lippincott, Williams, and Wilkins; 2004. Serafini AN. Therapy of metastatic bone pain. J Nucl Med. 2001;42:895–906. Bauman G et al. Radiopharmaceuticals for the palliation of painful bone metastases- a systematic review. Radiother Oncol. 2005;75:258–70.

33. The correct answer is D. Samarium-153 and strontium-89 are radionuclides employed in the treatment of painful, blastic bone metastases. To be considered for radionuclide therapy, a patient must have a life expectancy of >6 weeks, have multiple painful blastic metastases which show uptake on bone scan, and

have leukocyte count >3,000 per μL and platelet count >60,000 per μL. Factors that typically preclude radionuclide therapy are the following: impending pathologic fracture, spinal cord compression, index lesions with poor uptake on bone scan, large extra-osseous component of disease, and extensive areas of bone destruction. U.S. Nuclear Regulatory Commission: Part 35- Medical use of byproduct material. http://www.nrc.gov/reading-rm/doc-collections/cfr/part035/. Perez C, Brady L, Halperin E, et al., editors. Principles and practice of radiation oncology. Philadelphia: Lippincott, Williams, and Wilkins; 2004. Serafini AN. Therapy of metastatic bone pain. J Nucl Med. 2001;42:895–906. Bauman G et al. Radiopharmaceuticals for the palliation of painful bone metastases- a systematic review. Radiother Oncol. 2005;75:258–70.

34. The correct answer is A. The phase III randomized ALSYMPCA (Alpharadin in Symptomatic Prostate cancer) trial of 922 men with symptomatic castration-resistant prostate cancer to bone, ineligible/intolerant/ineffective to docetaxel, showed improved median overall survival, improved time to PSA progression, and increased time to skeletal-related events with alpharadin (radium-223 chloride) versus placebo. Alpharadin targets bone metastases with high-energy alpha particles of short range. Median survival was increased from 11.2 to 14 months ($p=0.00185$), and time to skeletal-related events increased from 8.4 to 13.6 months ($p=0.00046$). Bone pain was the most common grade III/IV adverse event (18 %), and 15 % experienced anemia. Due to the results of this trial, radium-223 was granted "fast-track designation" by the FDA, with FDA approval expected by the end of 2012. Sartor AO et al. Radium-223 chloride impact on skeletal-related events in patients with castration-resistant prostate cancer (CRPC) with bone metastases: a phase III randomized trial (ALSYMPCA). J Clin Oncol. 30, 2012 (Suppl 5; abstr 9).

35. The correct answer is A. In a review of 52 patients undergoing re-irradiation (median dose 30.6 Gy) for recurrent rectal cancer (median initial RT dose 50.4 Gy), mass effect was the least palliated system, with a 24 % complete palliation response. Ninety percent of patients received concurrent 5-FU chemotherapy. Bleeding was the best palliated symptom with a 100 % complete response rate; pain was completely palliated in 65 % of patients. Lingareddy V et al. Palliative reirradiation for recurrent rectal cancer. Int J Radiat Oncol Biol Phys. 1997;38(4):785–90.

36. The correct answer is B. In a review of 52 patients undergoing re-irradiation (median dose 30.6 Gy) for recurrent rectal cancer (median initial RT dose 50.4 Gy), mass effect was the least palliated system, with a 24 % complete palliation response. Ninety percent of patients received concurrent 5-FU chemotherapy. Bleeding was the best palliated symptom with a 100 % complete response rate; pain was completely palliated in 65 % of patients. Lingareddy V et al. Palliative reirradiation for recurrent rectal cancer. Int J Radiat Oncol Biol Phys. 1997; 38(4):785–90.

37. The correct answer is D. In a small series of 12 patients undergoing palliative radiotherapy (30 Gy/10 fractions), 75 % experienced pain response. Half of the patients sustained pain control with radiotherapy alone, not requiring pharmacological therapy; three patients (25 %) reduced their use of analgesics. Morganti AG et al. Pain relief with short-term irradiation in locally advanced carcinoma of the pancreas. J Palliat Care. 2003;19:258–62.

38. The correct answer is B. In a prospective randomized study comparing radiation therapy +/− misonidazole for hepatic metastases in 214 patients, misonidazole was not found to confer any additional benefit. Radiation (21 Gy/7 fractions) resulted in excellent (80 %) symptomatic improvement in pain from liver metastases, with complete pain relief in 54 %. The median duration of pain relief was 13.0 weeks, with performance status subsequently improved in 28 % of patients. The median time to relief was 1.7 weeks, and colorectal cancer metastases were best palliated versus other tumor types ($p = 0.02$). Leibel SA et al. A comparison of misonidazole sensitized radiation therapy to radiation therapy alone for the palliation of hepatic metastases: Results of a radiation therapy oncology group randomized prospective trial. Int J Radiat Oncol Biol Phys. 1987;13(7):1057–64.

Index

Printed by Printforce, the Netherlands